# Music Measures M

## The Diaries of a Me

**Jamie '*Boomerang*' Robertson**

Inter/Connexions

Oxfordshire, United Kingdom

© Inter/Connexions
https://inter-connexions.net/

First edition 2024

*Inter/Connexions* is a global, inclusive not-for-profit publishing research network. Our books aim to encourage and promote work which is collaborative, innovative, imaginative, and which provides an exemplar for inclusive interdisciplinary publishing.

Reprints and Permissions
Contact: publish@inter-connexions.net

All rights reserved. Mechanical, photocopying, recording or otherwise without either the prior written permission of the publisher or a license permitting restricted copying issued in the UK by The Copyright Licensing Agency and in the USA by The Copyright Clearance Center.

Any opinions expressed in the book/chapters are those of the author or authors. Whilst Inter/Connexions makes every effort to ensure the quality and accuracy of its content, Inter/Connexions makes no representation implied or otherwise, as to the chapters' suitability and application and disclaims any warranties, express or implied, to their use.

British Library Cataloguing in Publication Data.
A catalogue record for this book is available from the British Library.

ISBN: 978-1-84888-549-3

Inter/Connexions, Priory House, Wroslyn Road, Freeland, Oxfordshire. OX29 8HR, United Kingdom.

First published in the United Kingdom in Paperback format in 2024.

# Music Measures Memories

# Inter/Connexions

**Series Editors**

Robert Fisher  Teresa Cutler-Broyles
Lorraine Rumson  Petra Rehling

*Inclusive Global Interdisciplinary Publishing*

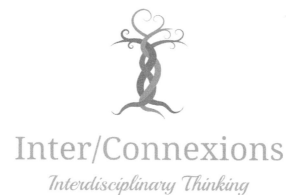

**2024**

# Contents

| | | |
|---|---|---|
| **Introduction** | | vii |
| **What's a Melomaniac?** | | x |

## VOLUME ONE: 1954-1981

| 1 | Da Capo | 1 |
|---|---|---|
| 2 | School Days | 13 |
| 3 | Break on Through (To the Other Side) | 27 |
| 4 | Nothing is Easy | 39 |
| 5 | Changes | 57 |
| 6 | And You and I | 77 |
| 7 | The Cinema Show | 97 |
| 8 | Show Me the Way | 113 |
| 9 | It's a Long Way to the Top | 125 |
| 10 | Solsbury Hill | 139 |
| 11 | Free Bird | 155 |
| 12 | Kashmir | 171 |
| 13 | The Kids Are Alright | 185 |
| 14 | Prove It All Night | 197 |
| 15 | Even in the Quietest Moments | 215 |
| 16 | London Calling | 229 |
| 17 | Comfortably Numb | 249 |
| 18 | Tunnel of Love | 267 |

# VOLUME TWO: 1981-1997

| 1 | History Never Repeats | 283 |
|---|---|---|
| 2 | Great Southern Land | 301 |
| 3 | Reckless (Don't Be So) | 313 |
| 4 | All Lovers Are Deranged | 329 |
| 5 | Give Me Love, Give Me Life | 341 |
| 6 | Let's Go Crazy | 353 |
| 7 | Now We're Getting Somewhere | 365 |
| 8 | Welcome To The Jungle | 383 |
| 9 | Rock And A Hard Place | 399 |
| 10 | Hold On To Me | 415 |
| 11 | Never Tear Us Apart | 429 |
| 12 | Before You Accuse Me | 439 |
| 13 | My Country | 453 |
| 14 | Time To Move On | 469 |
| 15 | For All The Cows | 483 |
| 16 | Full Circle | 497 |
| | **Coda** | 513 |
| | **A-Z List of Concerts** | 517 |
| | **Quote Sources** | 535 |
| | **Acknowledgements** | 537 |

*A life lived with integrity, even if it lacks the trappings of fame and fortune,*
*is a shining star in whose light others may follow in the years to come.*

Denis Waitley

## INTRODUCTION

So, who the hell am I and why would you want to read about someone who isn't rich and famous and never sought to become either? And why should you believe reading my words might make a difference to you? Well, it rather depends on how you measure success.

If you measure how successful you are by how much money you have in your bank, or how well-known you are on social media, or how much better you are at something compared to others, my story might not appeal to you. But if you are someone who measures your success by how happy you are because you are doing what you love for a living, or by how much freedom you have to satisfy your love of travel, or you believe music is a universal language, which helps connect you to other people, you might enjoy reading about my serendipitous mistakes and music-inspired adventures. My words might even inspire you to become more proactive and hopeful, so you can make your own dreams come true.

The idea started as a simple A-Z of all the musicians I have ever seen perform live but who are now dead. The trigger for making this list came on the 10th of January 2016, the day David Bowie died. While mourning his tragic loss to the music world and discussing what a wonderful artist he was with some of my friends, I was asked if I had ever been to any of his concerts. I was lucky enough to see the Thin White Duke three times at different stages of his career. The first time was with The Spiders from Mars at Starkers Royal Ballrooms in Boscombe in 1972 on the *Ziggy Stardust Tour.* I still have the ticket and it only cost a pound! I also saw him in Sydney on his *Serious Moonlight Tour* in 1983 and on his *Glass Spider Tour* in 1987.

My mates then asked me who else I had seen who were no longer with us, so the next day I wrote down the names of a few other music legends like Jimi Hendrix, Jim Morrison, Keith Moon, John Bonham,

Stevie Ray Vaughan and Freddie Mercury. Fortunately for us, their wonderful music lives on long after they are gone and whenever we hear one of their songs, we can be transported back in time to a specific moment in our lives. That's how powerful music can be.

As this *triste* list grew longer, I became increasingly dejected so decided it might be better and less gut-wrenching if I made a list of all the rock bands, blues guitarists, folks singers and jazz musicians I have seen whether now dead or alive. I went through all my old diaries and wrote down when and where I had seen each band or artist perform next to their names. While I was verifying the dates and locations, I played my favourite songs by each of them and as I went down memory lane many meaningful musical experiences came flooding back and I began to appreciate how important music has been to me throughout my life and perhaps even helped shape my identity. Music has motivated me, relaxed me, moved me and inspired me. It has been my constant travelling companion throughout my life and most importantly it has been my safe place, especially when I have felt lonely or depressed.

Writing about the vital role music has been for my well-being has allowed me to travel back in time, evoking memories stimulated by a diverse range of music from major events in my life and acknowledge how the social and cultural changes of each era affected the decisions I made along the way.

My first ever rock concert was the Isle of Wight Festival in 1970. Since then, I have attended hundreds of other gigs and loved every one of them. Along the way I was able to meet a few of my heroes, including The Who's charismatic drummer Keith Moon, while I was working on the movie *The Kids Are Alright*, and the artist formerly known as Prince Rogers Nelson when he was editing the video of *Let's Go Crazy*. ABBA also get an honourable mention, as they indirectly helped me get a job in the Australian film industry.

I have spent over 45 years working in the Film and TV industry, mainly as a freelancer, which is not the best path to take if your goal is to have financial security, but what freelance work does give you, or gave me at least, is freedom.

The idea of having a secure full-time job but only having a couple of weeks off each year and then trying to cram as much adventure into a such a short time frame didn't appeal to me at all. Living life like one long working holiday sounded like much more fun, so that was what I decided to do. To achieve this rather Bohemian lifestyle, I have had to live a slightly nomadic life, often on the smell of an oily rag, especially when there were long gaps between jobs, which I appreciate isn't for everyone, but it worked for me... most of the time.

Measuring my life with music helped me recall experiences both good and bad. It made me re-examine how I dealt with triumph and disaster and question whether I treated those two imposters just the same. It also allowed me to re-experience immense joy and incredible sadness, but more importantly, it enabled a healing process that I hadn't realised I needed until I began writing this book The result might best be described as **The Diaries of a Melomaniac.**

## WHAT'S A MELOMANIAC?

Could you be one too? Here is a quick test to find out.

1. Do you have a compulsive need to hear new music?
2. Do you like to change the music genre to suit your mood?
3. Do you have a playlist for every occasion?
4. Do you feel immense joy when you hear a new artist?
5. Do you spend money you should be saving on new music?

If you answered YES to all 5 questions, then you are a melomaniac like me but fear not, just because you have Music Addiction Disorder does not mean you are MAD! However, it might mean that you will enjoy my story…I hope so anyway.

Thank you for taking the time to read it.

Jamie '*Boomerang*' Robertson

# Volume One: 1954-1981

*Where am I? Who am I? How did I come to be here? What is this thing called 'the world'? How did I come into the world? Why was I not consulted? And If I am compelled to take part in it, where is the director? I want to see him.*

Søren Kierkegaard

## CHAPTER 1: DA CAPO
(An Italian musical term that means 'from the beginning'.)

This was the third time I had been mortally wounded and the day was far from over.

A nine-note trumpet fanfare was followed swiftly by the sound of an arrow embedding itself into a tree. With the theme song of *The Adventures of Robin Hood* still playing in my head, I dusted myself down and continued swooshing, swerving and swiping with an imaginary sword in hand fighting the Sheriff of Nottingham's men. Earlier that morning, my two friends and I had made swords out of sticks and twine and since then many duels had been fought by swashbuckling musketeers and battles won by knights of valour, or in my case lost. My lack of hand-to-eye coordination and motor skills made me an easy target but I never remained dead for long. After each noble death I would re-incarnate into another of my favourite fictional heroes.

Every little boy needs a hero and the first one for me was my father. I was only three when he died and the psychological harm of his absence during my childhood remains with me to this day.

During the Second World War, my father was a fighter pilot and rose to the rank of Lieutenant Commander in the Fleet Air Arm, a branch of the Royal Navy operating planes from aircraft carriers, including the rugged Fairey Swordfish, a biplane torpedo bomber, and the Supermarine Seafire, the naval version of the Spitfire. He met my mother when she was based at H.M.S Heron, an airbase in Yeovilton, working as a Night Vision Tester. Before the war she had been sent to a finishing school for young upper-class women where they taught her all the social graces needed to enter society, eventually joining the W.R.N.S to do her bit for the war effort.

After the war was over, they moved to Scotland so my father could finish his studies at the University in Edinburgh before working for the Forestry Commission. He loved nature and really understood the importance of ancient woodland, wanting more than anything to protect the wildlife that relies on their existence. Being connected to nature would play a vital role in my well-being and mental health for the rest of my life. That was his legacy to me.

In 1954, my family lived in Pitlochry, a town less than ten minutes away from the site of The Battle of Killiecrankie - one of the bloodiest skirmishes in Scottish history. I was born 265 years later on the 3rd of November at Aberfeldy Cottage Hospital, less than half an hour from the spectacular gorge where the Jacobites secured their first victory of the rebellion.

The doctor who delivered me told my mother it was the first time he had ever seen a baby born with its hands in prayer. I had been due three weeks earlier, so perhaps I was praying for forgiveness for being a tad late.

On the same day I entered the world, French artist Henri Matisse departed it and the movie *Godzilla,* directed by Ishirō Honda, was premiered in Tokyo. Both these men would have an influence on me many years later. One inspired me with his unique art and the other with his calm way of directing movies.

When my father was promoted to Chief Education Officer, the family moved to London and rented a house in Drayton Gardens in Kensington. I was the youngest of three. My sister Nicolette was nine years older than me and my brother Niall was seven years older.

My earliest memory is of my mother taking me into the street each morning to look at the horse-drawn milk float. When it got close to our house, the milkman, perched on the side of the float, would jump off, grab a handful of glass milk bottles and deliver them to each doorstop in turn. While he did this, my mother would hold me up to pat the horse's nose.

I only have a few memories of my father. One is of being picked up and put on top of his broad shoulders to get a better view of the Horse Guards Parade at St James Park. I can still smell the horses, see the shine of the breastplates and hear the rhythmic beat of the kettledrums. Another is being taken for long walks in Kensington Gardens to look at the statue of Peter Pan and feeding the noisy ducks in the pond. I also have a strong recollection of watching him sitting at a small table where he was building a Viking longship out of matchsticks that he had carefully cut into equal lengths with a sharp knife, and glued together to form the hull. I don't know if he ever got to finish it.

Near the end of the war, my father had to make a hasty escape from the cockpit of his plane and parachute into the Indian Ocean. Although he badly injured himself as he fell, he somehow managed to inflate a small rubber dinghy after he had landed in the sea. He then poured a bottle of coloured dye around the lifeboat, so that the rescue plane could spot him from a distance, which they eventually did more than 24 hours later. As he had survived in the ocean for so long before being rescued, he was made a member of the Goldfish Club, an association made up of pilots who had either had to parachute into, or whose planes had crashed into, the ocean and who had only survived because they had inflatable dinghies or life jackets. Unfortunately for my father, some of the dye had splashed into his wound and infected it, so by the time he got back to England it had become gangrenous and he had to have his left leg amputated.

The prosthetic limb they gave him was made of tin, which he found heavy and very uncomfortable. At weekends he used to take his artificial leg off and use it like a bat to play cricket with me in the garden while balancing on his good right leg. After he died, my mother's brother Peter tried to take over cricket duties, but apparently, I became upset with my uncle when he wouldn't take his leg off to hit the ball with it as my father had done. I must have assumed that every grown-up could do it.

I only have three photos of my father and he looks like a movie star in all of them.

Many years later, one of my girlfriends, seeing a photo of him on my bedside table, remarked on how handsome he was and then added rather unkindly, 'You don't look anything like him!'

I have no memory of being told my father had died. Being so young, perhaps my mother thought that I wouldn't have understood what death meant, but at some stage I must have realised what had happened or at least accepted the fact he was never coming back and I had lost my hero.

After the funeral, my siblings went back to their respective boarding schools, which must have been a very harrowing time for them. I was too young to know what grief was or how to deal with it at the time, but sadly I would get other opportunities when I was older.

My mother and I went to stay with her parents who lived in a large house in Forest Row in East Sussex. My grandmother had been a volunteer ambulance driver in WW2 and my grandfather had been in the Royal Horse Artillery in WW1. He lost a lung due to gas poisoning in the trenches at Ypres and had difficulty breathing normally. I have little recollection of the period except for my first awareness of music. To help her grieve, my mother played records when her parents were out. Listening to Gabriel Fauré's *Requiem* made her cry and even though I was so young, I instinctively knew this melancholy music was somehow connected to my father not being there anymore. One of the many benefits of music is how it can make us feel close to another person, which might explain why the bond with my mother would remain so strong forever.

The first Christmas without my father was a sad time for my mother and my siblings. All I can remember is being given a drum as a present, which must have driven them all crazy during the day, but hopefully, I was silent at night so that they could sleep in peace.

We moved to Lymington in Hampshire at the end of 1958. The town was close to both the Solent and the New Forest, so it was an idyllic spot for children to grow up.

My sister and brother continued going to their boarding schools while I stayed at home with my mother until I was old enough to go to a local kindergarten, where I first met Mark, Phil, Harry and Richard who are all still friends of mine to this day.

Down House was run by an elderly spinster called Miss Mac who was strict but kind. We were taught how to write the letters of the alphabet, which I would often write down in the wrong order, and how to draw with coloured crayons, which I was much better at and even created some recognizable images. We also had a class called Music and Movement, which was a way of giving us some daily exercise and a way of learning about coordination. Miss Mac would place a 78rpm (revolutions per minute) record onto her turntable, something like the uplifting instrumental *Da Capo* by Georges Boulanger and his Dance Orchestra. When the music started, she would tell us to raise our arms in the air and pretend we were trees bending in the wind and imagine we were leaves slowly fluttering back to the floor. My coordination was all over the place but I loved every minute of it. My passion for music had begun.

In 1959 we moved to a bigger house in Daniell's Walk, which was very close to the town centre. It had a long lawn at the back with several fruit trees and a vegetable patch at the end of it, so most of the food we ate was from our own garden. I can remember picking strawberries off their stems in an area that was netted off to stop the birds from eating them and helping my mother pod peas in the kitchen.

As there weren't any supermarkets in those days, my mother went shopping every day and took her own basket to bring everything home. Meat was wrapped in paper, bread was wrapped in paper tissue and fruit and veg were sold loose and put in paper bags, which would either get used again, burnt on a bonfire or used to light our coal fire in the winter. We also had a compost heap in the garden where we threw away any food waste and left it to rot. I still remember the dustman collecting our steel dustbin from the side of the house, carrying it on his back to his dustcart and emptying it before bringing it back but I can't remember how often he came. I don't think it was weekly back then as we had so little to put in it.

Sometimes my mother left me with our elderly neighbours when she went shopping or to see friends. The Bardells were French and tried to teach me a few words in their language. When my mother came to collect me I attempted to name each food item in French. Côtes de porc, patate, carotte et petite pois were easy peasy, as they didn't sound very different from the English words but trying to learn *bâtonnets de poisson* meant fish fingers or *fèves au lard* meant baked beans was a bit harder. They then taught me the French lullaby *Frère Jacques* and I found it much easier to learn the lyrics having a tune to go with the words. I also learned to sing *Alouette* but at the time I had no idea that it was a song about plucking a lark. If I had I might not have been quite as keen.

That winter I caught pneumonia and had to stay at home in bed for six weeks. To keep me entertained, my mother let me listen to *Children's Favourites* on BBC Radio every morning. A man called Derek McCulloch, better known to children as 'Uncle Mac', played a variety of songs suitable for children of my age. I loved this radio programme; it stimulated my imagination and triggered my ongoing love for music. *Nellie the Elephant* and *Tubby the Tuba* were my favourite songs at the time followed closely by *Puff the Magic Dragon* and *Sparky the Magic Piano.*

I must have completed a dozen jigsaw puzzles during my convalescence, including at least one with the image of *Rupert Bear* on it, but as most of them only had 80-100 pieces they didn't take very long for me to finish, which meant my problem-solving skills and spatial awareness must have been improving along with my health.

Once I was well again, my mother bought me the book *A Bear Called Paddington,* a wonderful children's story about an unusual bear who had travelled to England from Darkest Peru with only an old suitcase, a stained hat and a solitary jar of marmalade in his possession. Reading Michael Bond's delightful books taught me about the importance of being polite and to remember to always say 'Yes please… and thank you.'

When I was a bit older, my mother told me she thought all children should be taught manners and morals before they can read and write, as good manners and etiquette show compassion and respect for others, which is the key to interacting with other people and having a successful life. She was quite right of course, as mothers usually are!

The day my mother came back from the shops with a black and white television set, my life changed completely, as it must have done for anybody else fortunate enough to have one. I loved watching a children's programme called *Watch With Mother,* which featured different puppets each day of the week. My favourite ones were Andy Pandy, Bill and Ben the Flowerpot Men and Rag Tag and Bobtail. A short tune was played on the piano at the beginning of each programme to the rhythm of the words *quarter to two*, which was the time the broadcast started. Along with hundreds of other children, that was most probably how I learned to tell the time.

As my friend Mark's father owned a toy shop, he usually got the latest toys first. When he was given one of the very first sets of self-locking coloured plastic bricks, I naturally wanted one too so my mother took me to H.E. Figgures, a traditional toy shop in Lymington that had been family-run since 1904, to buy a set. Playing with Lego kept me busy for hours, which must have been a big help to my mother, as she had recently decided to set up a nursery playgroup looking after young children to give her a modest income to supplement her widow's pension.

After I had turned six, my mother started taking me to Sunday school at her local Christian Science church. While she attended the service for 'grown-ups' I went to the children's class in a room at the rear of the church, which mainly consisted of listening to stories about Jesus and singing a couple of hymns. I wasn't interested in doing either and preferred staring at the passing clouds through the window. I often saw recognisable patterns in the sky that resembled the faces of people and shapes of animals or objects. One day, the teacher must have had enough of my constant cloud gazing and asked me.

'What are you staring at this time, or perhaps I should ask, who?'

'Jesus!' I said, as that was what the face in the clouds looked like to me. After that, she never stopped me doing it again.

My next experience of religion was at Walhampton, a preparatory school in Lymington where they promoted the importance of moral, spiritual and Christian values but I wasn't interested in the religious aspect at all. What I did enjoy was singing hymns as part of a group as it gave me a sense of belonging. My favourite song was *All Things Bright and Beautiful* but one day after singing the words 'All creatures great and small,' I added, 'except poodles', which made the other boys in my pew laugh and that was the first time I realised that by making jokes you could also make friends.

The 18th-century country house was Grade 11* listed and had grounds of about 90 acres, including a series of ponds and lakes, which I couldn't wait to explore. There were no enforced rules for health and safety in those days and playing outside for long periods without any supervision was considered completely normal. Fighting with swords made from sharp sticks or playing conkers or with toy guns with caps wasn't considered a problem, and neither was riding a bicycle without a helmet.

I was initially sent there as a day boy. Our teacher was a middle-aged woman called Miss Fisher who we nicknamed 'Fishcakes' behind her back. I liked her a lot as she was 'jolly', a word seldom used these days, but accurate in her case. After I had got over the anxiety of being separated from my mother and into a routine, I became a boarder.

The following conditions had to be met before being allowed to board. Each boy had to be able to dress and undress himself, tie his tie, lace his shoes, wash, bath and brush his hair, make his own bed and hold his knife, fork and spoon properly.

The 200 boys were broken down into smaller groups known as houses, including Scott, Shackleton and Mallory. I was put in Mallory and given the number 9. My poor mother then had to sow tags on all my items of clothing with that number marked clearly on them, so that once they had been sent to the school laundry with all the other boys' dirty clothes they could be returned later to the correct owners.

At eleven o'clock every morning we were forced to drink a half pint of milk, which I wasn't keen on as it made me feel unwell, as did anything with cheese or cream in it. (Many years later, I discovered that I was lactose intolerant but at that time I was just considered 'difficult'.) The crates of milk usually sat outside for a few hours before we got them and if it had been a particularly chilly morning the teachers would warm the bottles up next to the radiators before handing them out and by then the milk would taste sour but we still had to drink it. Our lunches and suppers consisted of meals like minced beef, mashed potatoes and carrots or a stew with boiled cabbage that you could smell in the school corridors for hours afterwards but on Fridays, we always had fish with a white parsley sauce, tinned peas and potatoes, which was a bit of a treat. The best course was usually the puddings. Spotted dick, jam roly-poly or apple crumble served with hot yellow custard were my favourites but I wasn't that keen on tapioca, blancmange or prunes. However, we were expected to eat everything on our plate and couldn't leave the table until we had.

In the 1960s the teachers used to stand in front of the class, which consisted of about twenty of us sitting at individual wooden desks facing a chalkboard, and talk to us while writing facts on the board, which we would then have to copy in our best handwriting into notebooks. I always placed my ink, pen, pencil, rubber and ruler in the same order on my desk in the classroom and if I saw anything that wasn't properly aligned I had to immediately rearrange it to restore order...at least to my eyes. The school library was organised in alphabetical order by author but from time to time I would find a book, which had been replaced incorrectly, so I would then have to move it back to its correct place before being able to continue with my own search. This simple action often took me ages to complete as I found it hard to see the author's names on the spines of the books unless I was standing right in front of them. When one of the teachers noticed that I was having trouble reading the blackboard from a distance, I was sent for an eye test and that was when I discovered that I was short-sighted and would have to wear glasses for the rest of my life.

The National Health glasses at the time were rather ugly and because my eyesight was so bad the lenses were thick and heavy. It didn't take long before other boys started calling me 'Four-Eyes!' When one of the school bullies grabbed my specs and snapped them in half, I fixed the problem by sticking the two halves together with Elastoplast. Luckily the temporary repair lasted until my mother was able to get me a new pair.

After a bit of trial and error, I eventually found an innovative way of using the broken spectacles to my advantage and used them to help me put on a film show in the dormitory after lights out. I made my *movie* using Sellotape, which was normally used to repair tears in paper because it had a kind of rubber adhesive on the back. I spent many hours rubbing this gluey substance off to create a clear cellophane strip before marking frames at equal intervals and drawing images of two men firing guns at each other followed by a car chase, carefully animating the movements frame by frame.

The *projector* was constructed using the cardboard core of an empty loo roll and attaching the lenses from my old glasses with Sellotape to it at one end and a bulb connected, using chewing gum bought from the Tuck shop, to a small battery at the other. I wound the cellophane strip tightly onto a pencil that I held firmly in my left hand and then wound it frame by frame onto a second pencil held in my other hand while twisting clockwise, so that the image passed directly in front of the loo roll and the backlit lenses onto the screen, which was a white sheet hung on two hooks on the back of our dormitory door.

The focusing process took a bit of time to perfect but after a while I found the correct distance between the cellophane strip and the lenses to keep the images sharp. It was then just a matter of twisting the pencils in sync with each other to bring my amateurish animation to life. As the *movie* appeared on our makeshift screen, I used my voice to create the sound effects, which consisted of gunfire, explosions and screeching tyres. Unfortunately, the school matron was woken up by the noise, which resulted in a strict telling-off followed by the threat of being sent to the headmaster.

I slept very little that night worrying that I might be in for my first encounter with the cane or the butter paddle, which JB our headmaster was also known to use. My fears were justified and sure enough, I got six of the best on my backside with the cane the following morning.

JB, the headmaster, informed me that it was for my own good, which I thought, as I dropped my trousers and bent over as instructed, seemed highly unlikely. Oh, and by the way, if you ever hear the expression 'This is going to hurt me more than it's going to hurt you,' it's a lie.

As I was pulling my trousers back up and holding back the tears at the same time, JB told me I should concentrate on my school studies a bit more and stop dreaming about making films in Hollywood. Naturally, all I wanted to do from that day on was exactly that.

*Go confidently in the direction of your dreams and live the life you have imagined.*
Henry David Thoreau


## CHAPTER 2: SCHOOL DAYS

Our art teacher, Miss Le May was a wonderful motivator who always encouraged me to use my imagination. When I told her I hoped to learn how to make films one day, she said, 'Then it will happen... as hope is the will and the way to success.'

At the end of term, I won the school art prize and to my surprise, JB was the first to congratulate me. The fact he had recently started dating our attractive female art teacher might have had something to do with that.

Telling stories in my paintings came naturally to me but writing them down was a lot harder. I knew the correct letters for each word but wrote them down in the wrong order or as *Winnie the Pooh* said in one of A.A. Milne's wonderful stories. 'My spelling is Wobbly. It's good spelling but it Wobbles, and the letters get in the wrong places.'

I was also terrible at maths and would often write the numbers down back to front. If it had been today, I would probably have been diagnosed with dyslexia and dyscalculia but those terms weren't in common use back then and I was just considered a bit slow. The school's answer to my problem was for me to spend some time with Mr Gordon for extra tuition.

Luckily for me it was a good decision. 'Gordo', as everyone called him, had been such a popular teacher that after retiring the school kept him on to mentor the younger boys. He was a kindly old man who immediately put me at ease by telling me he had taught many other boys how to spell and he would help me too.

After I told Gordo that some of the boys were taunting me and calling me names like 'Spaz, Moron and Dumbwit,' he frowned and said, 'Oh dear, I wish they could act with a little more kindness and a little less judgement.'

Gordo then asked me if I knew what the three Rs were, which I did, so I told him, 'Reading, writing and arithmetic sir.'

'You are quite right young man, but as only one of those words actually begins with an R, I don't think they are the best examples to teach you how to spell correctly, do you?'

He then chuckled before saying, 'So, let's choose some words that are spelt exactly how they sound and you will get better at it in no time… Tick Tock… goes the Clock!'

Gordo had an old-fashioned Albion printing press in his study and after I had finished my weekly tutorial with him, he took the time to teach me how to use it. Setting the 14-point Kennerly Old Style serif typeface involved selecting a series of metal keys that had each letter of the alphabet or punctuation mark at the tip and placing them in the right order to spell words and create sentences. It soon became clear I didn't have any problem with spelling and I was placing the letters in the correct sequence when I was using these keys but when I attempted to write essays in pen and ink on paper I struggled with the order of the letters, for example, writing *aminal* instead of *animal*, *silnaig* instead of *sailing* or more confusingly words like *reserve* instead of *reverse* which were correctly spelt but had different meanings. This hands-on experience was very helpful as Gordo was able to reassure me that I wasn't *slow*, as one of the other teachers had called me. In fact, he thought the problem was my brain was working too fast, especially when I was writing things down on paper and I should try to do everything slower from now on.

When my extra tuition was over, he gave me a small book about butterflies and moths as a present and signed it 'From your friend Gordo'. It is still one of my most prized possessions.

Every morning Gordo would amble to the nearest lake on the school grounds to feed the ducks and geese. A handful of us would walk with him whenever we had the chance. The boys all felt completely safe with him but he did have one rather quirky habit we thought was amusing and our parent's thought was 'quite disgusting'. When any of the boys lost a primary tooth, he would ask us to give it to him and glue the dead tooth into the top of his walking stick next to a dozen or so others to decorate it. When asked why he did this, he explained he was simply replacing the whalebone inlay that had adorned his stick when he first bought it.

During the next school holiday my mother allowed me to have a pet - a tortoise my brother named Fangio but unfortunately, he came to an untimely end. Cause of death unknown. He was quickly followed by a white rabbit predictably named Snowy. Having now shown I could care for a pet I was also allowed to have a goldfish, or possibly a series of goldfish, as I seem to recall Goldie appeared to change his markings and shape every few weeks. I suspect my big brother was asked, or perhaps bribed, by my mother to find a replacement at the local pet shop each time the previous goldfish was found floating on the surface.

My interest in animals started a couple of years earlier while watching *Animal Magic* for the first time. This wonderful BBC TV show was presented by Johnny Morris who educated and entertained children by pretending to be one of the Zookeepers at Bristol Zoo and used funny voices to make it sound as though the animals were talking to him. He was later unfairly criticised for anthropomorphising the animals but I will always be grateful to him for inspiring me to learn more about the natural world.

The following term I was given permission by my mother to learn to ride a horse, as the school had its own stables with a few small ponies suitable to be ridden by young boys. But once I had met Bob, a tall grey Shire horse, I was smitten and whenever there was an opportunity to sit on this gentle beast's back I did so. During one of the school holidays, Miss Kemp, who was in charge of the stables, took a small group of us on a gypsy caravan trek through the New Forest. It is one of the happiest memories of my childhood.

Every year the school would put on plays like *Androcles and the Lion*, which would be seen by our parents as well as the rest of the school. I usually only got a bit part such as 'third centurion' as I could never remember my lines but my paintings were often in demand, especially if any of the productions required images of animals. When the school decided to do *Noah's Ark*, I was doubly busy.

During the school holidays, I spent most of my spare time watching children's science-fiction marionette puppet shows like Gerry and Sylvia Anderson's *Fireball XL5* and *Thunderbirds*. I must have liked glamorous women even at that young age, as I remember taking a fancy to Doctor Venus in the first show and to Lady Penelope Creighton-Ward in the other. My favourite character was her butler and chauffeur, Parker, a loveable rogue with a heavy cockney accent who would try to sound posh by adding an 'h' to words that didn't need them.

Parker: 'Er, yes, m'lady. I h'understand he's been on his way now for two weeks.'

Many years later, I discovered Gerry Anderson had taken the gifted character actor David Graham to dinner at a pub one evening to tell him about a new puppet series he was planning and to ask him if he would provide some of the voices. Shortly after they had sat down at their table, an elderly waiter who they could tell was from the East End of London came up to them and asked 'Would you like to see the h'wine list Sir?' and that was the moment when the voice of Parker was born.

Another wonderful fictitious character entered my life on the 21st of December 1963 in the form of *Doctor Who*, played by William Hartnell, who travelled through space, time and matter in an old police box called the Tardis. As soon as I heard the theme music written by Australian composer Percy Grainer, I was hooked. This episode was actually the second story broadcast on TV but the first with the Daleks, which is what really won me over to the science-fiction series along with many other children.

My other Sci-Fi hero was *Dan Dare: Pilot of the Future* who featured in the comic periodical the *Eagle*. Dan's arch-enemy was *The Mekon*, who had a truly massive head and whose sole goal appeared to be the conquest of Earth.

I spent an excessive amount of time daydreaming, immersed in my own imagination, but was also becoming a compulsive reader. The books I enjoyed the most at that time were *Robinson Crusoe* by Daniel Defoe and *Kidnapped* by Robert Louis Stevenson.

Both novels had heroes with qualities I admired. After being shipwrecked and stranded on a remote island, Crusoe manages to succeed against the odds by being self-reliant and resourceful. In the other story, a naïve young boy called Davie Balfour, goes through all kinds of misfortunes but through sheer determination and willpower survives everything that is thrown at him to regain his identity and get his inheritance back.

The school library also had a few books about a fictitious pilot and adventurer called James Bigglesworth, better known to his 'chums', Algy and Ginger, as Biggles. The stories of his adventures written by W.E. Johns had titles like *Biggles Flies North* or *Biggles Flies East*. My 'chum' Fish thought the next book should be called *Biggles Flies Undone*, which being young boys we thought was hysterical.

Books played a larger role than music for me initially but once I was taught to appreciate how listening to music would allow me to visualise my own stories in my head and create my own characters or even include myself in some of my imaginary adventures, I fell in love with this emotional form of storytelling and from that moment on music was the key to my happiness.

We were lucky to have a charismatic music teacher called Mr Hutchinson who taught us music was a way of telling a story and immersing ourselves in music would help unleash our creativity. He encouraged us to really concentrate when we listened to the 33rpm records he played in our classes and to allow our imaginations to go wild. *The Young Person's Guide to the Orchestra* by Benjamin Britten was an immediate favourite. It was a wonderful way to be introduced to all the instruments in an orchestra and has some of the most memorable melodies I have ever heard. I also loved Gustav Holst's *The Planets,* especially *Mars, the Bringer of War* with its relentless repetitive and dramatic phrase, which fuelled my imagination. Every time I heard it, I visualised a wicked alien warlord sending hundreds of spaceships into battle. However, it was the *1812 Overture* by Tchaikovsky I liked the most, as the dramatic music helped me form images in my head of the desperate Russian soldiers defending their country against Napoleon's army. 'Hutch' had his own favourites, including Rossini's *The William Tell Overture*, which I had already heard because it was also the theme for the TV show *The Lone Ranger*.

Hutch gave me a few piano lessons but because I couldn't get my fingers to stretch as far as an octave I became frustrated. He then gave me some exercises to stretch my small hands and short fingers but they weren't flexible enough and eventually I just gave up.

My next instrument was the cornet, which was similar to a trumpet, but it didn't take long before I realised that I would have to stay indoors and practice every day to become any good at it. Playing football outdoors with my friends, using our jumpers as goalposts, was far more appealing, or playing conkers, taking turns to strike each other's horse chestnuts as hard as we possibly could until one of them broke.

My introduction to what was considered popular music at that time began when my siblings listened to their 45rpm singles on our record player at home, which included *Glad All Over* by The Dave Clark Five, *I Only Want to Be with You* by Dusty Springfield and *Twist and Shout* by The Beatles, which was actually an extended player (EP) that also had *A Taste of Honey, Do You Want to Know a Secret* and *There's a Place* on it. These songs stayed in my musical memory bank for ages because the titles were in the lyrics, which made them easy to remember.

My brother Niall was lucky enough to see The Beatles play in Bournemouth, which I remember being rather envious about. But it was an old single from 1957 that one of my friend's fathers had in his collection that I liked the most called *School Days* by Chuck Berry, which grabbed my attention because of the way he got his guitar to echo each of his lines. The B-side was a pedal steel guitar instrumental called *Deep Feeling* which completely blew my mind. I had now officially been introduced to Rock and Roll and the Blues for the first time courtesy of Mr. Charles Anderson Edward Berry.

Thanks, Chuck!

My sister watched the rock/pop music show *Ready Steady Go!*

presented by Keith Fordyce and Cathy McGowan on television every Friday evening, so I would often sit on the sofa next to her and look at the artists miming their hit songs in front of a studio audience.

Top of the Pops first appeared on the BBC on the 1st of January 1964. It was introduced by Radio One DJ Jimmy Savile. The Rolling Stones opened the show with *I Wanna Be Your Man* and were then followed by Dusty Springfield singing *I Only Want to be With You*, the Dave Clark Five performing *Glad All Over*, The Hollies with *Stay* and The Swinging Blue Jeans with *The Hippy Hippy Shake.* The show also featured film clips of Cliff Richard & The Shadows, Freddie & The Dreamers and The Beatles, currently Number 1 with *I Want to Hold Your Hand.*

A few weeks later, my sister bought the album *With the Beatles*, which featured Robert Freeman's iconic black and white photo of the band's floating heads on a black background on the record sleeve. It was the first time I had really taken notice of a cover on an LP. It caught my attention simply because it was so eye-catching.

At the start of the next term, I had to move to a larger dormitory, which had 15 other boys in it and the only way I could get to sleep was to compulsively repeat the lyrics of the songs which had recently been in the singles charts in my head every night. *Needles and Pins* by The Searchers, *Bits and Pieces* by the Dave Clark Five and *Not Fade Away* by The Rolling Stones all helped relieve my nocturnal anxiety. I rarely needed more than three songs before I felt safe and nodded off.

It was at about this time I started listening to comedy shows like *The Navy Lark, Hancock's Half Hour* and best of all *The Goon Show* with Harry Secombe, Peter Sellers and the wonderful Spike Milligan. *The Ying Tong Song* still makes me smile today.

As a special treat, my mother took me to see the Bernard Miles production of *Treasure Island* at the Mermaid Theatre in London. Spike played the part of Ben Gunn brilliantly. A few weeks later, my godmother Puck took me to Covent Garden to see the ballet *Cinderella* starring Robert Helpmann and Frederick Ashton as the Ugly Stepsisters, which was mesmerising as their comic timing was perfect.

The combination of Ashton's brilliantly choreographed visuals and Prokofiev's memorable melodies really captured my attention.

On Saturday evenings we would sometimes be allowed to watch a movie on a huge screen in the main hall. We would sit on the floor in neat rows and be treated to whatever films the school had been able to acquire. The most memorable being *Spartacus, The Great Escape* and *The Magnificent Seven.*

When the James Bond movie *Goldfinger* starring Sean Connery was released during the school holidays, my mother took me to see it at a cinema in Southampton. Although Goldfinger's henchman Oddjob with his razor-edged bowler hat stole the show, it was the superbly designed Aston Martin DB5 with its retractable machine guns, rotating number plate and ejector seat which triggered my imagination. For my birthday I was given a tiny replica of Bond's Aston Martin complete with all the accessories including the ejector seat. It was created by Corgi Toys and I took it with me everywhere. I also got an extra carriage for my Hornby's Pullman train set. During the previous holidays, I had created mountains out of chicken wire and Papier-mâché and built tunnels in them, which allowed my train to travel between different countries and time zones. I could make the train stop at the Wild West Frontier where I had placed miniature cowboys and Indians fighting each other or stop at The Battle of the Somme where I had English and German soldiers fighting in muddy trenches complete with barbed wire fences made with insulation wire wound around a pencil a dozen times. Making Airfix models was a great hobby for a while, but when it started to become a bit boring, as everything eventually does when you are young, we decided to upgrade our means of time travel using real steam engines.

In those days the trains were driven by steam and as Alias lived near a station we decided to play our new game there. The rules were simple. We both had to stand on the bridge which separated the two platforms just as the next train passed underneath and as the steam engulfed us, we had to shut our eyes and whoever's turn it was would shout out a specific year. After the train had gone, we would open our eyes and pretend we were now living in that particular year until the next train was due. When we encountered other people, we had to remain in character and speak the way we thought they would have done in the era we had chosen. If it was 1066 then we were Anglo-Saxons fighting William's Norman-French army, if it was 1642 we were Cavaliers fighting Cromwell's Roundheads and if it was 1914 we were a couple of Tommies fighting the Hun. It was fun pretending to be a time traveller like *Doctor Who*.

There were many other TV shows which also had a profound influence on me at this time. I was a huge fan of *The Avengers, The Man from Uncle* and *Dangerman.* The TV series *Mission Impossible* was also a great source of inspiration. Alias and I loved creating our own missions but on one occasion we got more than we bargained for.

A famous author called Dennis Wheatley lived in a two-storeyed Georgian house less than a mile from our family home. He had written many books about witchcraft and the occult and his best-known novel was called *The Devil Rides Out*, which mentions a blue Rolls-Royce, a green Daimler and a yellow Sunbeam. We had heard these amazing cars were locked in his large double garage so wanted to find out if it was true.

Wheatley had devised a number of board games including one called 'Invasion', which was rather apt for what we were about to do next. Because he had written a few books about the occult, he occasionally received anonymous threats from groups who sought to 'rid our planet of his type'. This meant he had to protect his property more than most, so he had put broken glass on the top of all the high wavy walls surrounding his home. Apparently, he had done the bricklaying himself in the form of a serpentine wall, which was very impressive but getting over the crinkle-crankle fortification was exactly the sort of challenge young boys thrive on.

Alias and another friend who we nicknamed Fish, as his surname was Gill, came to our house to play with my train set one day but we had another activity in mind. Using burnt cork to blacken our faces to blend in with the darkness of the night, or in our case bright afternoon light, as it didn't get dark until late in the summer, we walked the short distance to Wheatley's house taking turns to carry a small ladder, a picnic rug, a pillow and a small bag which contained our secret weapons, which were all vital for the mission we had all just agreed to accept. When we arrived at our destination, Alias put the ladder against the wall and Fish climbed up to place the pillow over the shards of broken glass. After I handed him the rug, he draped it over the pillow so when we climbed over the wall, we wouldn't cut ourselves. The intention was to then abseil down the other side, or would have been if we had remembered to bring any rope. What we actually did was jump down and fall flat on our arses.

Having got into the grounds, we then made our way to the garage. As we expected, it was locked. This is when our first secret weapon was deployed. Runny honey. After making sure nobody had seen us, Fish poured a little of the clear honey into the lock of the garage door before adding some more all the way down the crack between the double doors and finally along the ground to where we were crouching trying not to be seen by the inhabitants of the house. Our second weapon was gunpowder. Before we left home, we had pooled all our penny bangers, which were small fireworks easily purchased at the local toy shop. Alias sprinkled the gunpowder onto the honey just as we had seen done on a certain TV show recently, which we all presumed would create the perfect slow-burning fuse. The remaining bangers were placed around the lock and stuck on with chewing gum, which we hoped would create a mini explosion and break the lock. Our final weapon was a sparkler to act as the detonator.

What was supposed to happen was the lit sparkler would ignite the gunpowder-honey mix nearest to us and the flame would continue along the honey trail until it finally got to the keyhole and finally a small bang would occur, destroying the lock and enabling us to be able to open the doors and finally see the cars which were kept in there.

What actually happened was that after we lit the sparkler it just fizzed out, so Plan B was put into action. A box of matches solved the problem and suddenly our homemade fuse was working a bit too well and burning brightly towards the garage doors. When the flames got to the penny bangers, we had quite a shock, as instead of the little bang we had expected, a series of rather large bangs took place. This was quickly followed by the doors of the garage being almost blown off. Three small and rather frightened little boys quickly ran for their lives.

We were worried the police would be called in to look for the terrorist group who had destroyed Dennis Wheatley's garage but thankfully there was no mention of anything in the local newspaper, so it looked as though we had got away with our misguided mission. I must admit I was more than a wee bit disappointed not to see his Rolls-Royce or any other fancy car for that matter but it is quite possible there were none there anyway, as I was told at a later date the novelist preferred riding a motorbike and it was his wife Joan who did most of the driving.

The next opportunity to see some impressive cars came sooner than expected. Filming scenes for *The Avengers* TV series was about to take place at Lord Montagu's Motor Museum so my mother found out exactly when and drove me there on the day of the shoot. Patrick Macnee as *Steed* and Diana Rigg as *Emma Peel* spent the whole day doing 'drive-offs' in an assortment of vintage cars. The theme music by Laurie Johnson was absolutely perfect for the show and when I hear it today it takes me right back to Beaulieu.

As my siblings were so much older than me and had their own friends, we didn't spend a lot of time together during the day but would often eat together in the evening when they were home, so I knew what they were up to. My sister was now studying fashion at Saint Martins in London and my brother had followed in our father's footsteps and was studying to be a land agent at the Royal Agriculture College in Cirencester.

My sister loved music and introduced me to The Beach Boys. She had a copy of their album *Pet Sounds,* which I liked because it was different to anything else I had heard and contained a collection of songs which combined elements of pop, jazz and classical music together with various sound effects added to the mix and the band's fabulous vocal harmonies were layered on top. *God Only Knows* remains one of my favourite songs of all time.

Later that term, I passed my Eleven-plus exam, which meant I would be sent to a public school in the autumn. I wasn't looking forward to it at all but at least we had the summer holidays to enjoy first. Mum had promised we could go to Lyme Regis on the Jurassic coast in Dorset to hunt for fossils on the beach. It took patience but eventually I found a small spiral-shaped ammonite and holding something millions of years old was very exciting.

After we had finished our fish and chips, Mum said she was going to buy me a pair of sensible shoes to wear at my new school. When we were inside the shop, I saw a boy of about the same age as me standing next to a strange-looking contraption. He looked at me and said he could see the bones in his feet. I thought he must be fibbing, so asked if I could have a go and to my surprise discovered he had been telling the truth. I was told by the sales assistant it was a shoe-fitting fluoroscope device which would help him determine the correct shoe size I should have. After telling me to place my feet in the space provided, he then said I should look down one of the ports at the top and he would look down the other. I was amazed I could now see x-rays of both my feet. What I didn't know at the time was despite being shielded by the wooden exterior of the Pedoscope, a significant amount of radiation was now bathing my entire body.

Just before midday, the manager walked up to us and said they were closing early because they were going to watch the 1966 World Cup Final between England and Germany, which was about to be screened live on both the BBC and ITV. They had brought a black and white television into the store so all the staff could watch the football match. I asked if I could stay and watch it with them and after being reassured by the manager they would look after me, my mother agreed I could stay and told me she would go shopping until it was over. Kenneth Wolstenholme's words as the fourth goal was scored became etched in my and millions of others memories forever. 'They think it's all over! It is now! It's four!'

The final score was 4-2 to England and like many other young boys, I became a huge football fan from then on and for the rest of the holidays all I wanted to do was play in the garden with the heavy leather football my mother had bought me before we left Lyme Regis.

On the same day as the World Cup Final, a song written by Jerry Samuels but billed as Napoleon XIV, became a huge hit on the radio and as I was about to be sent away to a new boarding school in Gloucestershire, I thought it couldn't have been more appropriately titled. *They're Coming to Take Me Away. Ha Haa!*

The public school I was about to attend had been established as a facility for 'wayward and orphaned children', so quite why I was being sent there was a mystery. Perhaps it was to toughen me up? It didn't help matters it had the rather unfortunate nickname of 'Borstal on the Hill'. The grounds were surrounded by tall fences with barbed wire at the top reminiscent of POW camps in the Second World War. Instead of having a headmaster in charge there was a Warden, so it was evident this was going to be more a place of correction than of education.

The thought of being sent to such a strict school so far away from my mother was more than a little frightening, especially as I was only eleven. I had been rather mollycoddled up until now but it was all about to change.

*Sticks and stones can break your bones, but words can never hurt you…unless you believe them. Then, they can destroy you.*

Charles F. Glassman

## CHAPTER 3: BREAK ON THROUGH (To the Other Side)

I was the youngest boy at my new school and the bullying started on day one.

There was a system called Fagging, which had been a traditional practice at most English public schools for many years, where the younger boys acted as personal servants to the older prefects. We were expected to make them cups of tea, polish their shoes or do any other menial task they ordered us to do. Most of the time it was fairly harmless but from time to time we would hear a Chinese whisper one of the boys had been forced to do sexual favours, so we lived in constant fear of similar abusive coercion. Older boys getting crushes on pretty boys who looked like girls was quite common. Thankfully, I was never targeted this way but as I was small and wore National Health glasses it didn't take long before the school thugs were lining up for a go at me.

During my first week, three older boys forced me to scrub the filthy urinal in the house lavatory with my toothbrush and then made me use it to brush my own teeth. But this wasn't enough for this sadistic trio. The largest of them said, 'You are a useless piece of shit Robertson'. The other two then held me upside down by my legs and lowered my head slowly into the toilet bowl, which was full of steaming excrement before pressing the flush, drowning out their laughter as well as nearly drowning me. They then told me if I reported them, I would be given more of the same treatment or worse. The fear of the potential consequences was enough for me to stay silent.

Being bullied so often made me feel completely worthless. It was a struggle to get through each day without feeling sick with fear. I had made friends easily at my last school so why couldn't I do the same here? I couldn't understand why I was hated so much and presumed I must be unlovable. After one particularly brutal bashing, I experienced suicidal thoughts for the first time in my life. Thankfully, being so young, I had no idea how to 'do myself in' and the thought of how my mother would feel if I died by my own hand was enough to stop me from taking this drastic course of action. As I cried myself to sleep each night, I told myself I would just have to learn to cope.

Bullying wasn't only done to me by my fellow pupils. One of our teachers, Mr Gadd had recently been transferred from one of the country's toughest Borstals, which were youth detention centres run by the HM Prison service with the aim of reforming problem boys aged between 16-21. It soon became clear he intended using the same bullying tactics he had perfected there on us.

One day I made the unpardonable mistake of using the word 'nice' in an essay, so Gadd decided to make a mockery of me in front of the rest of the class. Instead of just throwing the chalkboard rubber at me as he usually did, he tweaked my sideburns with his podgy little fingers and pulled my head down so my body was bent in half and then dragged me all the way from my desk to the chalkboard at the front of the class. He then recited a story about 'Noddy and Big Ears' using the word 'nice' as many times as he could, and each time he pronounced it as though it was the most stupid word in the world. When he had finished humiliating me verbally, he dragged me nearer to the wall so my head was right next to it and while I was still bent in half, kneed me in my bum so hard my head cracked against the classroom wall.

'The problem with you Robertson is that you think too much!' he bellowed. 'It's a jungle out there boy, so it's every man for himself. Survival of the fittest. Those that can't survive on their own have to perish. It's Nature's way of weeding out the weaklings. Are you a weed or a weakling Robertson?'

There were a few nervous titters from the class, as my eyes began to well up.

'I think perhaps you are both. What do you say, boy? Are you a man or a mouse?' Gadd said with an unpleasant smile.

I made a squeaky mouse sound hoping that my sense of humour would make me appear braver than I really felt in front of my classmates. They dutifully roared with laughter but this just incensed the teacher even more.

'I'll make you laugh on the other side of your face boy!' He then proceeded to force me back to my desk, opened the heavy wooden desk lid, placed my head inside the open desk and banged the desk lid down hard. It hurt like hell.

'Sticks and stones may break my bones, but words will never hurt me,' I silently repeated in my head that night in bed. But the truth was they did hurt. A lot. After a while, I became disheartened and didn't want to join in with the other boys when they suggested playing a game. The bullying also affected my studies. Up until now, I had been in the top three in my class but I now feared standing out from the others in case I was picked on for being a 'smart-arse'. As a result, my grades began to drop and I no longer had any ambition to be the best in any of the subjects I had previously excelled in. Having had such a happy experience at my previous school where I was encouraged to read books, appreciate music, use my artistic skills and make friends, I was now in an institution where the oppressive culture negated almost everything which I was familiar with and as a result, I felt totally alone, completely powerless and utterly miserable.

The abusive behaviour of the teachers was copied by some of the prefects and if one of them took a dislike to a junior boy he could make their life a living hell. The prefects in our house had taken it upon themselves to come up with a punishment of pure sadism.

'The Mill' was a cruel ritual that took place in the dormitory just after Bible reading and was a team effort. Six prefects would stand in line, one hand behind their backs, the other wielding a hard-soled slipper. The victim would then have to crawl on his hands and knees in their pyjamas along the splintered wooden floor through the tormentor's legs. When you were halfway through the first pair of legs the prefect would use his knees to hold you in place while he gave you 'six of the best' and this was then repeated by each of the other prefects, as we tried desperately to get to the other end as quickly as possible.

This punishment was given for 'crimes' such as not cleaning your shoes properly, leaving your shoelaces done up or walking with your hands in your pocket, but more than once for not succumbing to their wishes in giving them sexual gratification. It was a barbaric practice and part of the fear was not knowing which night it was going to happen or if at all and whether you would be one of the victims that particular night or not. These 'nights of fear' scarred me both physically and mentally for a long time. After each thrashing through the Mill, I would pull my pillow over my head and bury my face in the horsehair mattress as hard as I could so that no one could hear me weeping.

There were fifteen of us in each dormitory and we were woken every morning by the housemaster clanging an old school bell and shouting, 'Five to seven, time to get up!' We would then go downstairs and take turns in the bathroom to wash our face and brush our teeth before getting dressed in the changing room and going back upstairs to make our beds, complete with hospital corners. We then had different jobs of housework to do for the next twenty minutes like polishing the floors, hoovering the carpets, cleaning the windows and scrubbing the showers. These were administered on a rota system. Once our allotted time was over and we had finished our chores another bell would be rung, which was the cue to walk up to the main school building for breakfast. This usually consisted of runny tasteless porridge or a hardboiled egg with a slice of bread and a cup of tea. But one day, the Warden came into the dining room with a box of windfalls. As he got the kitchen staff to hand them out to us he said, 'Now don't waste them boys, apples don't grow on trees you know!' It was the only time that I ever saw him smile.

At this school, the 'chalk and talk' system of teaching was still being used, which meant the teacher stood at the front of the class and we all sat at individual wooden desks facing him while he spoke. But our Maths teacher, Mr Boseman had his own version, which we called 'chalk and chalk' because he often spent an entire lesson writing formulas and equations in white chalk on the blackboard without uttering a single word to us. To make matters worse, he wrote so fast he often got to the bottom of the board and wiped it clean with a chalk duster so he could start again at the top before we had finished writing down the first set of equations.

I made the mistake of asking him if he could slow down a little one day and got the harsh response, 'Why? Are you a bit slow boy? Are you a slowpoke?'

Boseman's cruel comment was an unexpected gift, as I was able to mimic this teacher perfectly and repeated those words using the same tone of voice and facial expressions as he had in front of the other boys later in the day. This made them laugh out loud and it didn't take long before I received requests to imitate other teachers, which I did with great aplomb. This previously unused talent made me quite popular with my class for a while but when Boseman caught me doing what I thought was a rather reasonable impression of him, he decided to be unreasonable and sent me packing with the words, 'You are completely hopeless at Maths, so leave my class immediately and don't come back. I suggest you go to the Art room, as that is obviously where your talent lies!' He had a point.

When I went home for the winter holidays, the first song I heard on the radio was called *Night of Fear* by The Move. But hopefully I would have no more of those for a while now I was safe at home with my family for Christmas.

1967 began well when during the holidays my mother agreed to take me to a cinema in Southampton to see *One Million Years B.C.* If I had watched the movie a year earlier, I would most probably have only been interested in the dinosaurs but as I was almost a teenager my testosterone levels had begun to soar so the velociraptors now took second place to the voluptuous actress Raquel Welch. My mother bought me the iconic movie poster which I hung on my bedroom wall as soon as we got home. It featured Raquel in a fur bikini, which showed off her ample cleavage to maximum effect and so began my interest in the opposite sex. It was at about this time I started smoking. Most of the boys at school smoked one brand of 'ciggies' or another. Embassy was the most common, as it was the cheapest but Player's

No. 6 was also in demand. I chose Benson & Hedges special filter simply because I liked the gold packet, which had the Royal Warrant on it.

During the next term, we were told we had to either join the Combined Cadet Force (CCF) or the Scouts. Before having to make a decision, I was given a quick lesson on how to shoot with a Lee-Enfield rifle, more commonly known as a 303. They were a bolt action, magazine-fed rifle the British used in both world wars. Lying on my front, I took aim at the target and then shot five rounds at it in quick succession. To my surprise, I had not only hit the target every time but also got two bullseyes, so I was tempted to join the CCF. However, when I discovered this meant wearing a uniform and doing drills every week, I wasn't prepared to do that, so decided to join the Scouts instead and just 'be prepared'.

On the 26th of May 1967, the Beatles released *Sgt. Pepper's Lonely Hearts Club Band*, which was a real game-changer as far as record production was concerned. It was full of joyful songs so despite feeling incredibly lonely and unhappy at the time, I also had a sense of optimism because of the uplifting music. *Lucy in the Sky with Diamonds* was my favourite track: it allowed my imagination to wander freely but it was *Getting Better* I identified with the most because *'the teachers who taught me weren't cool'* either and when John Lennon sang *'it can't get no worse',* it made me laugh, as of course it could, and did.

The following term I managed to get into the school rugby team, which says more about their lack of options for a better hooker than my ball skills. We usually played against another school most Saturday afternoons but sometimes we would play a team made up of boys at our own school instead. For these games, one team would wear the school colours, which had two shades of blue horizontal stripes and the other team would wear their house colours. Each house had a different colour and my house colour sports shirt was green. This usually worked perfectly but one day I was selected to play in school colours but couldn't wear my school shirt as it had been torn in the previous week's match and I was still waiting for a new one. The normal outcome would have been for me to borrow one of the other boys' school shirts they weren't using but Gadd was our referee and wouldn't allow me to swop shirts with one of the other boys. Instead, he made me play bare-chested. Being winter it was freezing and the ground was covered in a fine layer of snow, so it was hardly surprising the following day I caught a nasty cold and was sent to the San to recover. I was so unwell I had to stay in bed for the next ten days but on the plus side, Matron allowed me to listen to her radio. Procol Harum's *A Whiter Shade of Pale* had recently been released and I had to admit the title seemed rather appropriate considering my current complexion.

The actual physical abuse was left to my Housemaster Mr Hyde who seemed to take sadistic pleasure in spanking our bare bottoms until they bled. After he caught me smoking a ciggie on one occasion, he took me into his study and told me to lower my trousers. After I had complied, he then told me to take my pants off as well, which I thought was a bit odd as when I had been caned at my previous school, I had been allowed to keep both my trousers and underwear on. He then slapped my buttocks as hard as he could with his bare hand six times, which hurt like hell. After the final slap, he left his hand on my bottom for a while, which made me feel very uncomfortable.

After I had told one of the other boys what had happened, he warned me Hyde's favourite punishment was reserved for the really young boys who he made take early morning cold showers while he watched them. Closely, much too closely.

I decided that my only option to get away from the constant physical and mental abuse would be to run away but also realised if I got caught the punishment would be worse than I had already experienced so delayed my escape until I had a foolproof plan.

Every week we had to do a five-mile cross-country run within a certain time limit, which I loathed as it involved running through a particularly muddy section known as 'the porridge'. I lost one of my running shoes in the deep sticky grey mud once and had to complete the run with only one shoe. If I had tried to recover it, I would have lost precious minutes and got to the finishing line after the time limit, which would have meant being given the forfeit of doing the entire run again. I decided to bypass 'the porridge' on the next run and took a slight detour just before getting to that spot. After making my way through a wooded area I found a dismantled railway track. I wondered where it led to and whether this would be a potential escape route. The following week I found out the railway line had only been dismantled two years earlier and that hardly anyone went near it anymore. This was exactly what I needed to know.

The distance to the nearest big town with a working railway station was just over five miles away, about the same length as our weekly cross-country run, so if I made my daring escape during the next one I should get there at much the same time as everyone else was crossing the finishing line. I was nearly always last back so I doubted that anyone would notice or care I hadn't returned and when they did eventually discover I was AWOL, I should have had enough time to get to the station to purchase a train ticket back to within a bus trip to my mother's home.

When I confided with Thompson, one of my housemates who had also suffered bullying, he asked me if he could come too which I readily agreed to. During the next run, we lagged behind the others until we got to the farm where we normally turned left to run up a hill along the side of one of their fields. We turned right instead and after crossing a meadow, climbing over a style, across another field and through woodland we found ourselves at the railway track. From there it was simple. All we had to do was walk along the old track all the way to our destination. We walked as quickly as we could until we saw the chimney of the Tweed Mill, which signified that we were close to the end of the track. Thompson looked at his watch and told me were 'running' behind schedule. The irony of his words made us both laugh and we then both broke into a sprint.

Just as we got to the main road, a red sports car sped past us and suddenly screeched to a halt. I asked my fellow escapee if he thought we had been reported missing already and wondered whether this was someone out searching for us. Thompson didn't think so as the car was too flashy. In fact, neither of us recognised the make. To us, it looked more like something from the future. The car slowly reversed and when it was level with us the driver leaned out of his window and asked us if we wanted a lift. The driver had an American accent and I noticed he wore a uniform but couldn't tell what service he was in. We couldn't believe our luck. If this kind 'Yank' was willing to take us to the station then we would be ahead of schedule and have plenty of time to buy our tickets before boarding our train. Thompson asked him if he was in the American Air Force. He didn't answer the question directly and just said that he was based in Huntingdon, which neither of us had ever heard of. I wanted to know what kind of car it was and he proudly told us that it was a Pontiac Firebird.

The car only had two doors, so we presumed that it must only have two seats as well and that one of us would have to sit on the other's lap but when we looked through the passenger side window, we could see that it had a black leather bench seat with an armrest in the middle. The man raised the armrest so that we could squash up side by side and told us to get in. As I opened the door, I must have done it too quickly as the sharp edge of the door frame hit my glasses hard enough to shatter one of the lenses and I started to bleed profusely. The man yelled at us to get in and said that he would take me to the nearest hospital, which he did but as soon as we arrived, he ordered us to get out of the car and sped off without another word.

I was in too much pain at the time to think about why the man had sped off like that and was just grateful to Thompson for finding a nurse to come and tend to my wounds. She made me put my damaged eye over a small glass of lukewarm water and tilt my head back and open my eye to flush any fragments of glass out. I must have managed to close my eyes in time before any real harm was done as she didn't ask me to rinse twice but instead picked up some tweezers and plucked out the tiny shards that had entered the skin near my eye. The nurse told me how lucky I had been but my luck was about to run out.

While we were at the hospital, one of the matrons must have guessed we were schoolboys on the run and told us to sit and wait in reception while she rang our school to report us. An hour later we were both back where we had started our failed escape attempt.

The caning took place just before bedtime, which meant we were only in our pyjamas when we received our punishment. I could hear Thompson cry out as he received six of the best from our housemaster and when his torment was over my partner in crime rushed out of the study and headed straight to the lavatory, presumably to have a good cry. When it was my turn, Hyde stood right behind me and put one hand around my body to pull the cord at the front of my pyjamas making them fall to the ground. He then told me to bend over. It felt like an eternity I was bent in this unnatural position but eventually he administered six strokes of the cane on my backside and the pain was unbelievable.

The one positive thing about being caned at night was by the time I got back to the dormitory the lights were already out so the other boys couldn't see my tears but the welts from the beating remained visible for days. The only thing that got me through this rather dark period of my life was listening to music.

After our last class of the day, we usually had sports practice but two days a week we were free to do what we liked for an hour before supper. I made the most of that freedom listening to LPs in a tiny soundproofed room next to the lavatories, which had psychedelic designs painted on the walls by some of the pupils and had the rather unfortunate nickname, The Glory Hole.

Playing records as loudly as possible kept me sane when I felt I had nowhere else to go and instead of amplifying my anger actually made me feel calmer, so every time anything bad happened to me I would listen to my records, which would help me relax.

*Are You Experienced* by Jimi Hendrix, *Disraeli Gears* by Cream and The Doors self-titled album were my go-to albums at the time. I particularly liked Hendrix's *Manic Depression,* Cream's *World of Pain* and The Doors' *Break on Through (To the Other Side).*

Sometimes it felt like the lyrics were speaking directly to me. A good example was *Waterloo Sunset* by The Kinks, which had recently come out as a single. Apparently, Ray Davies had initially called the song 'Liverpool Sunset' but changed the title after hearing The Beatles song *Penny Lane,* as he didn't want to be thought of as a rip-off merchant. Although it initially sounded like a happy song, after listening more closely to the words, my tormented teenage mind interpreted it to be a melancholic song about someone who chose to be alone. This was mainly due to the line 'I don't need no friends', which I could identify with as I felt totally detached. The prolonged separation from my mother combined with the daily bullying put me under intense emotional stress and if it hadn't been for my meagre record collection I may not have survived as I did. Music was now so vital to my well-being that it had become my safe place.

*Where words fail, music speaks.*

Hans Christian Andersen

## CHAPTER 4: NOTHING IS EASY

In August, I flew to Mallorca to visit my sister Nicci, which allowed me the chance to heal from the mental stress my boarding school had inflicted on me, albeit temporarily.

As she was pregnant with their first child, she wasn't feeling like doing much because of the intense heat so I went on adventures each day by myself. Although I didn't speak the local language, I had learnt a smattering of schoolboy Spanish and was fairly sure I could get the bus into Palma and back without getting lost. I walked down numerous narrow alleyways until I came upon a huge indoor market called Mercat D'Oliver, which is where the locals buy their fruit, veg, meat and fish. I was overwhelmed by the many colours and smells. It was a visual and olfactory feast for the mind.

This was the first time I had travelled alone and all my senses were on hyperdrive. After wandering through the market for about five minutes, I went down some steps into a stunning tree-lined boulevard called La Rambla, which I immediately fell in love with. I had never seen so many stalls selling fresh cut flowers. My sense of smell was working overtime but at the expense of my sense of direction. I was lost.

I eventually plucked up courage and asked one of the flower sellers how to get to the Cathedral in Spanish, 'Puede … decirme dónde… está la Catedral… por favor?'

'Oh yes, it's in that direction,' he replied in perfect English, 'It will only take you about ten minutes to walk there.'

The Cathedral of Santa Maria is known locally as La Seu. I was fascinated by the Gothic architecture and loved seeing how the sun shone through the stain-glassed windows to create colourful patterns everywhere but it was becoming extremely hot so after a short walk to the nearby beach I then took my first swim in the Mediterranean. I had never swum in such clear water before so decided to spend the rest of the day there. By time I got back to my sister's flat, my lily-white

English complexion was now red and blotchy. Nicci advised me to stay indoors for the next two days, so while I was recovering from sunburn I read Ernest Hemmingway's *Death in the Afternoon,* which is where I first learned about the ceremony and traditions of the art of bullfighting. By the weekend I was ready to start exploring again and decided that I would like to see a real bullfight. If my mother had known I was about to go to the Plaza de Toros on my own to watch such a cruel activity she would not have been happy.

The bullring was very impressive from the outside and equally so on the inside. My sister told me to make sure I got a seat, *sombra* (in the shade), which I did but it was so high up I wished that I had brought some binoculars. I had entered the arena with a rather naive attitude towards bullfighting and had no idea of what to expect but was curious none the less. I enjoyed watching the drama unfold beneath me and the matadors almost ballet-like movements as they tossed and swirled their pink and yellow capes was breathtaking.

Interestingly, I wasn't the only young person there and noticed there were quite a few other children in the crowd. They were truly passionate and shouted 'Ole!' at every pass the matador Paco Camino made with his cape. I found out later he was considered one of the best bullfighters of his time and his mastery of the art was near perfection.

I could appreciate the artistic aspect, the incredible bravery of the matador and the courage of the bull but after the picadors had lanced the bull's neck muscle and I saw blood dripping from the wounded beast, I had an intense feeling of injustice and the reality of what I was seeing started to make me feel a little nauseous. Two banderilleros then plunged three sets of dart-like sticks into the bull's shoulders before the matador came back into the ring with a smaller crimson cape called a muleta and a sword. I could sense the excitement of the crowd build as each of Camino's passes with the cape exposed him closer and closer to the bull's horns. When he did finally kill the bull he did it by thrusting his muleta forward with one hand, which made the poor animal lower its head and as it then lunged towards the matador he sunk his sword between the shoulders blades and the bull then died almost immediately. The carcass was then dragged by horses out of the arena. Five more bulls were killed in similar fashion that day but I didn't stay to witness their slaughter.

My sister and I boarded a cruise ship called the T.S.S Hermes bound for Morocco a week later, as my brother-in-law was working as a tour guide for a German travel company and was allowed to take family members with him at a generously discounted price. We had short stopovers in Alicante, Spain and Gibraltar before getting caught in a severe storm.

The liner pitched and rolled for hours and I thought the seasickness would never end but of course it did and when we eventually docked in Casablanca, I was back to normal.

That night we ate couscous with a meat and vegetable tagine and a chicken that had been preserved in lemons and olives I had never eaten such delicious food in my life and it would be hard going back to the dreadful food my school served up when I went back the next term. 'Nutritious' meals such as undercooked mincemeat with overcooked cabbage and greasy gravy, which would require us to drink at least a gallon of cold water to force it all down and keep it there. Dark thoughts of my school were never far away but I was determined not to let them spoil my holiday, especially at mealtimes.

In Marrakesh, we stayed at the famous Hotel La Mamounia, which one of my favourite directors, Alfred Hitchcock, had used as a location in his film *The Man Who Knew Too Much*. Winston Churchill had stayed there once and is alleged to have told President Roosevelt that 'It is the most-lovely spot in the whole world.'

As soon as we had unpacked, I asked if it was possible for me to go up to the roof because I had read somewhere Winnie had called the views incomparably 'paintaceous', which I wholeheartedly agreed with once I had seen them for myself.

When Nicci's bump started kicking, she let me feel her large belly. My future niece was making her presence known. I knew absolutely nothing about the birds and bees at this stage and was more interested in exploring this fascinating city so as my sister wanted to sit by the pool, *The Boy Who Knew Very Little* took himself off on another adventure.

Nothing could have prepared me for Marrakesh. It most probably wasn't the best idea for me to wander around the narrow alleyways in the oldest part of the city on my own in the sweltering heat but I wasn't scared and had a marvellous time. The scenes I saw that day will forever stay in my mind. As I looked around me I noticed that the locals were all wearing traditional attire and there were never ending shops selling a wide array of colourful spices. I could smell the fresh nutmeg, cinnamon, paprika and turmeric filling the air but there were also many others that I didn't recognise. The multitude of aromas was overpowering. When I got to the main square, which is called the Jemaa El Fna, I walked past men selling huge rugs and beautifully made tea sets. I found the food stalls where they were making kebabs, tagines and various small pastries. The sights and smells of the food made me hungry but I wasn't brave enough to try anything. I was also thirsty so when I saw a group of water sellers, I was tempted to ask them for a cup but my sister had warned me to never drink the water here unless it was out of a sealed bottle, so I just stood and watched them go about their business. They wore bright red clothes and had large hats, which looked like lampshades. Metal cups were attached to chains hanging from their bodies and they filled them with water from a goat skin bag every time a customer approached them. I saw some Gnawa street musicians my sister had told me to look out for as she knew I would love to hear their music. One of them had a three-stringed instrument called a gimbri. The others either had drums and beat them with their hands to make a hypnotic rhythm or metal castanets they banged together like miniature cymbals. The repetitive beat of the percussion allowed me to switch my mind off completely for a while and not think about my problems at school at all, which was absolute heaven.

I felt completely safe walking around on my own but I was thirsty so headed back to the hotel, as they provided fresh bottled water for each room. On the way I found a stall selling mint tea and as the tea was boiling hot, I thought it would be safe to drink. I was soon refreshed and eager to do more exploring so instead of going back to the hotel I went the other way and wandered into a camel market where I saw a man auctioning camels for sellers to breeders and buyers. I saw a couple of tourists riding a camel and thought that could be fun so joined the queue. I was a bit nervous when I first got on the camel as it wobbled when it stood up but once it was upright it was very enjoyable and I could pretend to be Lawrence of Arabia for a while. I had seen David Lean's epic film a few years earlier and thought it was one of the best movies I had ever seen. Unfortunately, it was only a short ride as they were only doing it to get some publicity for the longer rides, which took place in the desert and cost considerably more.

My first overseas adventure not only gave me an appreciation of different cultures but also helped me become more in-tune with myself and build my self-esteem, which had been very low after all the bullying at school. Travelling alone in Marrakesh, had taught me to be responsible for myself; I didn't need anyone else to have a good time. I also discovered I liked my own company. These were invaluable experiences that would last a lifetime.

During the next term, my musical education took a huge leap forward when Jimi Hendrix's *Electric Ladyland* and Jethro Tull's debut album *This Was* were both released but it was the Beatles *The White Album* everyone at school was raving about because it had so many great songs on it. Everybody had their own favourite. Mine was *While My Guitar Gently Weeps,* as I loved George's guitar solo with its melancholic melody, as although it reminded me of times of despair and profound sadness, it also made me want to overcome those negative feelings and want to replace them with more positive emotions like love and hope.

When we broke up for Christmas, I bought a sampler album released by Island Records called *You Can All Join in.* The cover featured members from all the bands standing together and looking slightly awkward in Hyde Park. The LP was priced at 14 shillings and

6 pence. It included songs by Jethro Tull, Spooky Tooth, Free, Traffic, Stephen Stills, John Martyn and the Spencer Davis Group. I also bought my first ever single. *Albatross* by Fleetwood Mac. Peter Green's instrumental was sublime but it was the B-side, *Jigsaw Puzzle Blues*, I liked even more, as it made me smile every time I played it. Listening to Danny Kirwan's expressive way of playing his guitar when I felt unhappy was like having a re-set button putting me in a good mood instantly.

Later that month, we went to see Lindsay Anderson's anti-establishment movie *If,* starring Malcolm McDowell, which was advertised as a satire of life at an English boarding school but when I saw it felt more like watching a documentary as it was so true to life.

For Christmas, I was given another diary, which proved to be a much better present than I had appreciated at the time I received it, as 1969 was a year full of special dates to remember both musically and historically and I dutifully wrote them all down for posterity. What had previously been a minor fascination with dates was now becoming a major obsession.

On the 12th of January Led Zeppelin released their first self-titled album. Their fusion of blues and rock music really appealed to me and I became an instant fan of Jimmy Page whose style was so unique whether playing acoustic or electric guitars. The opening track *Good Times Bad Times* resonated with me as that was how my life was at that time. Good during the holidays and bad during term time. But my favourite track was *Babe I'm Going to Leave You*, which was a cover of a folk song by Anne Bredon that Joan Baez had covered and Jimmy Page had then re-arranged to suit Robert Plant's amazing vocals.

On the 30th of January, the Beatles played their last ever live performance on the rooftop of Apple Corps in London. I can still remember telling my mother how I wish I could have been there and her saying how cold it must have been for them. She was quite right. I found out many years later John Lennon had put on Yoko Ono's fur coat and Ringo had worn his wife's raincoat to stop them freezing to death.

On the 9th of April, we were in the middle of a history class when there was a sudden loud boom and some of the window panes in our classroom shattered. We screamed and ducked under our desks not understanding what had just occurred. Later that day we were informed by the Warden that veteran RAF pilot Brian Trubshaw had just done the first flight of a new supersonic airliner called Concorde 002 flying from an airfield near Bristol to another air base not far from our school.

On the 17th of May, The Who released a double album called *Tommy*, which included the brilliant songs *Pinball Wizard, The Acid Queen* and *I'm Free*. The music was thrilling and the drumming sensational. I thought Keith Moon was the best drummer I had ever heard and hoped I would get the opportunity to see him play live one day. But *Fiddle About* really disturbed me, as the fear of being sexually abused by one of the older boys or my creepy housemaster was never far from my thoughts every night.

On the 3rd of July 1969 Brain Jones, guitarist and founder of the Rolling Stones, died in suspicious circumstances. He was found motionless at the bottom of his pool, the official cause being 'death by misadventure', but foul play wasn't ruled out completely and there have been many theories doing the rounds ever since. He was only 27. The next day the band released Honky Tonk Women. Their producer Jimmy Miller's cowbell followed by Charlie Watts' drum fill made it the most distinctive intros of all time. On the 5th, the Rolling Stones with their new guitarist Mick Taylor performed a free concert at Hyde Park, which they dedicated to their former bandmate and released hundreds of butterflies as a tribute to him.

At 3.30am on the 20th of July, we were woken up by our housemaster and allowed to come downstairs in our dressing gowns to watch the moon landing on his TV. At 3.56am Neil Armstrong stepped off the Eagle's ladder onto the moon's surface and said those immortal words. 'That's one small step for man but one giant leap for mankind.'

A few days later, Jethro Tull released *Stand Up*. It was the first LP I bought with my own money. The album cover, designed by James

Grashow, was like a children's pop-up book and when I opened it up the woodcut style drawings of the band members stood up. This record was nothing like *This Was* and I really liked the different direction they had taken on their second outing. Although it still had a blues feel, especially on *A New Day Yesterday* with new guitarist Martin Barre showing off his ample skills, the rest of the songs were an eclectic mix. I thought Ian Anderson's flute playing was out of this world and Glenn Cornick's bass solo on the instrumental *Bouree* was pure genius.

The Woodstock Music Festival took place between the 15-18th of August that year and around 400,000 people went to Bethel, New York to see what was billed as: 'An Aquarian Experience: 3 Days of Peace and Music.' I could only read about it in the paper and felt envious when I heard which bands were performing there. The Who, Jimi Hendrix and Santana amongst them. I wondered if I would ever get the chance to see them.

Fleetwood Mac's *Oh Well* was released in September. The song was split into two parts with one section on each side of the disc. Peter Green played electric blues on his Les Paul on the first part and a Spanish influenced tune on a Ramirez guitar on part two. It was completely different to all the other music around at the time and that was its main appeal.

I also went to see Dennis Hopper's film *Easy Rider* at The Waverley Cinema in New Milton with some of my old friends from kindergarten who my mother had encouraged me to reunite with during the holidays. Having made no friends at my current school, it was quite a revelation to me that I could so easily reconnect with my old chums, some who I hadn't seen in years. Later in life, I would discover that true friendships always stand the test of time.

The story followed two long-haired hippies riding their motorbikes across America and depicted the adventures they had along the way, including taking drugs and having sex or 'free-love' as the papers were calling it. We had been informed they used real drugs in the scenes with the actors allegedly smoking real marijuana so we were interested to see what it looked like and after the film eager to try some for ourselves. But as usual, I was more interested in the music. I loved the way the movie's soundtrack had used particular songs to help tell the story rather than just using a traditional score. When I saw Peter Fonda and Dennis Hopper riding their customised 'choppers' on the highway and heard Steppenwolf's *Born to be Wild* I was hooked and wanted to buy the soundtrack as soon as I could afford to. Apart from *Easy Rider* I also bought Fleetwood Mac's *Then Play On*. *Rattlesnake Shake* was my favourite track on the album and despite being a teenager, I had absolutely no idea what the lyrics were referring to at that time. Honest!

In October, I heard *In the Court of the Crimson King* by King Crimson for the first time. The album featured the master of time signatures Robert Fripp on guitar. *21st Century Schizoid Man* really grabbed my attention but it was the title track composed by Ian McDonald I loved the most because of the magical sound of his mellotron and Greg Lake's impressive vocals. Led Zeppelin's second album was released a couple of weeks later. The song I played the most was *Ramble On*. The lyrics were inspired by J.R.R. Tolkien whose fantasy novel *Lord of the Rings* was being read by nearly all of the boys at school. Up until then, I had mainly listened to a song because it had a good beat, a catchy tune but now I was hearing music that not only told a story but also evoked an emotion.

At half-term, I went to see Southampton F.C play West Ham at The Dell. It was a 1-1 draw, which wasn't that exciting but as we waited for our train to take us home after the match, we saw the West Ham and England Captain Bobby Moore standing on the opposite platform. As we still had plenty of time before our train would arrive, we ran across the bridge and down the stairs so we could meet him. He was very friendly and signed his autograph on our match programme and then he introduced us to the player standing next to him. It was Geoff Hurst, the hattrick hero of the 1966 World Cup.

On the 15th of November, *Match of the Day* was aired on BBC 1 in colour for the first time. Liverpool beat West Ham 2-0.

Later in the month, I bought a sampler album by Island Records called *Nice Enough to Eat*. The front cover featured the names of the bands spelt out in alphabet sweets. The LP had tracks from the latest albums by some of my favourite bands like Jethro Tull, Traffic, Free, Mott the Hoople and King Crimson as well as artists I was unfamiliar with like Nick Drake, Dr. Strangely Strange and Blodwyn Pig. I also got *To Our Children's Children* by the Moody Blues. It was full of lovely gentle songs, which my mother told me she really liked as she didn't have to put her fingers in her ears as she did when I played some of my heavier music. It was John Lodge's *Eyes of a Child* that appealed to me the most. Listening to his lyrics made me vow to myself that even when I was a grown up, I would still try to see the world through the eyes of a child. I have kept that promise to myself and think it was the single most important decision I ever made.

One of my favourite albums released in 1969 was *Let It Bleed* by The Rolling Stones. *Gimme Shelter* was a powerful opening track and Merry Clayton's vocals were sensational but it was a song about a serial killer that really stood out from the rest. *Midnight Rambler* was loosely based on the life of Albert DeSalvo better known as the Boston Strangler. I didn't know it at the time but I later discovered it was the last time Brian Jones ever recorded with the band, playing congas on the track.

Over the course of the year, I had become increasingly obsessed with dates and times and found writing everything down in a diary also helped improve the mood swings I had been having recently, which I also kept a note of, along with how I appeared to get sudden bursts of positive energy shortly after hearing a new song that I enjoyed like *Spirit in the Sky*, a one-hit wonder released that December. I particularly liked the sound that Norman Greenbaum had got by building a fuzz box into the body of his Fender Telecaster.

As I was a bit disappointed when I didn't get given another diary at Christmas, I decided to buy one for myself as a gift, and have done so every year ever since. Recording important dates were important to my need for order, along with making sure my LPs were all lined up on the shelf alphabetically, prioritising the name of the artist rather than the album title.

When a record store manager asked me one day if I was 'OCD', I quipped 'No, I'm CDO!', as I felt it was a more accurate acronym in my particular case.

On Christmas Day there was no broadcast of the Queen's Speech for the first time since they had started doing it in 1957. The reason behind the decision was because there had been a documentary about the Royal Family shown on television earlier in the year and the Palace wanted to avoid too much exposure, so we watched *Top of the Pops* instead, which was a recap of all the year's hits, including songs by The Beatles, The Rolling Stones and Fleetwood Mac.

Although 1970 meant the end of the swinging-sixties, young people like me now had greater freedom than ever before and being a teenage rebel had become a rite of passage often expressed through music. We thought anyone over thirty would truly hate like Black Sabbath, who I thought at that age were the best thing since... sliced bread, which, just in case you were wondering, was first sold in 1928 and advertised as 'the greatest forward step in the baking industry since... bread was wrapped.'

On the 9th of February, The Doors released *Morrison Hotel.* I loved the distorted guitar riff on the opening track *Roadhouse Blues* and when I heard Jim Morrison's baritone voice singing 'Keep your eyes on the road, your hands upon the wheel' it was the first time I was aware a man's voice could sound sexy.

At the beginning of May, I was allowed a few days off from school to attend my mother's wedding. The previous year, my 5'2' Mum had met a 6'6' man called Robin who had two children from his first marriage - Mandy, a daughter two years older than me and John, a son one year younger. My real sister and brother had left home long ago, got married and started families of their own, so I was now going to have to get used to sharing my mother's house with three complete strangers. As we went inside my mother gave me a hug and told me to remember it wasn't going to be easy for them either.

A week after my mother's wedding The Beatles released *Let It Be,* their final studio album and about a month after they had split up. *Across the Universe, Let it Be, The Long and Winding Road* and *Get Back* were the tracks I liked the most and I remember being quite upset there would be no more albums from the Fab Four after that.

When I got back to boarding school, I played the album at every opportunity, which helped me cope with the stress of having to study for my O-Levels. Although the results weren't great, they were good enough for me to be accepted at the newly formed 6th Form College in Brockenhurst, which meant I would be able to leave the hell-hole on the hill and live at home with my mother... and my new family.

A loud knock on my door interrupted my train of thought. It was my stepbrother who asked if he could listen to some of my records with me. I was playing *Absolutely Live*, a double album by The Doors, which I thought was one of the best live recordings I had ever heard. John loved it just as much as I did and after talking for a little longer, we discovered we liked most of the same bands. We then put on *Deep Purple In Rock*. Ian Gillan's vocal range was rumoured to be 4 and a half to 5 octaves, which sounded implausible until we listened to the 10-minute epic *Child in Time* right to the end. Trying to imitate his high voice made us laugh so much we both had a fit of giggles and a lifelong bond was forged.

I was 15 and John was 14 when we persuaded our parents to allow us attend the 1970 Isle of Wight Festival, our first ever live concert. Two of my old kindergarten friends, Mark and Simon, came with us. I think the only reason we were allowed to go was because Mark's mother rented a flat in Freshwater for the duration of the festival so we had somewhere safe to sleep at night.

The festival was held between the 26th and 31st of August 1970 at Afton Down. I watched a documentary about the festival and there was an aerial shot showing 600,000 people had attended this memorable musical event. They looked like ants and it felt strange to think we were amongst the 'great unwashed' in the huge crowd. I can still remember the moment when some fans who had been sitting next to us got up and broke down fences, which allowed many others to enter for free and I recall the odd heckle but my main memory is of being overwhelmed by the diversity of the music on display…and the over-powering smell of dope.

We arrived just in time to see Black Widow, a band who sang songs about worshipping Satan, which our parents wouldn't have approved of. They were followed by The Groundhogs, another British band who we liked especially songs from their recent album *Thank Christ for the Bomb*. Up next was Terry Reid who two years earlier had allegedly turned down the opportunity to be the vocalist for Led Zeppelin. There was no doubt Terry had a fabulous voice and together with multi-instrumentalist David Lindley they put on an excellent show.

On the Friday morning, we managed to get right to the front of the stage to see Taste. Their Irish guitarist Rory Gallagher could really play the blues. They began with *What's Going On* and ended with a 14-minute version of *Catfish*.

'What do you think?' My stepbrother asked me.

'Cool!' I replied with a nod, adhering to the compulsory unspoken rule of using limited vocabulary common to most teenagers.

Tony Joe White was on next and although I loved his guitar style, I was more impressed by his drummer. When I asked the man standing next to me if he knew who he was, he replied, 'Colin Trevor Flooks. But you might know him better by his stage name. Cozy Powell!'

My friends and I were determined to stay close to the stage for the next band as we all loved Chicago. They played a terrific set, including a great version of *25 or 6 to 4*. Now feeling pumped and not wanting the day to end, we stayed put to see two more British bands before deciding to call it a night. Family with Roger Chapman and Procol Harum with Gary Brooker. At one point, Gary told the crowd, 'It's too cold to play anything slow,' so instead of playing some of their better-known songs they decided to give us some loud rock'n'roll instead. Cactus was the last band on stage, which allowed us to see powerhouse drummer Carmine Appice and bad-ass bass player Tim Bogart. We eventually made our way back to the flat with *No Need to Worry* still in our heads.

Saturday was a really big day. It started with an 80-minute set by John Sebastian who I wasn't familiar with at the start of his set but became a fan of his by the end of it. Later that morning Joni Mitchell came on stage but just after she had sung *Woodstock* a strange man who seemed to be under the influence of drugs interrupted her to make a speech but we didn't understand what he was saying at the time and became even more confused when the crowd started to boo Joni's manager for dragging him off stage.

'We've put our lives into this stuff. You're acting like tourists,' Joni said, visibly upset.

I wasn't sure what was going on but the mood of the crowd wasn't happy, so when Tiny Tim came on it was a big relief when everyone started singing along to *There'll Always Be an England*, which he sang in his instantly recognisable warbling voice through a megaphone. He followed it with *Tip-Toe Thru The Tulips With Me*, which got the crowd going and etched an everlasting memory in my mind.

Looking at all the smiling faces around us and feeling their positive energy was infectious. I had never smiled so much in my life but that might have just been the effect of absorbing dope second-hand. Here I was, standing with thousands of other like-minded people all enjoying the same bands and all thinking that nobody else understands us outside of these festival grounds. It was a wonderful sense of belonging and I felt that this shared magical musical experience would link us all forever.

Miles Davis came on next and did a very short set, which was slightly over half an hour without a break. The crowd were now back in good spirits and were ready to rock 'n ' roll, so it was just as well the next act could provide exactly that. Ten Years After with guitar maestro Alvin Lee played *Love Like A Man* followed by *Good Morning Little School Girl* and any residue of the negative vibes from earlier in the day were now truly gone.

Mark was looking forward to seeing Emerson Lake & Palmer, as he was a fan of Keith Emerson's previous band The Nice. It was only the newly formed Supergroup's second-ever performance and it felt pretty special to watch ELP wow the crowd with their half-hour interpretation of Mussorgsky's *Pictures at an Exhibition*. It was the first time I had seen a rock band attempt to play classical music and it was hard to believe such a huge orchestral sound could be created by just three men. When Keith Emerson started thrashing his C-3 Hammond organ around the stage and stabbing it with knives to sustain notes during *Rondo*, I realised this band were not just virtuoso musicians but also great showmen. Their set ended with *Nutrocker,* a unique version of Tchaikovsky's ballet The Nutcracker.

We nearly missed seeing The Doors, as they didn't start their set until around 1 am, by which time it was cold and windy and we were pretty tired. The lighting was terrible which was disappointing but when they finally began their set with *Roadhouse Blues* we were suddenly wide awake and ready to go again. Hearing Jim Morrison's powerful voice singing *When the Music's Over* and Ray Manzarek's outstanding keyboard solo on *Light my Fire* was exhilarating.

'What do you reckon?' John asked afterwards.

'Really cool!' I replied, my descriptive language now at full stretch.

It must have been well after 2 am when we heard a man's voice say, 'Ladies and Gentlemen, a nice rock and roll band from Shepherd's Bush, London. The Who.'

The passion of Roger Daltrey's vocals and the aggression of Pete Townshend's guitar playing with his trademark windmills were a sight and sound to behold. Keith Moon grinned like a Cheshire cat while thrashing his drum kit within an inch of its life and John Entwistle, wearing a black jumpsuit with a white skeleton printed on the front, demonstrated why one of his nicknames was 'Thunderfingers'. It was wonderful to hear *Tommy* played live, but the last three songs, *My Generation, Naked Eye* and *Magic Bus* are the songs I will always remember the most, as by then everybody was singing along with the band and it felt like we were all part of one enormous tribe.

Sunday started slightly subdued as we were all exhausted from the non-stop entertainment of the previous day. Sly and the Family Stone, Melanie and Kris Kristofferson were ideal acts to begin the day but when Free came on stage, we moved nearer to the front so that we could get a better view of Paul Rodgers on vocals and Paul Kossoff on guitar. *Be My Friend, Fire and Water* were standouts but it was *All Right Now* that got the biggest reaction from the crowd.

Donovan, Pentangle and The Moody Blues were all received well and then Jethro Tull took to the stage. Ian Anderson looked very scruffy, extremely hairy and had a grin like a lunatic who had recently escaped from the asylum, but as soon as they started playing, I realised I was witnessing a master flautist at work, especially on *My God,* which was exceptional. It was the first time I had seen Tull perform live, and I was impressed by their endless energy. Seeing Ian balancing on one leg like a demented flamingo while playing his flute so brilliantly on *Nothing is Easy* was something I will never forget. The song's lyrics suggested to me we shouldn't get overly stressed about the little things that happen to us, as they won't last forever so we might as well attempt to have a more optimistic outlook on life. I may have got the meaning completely wrong but at the time it was just the sort of encouragement I needed, so thank you Mr. Anderson for giving me a leg up… so to speak.

A nasty crackle suddenly came through the loudspeaker and then a man's voice said, 'Let's have a warm welcome for Billy Cox on bass, Mitch Mitchell on drums, and the man with the guitar, Jimi Hendrix.' After so much anticipation to see one of the greatest guitarists on the planet perform live, it was actually a little disappointing to start with. Jimi was obviously having some technical problems with his amplifier and from time to time it sounded like his guitar was out of tune. It wasn't until he did *All Along The Watchtower* that he started to sound a bit better and by the time they played *Red House,* Jimi was back to his best.

After Hendrix had finished, Joan Baez, Leonard Cohen and Richie Havens all gave great performances but by then I was far too tired to appreciate them properly.

When the music was over, and we were walking out of the festival grounds, I made a promise to myself my main goal in life would be to go to as many live gigs as I could and whatever career I eventually chose must enable that dream, as music was no longer just my safe place or a way to escape life's pressures, it was now as important to me as breathing.

*Music is the great uniter. An incredible force. Something that people who differ on*
*everything and anything else can have in common.*

Sarah Dessen

## CHAPTER 5: CHANGES

After the summer holidays were over, I bought a second-hand Honda 50cc moped so I could drive myself to and from home to the next village to catch the coach to Brockenhurst 6th Form College every day.

Having attended an all-male boarding school for so many years, it was a relief to now be in the company of both males and females. For some reason, I seemed to be popular with the girls, much to the amazement of Mike, one of my new friends, who was much better looking than me, or so he kept telling me, and Keith, whose nickname was Kipper, who constantly reminded me he was taller than me… much taller.

The main topic during the lunch breaks each day was which girls we fancied or who we had 'got off' with at a party over the weekend. I hadn't got off with anyone yet as I was quite shy and became a bit tongue-tied when I met a girl for the first time. It wasn't until I offered my seat to a girl on the school coach one morning, I discovered just how much I liked girls and how it would change my life forever.

Sue was a pretty girl with a lovely smile so I was attracted to her as soon as I saw her boarding the coach. As there were no spare seats left, I stood up and offered her mine but instead of taking it she pushed me down into a sitting position, made herself comfortable on my lap and then put both her around my neck and started kissing me. This was my first ever 'snog' and the effect it had on me was immediate, but fortunately wore off before we got to our destination.

The conversations on the coach trip to and from school each week usually consisted of who had appeared on *Top of the Pops* that week, repeating the funniest lines from *Monty Python's Flying Circus* and remarking how silly *The Goodies* were but we loved them anyway. We also liked to discuss our favourite bands and find out if they were going to be performing anywhere near us soon, so I started buying two weekly music newspapers, the New Musical Express, better known as

NME, and Melody Maker, which had details about upcoming gigs, interviews with a wide range of musicians and reviews of the latest albums.

Going to a record shop and flicking through album covers in alphabetical order was very therapeutic for me, as it appealed to all my senses. I loved the tactile act of trawling along the racks, looking at the artwork and reading the sleeve notes, while listening to whatever new LP was being played over the speakers but if there was a record that had been filed under the wrong letter, I would have to immediately take it out and put it in the correct place. Having found one mistake, I would then have to go through the entire shop checking there were no more. When I found an LP that I wanted to hear, I would take the empty sleeve to the front desk and then be shown to one of the soundproofed booths to listen to it.

I can still remember listening to The Rolling Stones *Get Yer Ya-Ya's Out!* for the first time and nodding in agreement with Mick Jagger when he said, 'Charlie's good tonight, ineee, 'just before the band went into *Honky Tonk Women*. I also loved a sampler album called *Fill Your Head with Rock,* which featured Jerry Goodman of The Flock on the front cover and had 23 tracks on it including songs by Chicago, Santana, Spirit, Blood, Sweat and Tears, Flock, Black Widow, Argent, Leonard Cohen, Janis Joplin, Taj Mahal and Johnny Winter.

After saving enough money from mowing lawns, washing dishes at the local pub and working as a petrol pump attendant during the holidays, I bought a second-hand Höfner cello electric guitar, which came with a small practice amplifier. My poor mother couldn't bear the noise in the house but fortunately the solution was close to home. We were lucky enough to have a large shed at the end of our garden, so were able to play loud music to our heart's content. My stepbrother John also had a guitar so we jammed together whenever we had the chance. I say 'jammed' but the truth was our amateur attempts were really no more than a mish mash of unpleasant sounds. As our garden backed onto the fields of the local dairy farm, the audience at our first 'gigs' comprised entirely of a herd of Friesian cows, so thankfully there were only moos and no boos.

I took my guitar and amp to school one day to have a jam at lunchtime with Mike who had a drumkit and another lad called Paul who had an acoustic guitar. We played *The House of the Rising Sun* by The Animals and *For Your Love* by The Yardbirds and became so engrossed performing the songs, we didn't notice the room had filled up with other students. They must have liked us though, as when we finished playing, they started clapping, which was a real boost to our self-confidence and made me realise how my interest in music could help me connect with others in a way that I could deal with.

After our jam, Mike told me he enjoyed music, football and girls just as much as I did, but not necessarily in that order. We soon became best mates and often went to Southampton to see The Saints together when they were playing at their home ground, The Dell.

During the week, we would listen to the latest LPs together in the common room where all the students would congregate at lunchtime and that is where we made friends with Judi, Sandra, Fiona and Penny, who were great fun to talk to and liked the same records we did.

Rock music helped me outgrow my shyness. Up until now, music had mainly been a form of escapism but now daring to share my thoughts about my musical tastes with the opposite sex helped me to open up and talk about my feelings for the first time in my life. It was exhilarating and gave me a sense of freedom, which up until now had been an unfamiliar experience.

We were fortunate enough to have some great concerts at our school from time to time, including an incredible double bill, which featured the ultra-loud space-rock band Hawkwind and British Blues band Chicken Shack whose guitarist Stan Webb had a style similar to the legendary Freddie King. The admission price was 50 pence. Later in the year we saw the Edgar Broughton Band who had a single called *Apache Dropout*, which was a mashup of The Shadows *Apache* and Captain Beefheart's *Drop Out Boogie.*

Although my modern music knowledge grew daily, the academic knowledge I was supposed to be learning in my chosen subjects wasn't going quite as well. History, which should have been fun and fascinating as we were learning about the dramatic Tudor era, was ruined by having a rather lacklustre teacher who either suffered from delusions of adequacy or was simply jaded having taught the same subject for far too long. English was also a little boring, as our lessons consisted mainly of sitting quietly and reading whatever books our elderly teacher thought would open our young minds. James Joyce's *A Portrait of an Artist as a Young Man* was a difficult one to connect with initially as it told the story of a boy growing up as a Catholic in Ireland in the 19<sup>th</sup> Century so I had no empathy towards the main character. But as Dedalus began to cast off his shackles, mainly in the form of his family's beliefs and started to think for himself, I realised I had underestimated both Joyce and our teacher's intention for us to do the same.

I thought Art would be easy for me because I had been quite good at it at both my previous schools and even won a couple of prizes. But my intuitive style clearly didn't suit the requirements of this particular art teacher. He told me that my portraits weren't realistic enough and he got quite angry if I didn't draw the models in exactly the same way he did. One day he yelled. 'Don't let your imagination run away with you,' so I simply stopped going to his classes and spent more time listening to my records instead.

On the 18<sup>th</sup> of September, we were at a BBQ having a great time listening to music around a campfire when we heard the tragic news that Jimi Hendrix had died. Like Brain Jones, he was only 27 when he died. Nobody said a word and we all just sat still in shock until the last of the embers had stopped glowing.

The first Glastonbury Festival was held that weekend but at the last minute we decided not to make the trip to Somerset, which was a real shame as we missed seeing Tyrannosaurus Rex and I never got another opportunity to see Marc Bolan and Mickey Finn perform live.

A month later, I went to Guildford to see a new band everyone was raving about. Their name was Yes and their complex music blew me away as the combination of their unusual time signatures, incredible musicianship and heavenly harmonies were all so fresh to my teenage ears. Although my friends were all talking about what an incredibly high voice Jon Anderson had after the gig, it was Chris Squire's distinctive bass sound that got me excited and their guitarist Steve Howe's virtuosity was equally impressive. *I've Seen All Good People* and *Yours is No Disgrace* were the songs I enjoyed the most and I couldn't wait to hear them again but it would be another four months before I got my hands on *The Yes Album.*

On the 4th of October, American singer Janis Joplin died of a heroin overdose in Hollywood at the age of 27.

All my male friends loved rock music. We each had our favourite band but were united in loving rock and hating disco music, which was a new genre that was taking over the radio airwaves at the time. But as all the girls we knew loved disco music and wanted us to take them dancing, we begrudgingly went with them. The closest venue was Chelsea Village in Bournemouth, which had previously been a bowling alley. The main reason we had agreed to go was in the hope of impressing the girls enough with our limited dancing skills for them to let us snog them during the slow songs.

The girls mainly danced on their own when the disco songs were played, while the boys hovered at the edges of the dancefloor eyeing up the talent. The DJ knew that the only way to get the boys to dance was to play something with a great beat like *Honky Tonk Women,* which always worked a treat. The more confident males would then stand next to the prettiest girl they could find and proceed to do a truly embarrassing impersonation of Mick Jagger, which looked more like a chicken flapping its wings by its sides in a series of uncoordinated myoclonic jerks and twitches.

The teachers must have felt that our music education was just as important as our other lessons because they allowed us to play records in the common room during our lunch breaks. Most of my male friends liked listening to The Doors *Morrison Hotel* or Pink Floyd's *Atom Heart Mother* but our female friends preferred hearing Simon & Garfunkel's *Bridge Over Troubled Water* or Elton John's self-titled

LP, which we affectionately named 'The Dwight Album' as a nod to The Beatles so-called White Album and because the singer-pianist's real name was Reginald Kenneth Dwight.

In November, my friend Jon G asked me to go with him to see Southampton play Manchester United. We were up against their very best team which included Bobby Charlton, Denis Law and the legendary George Best. On paper there was no way the Saints could win but they did. The only goal was scored by Jimmy Gabriel or 'Archangel' as we felt he should be called this great win. On the way home, Jon told me he and his younger brother Nick had been to a boarding school similar to the one I went to and were also taunted, being called 'Wog major' and 'Wog minor' respectively but certainly not respectfully. I was fascinated to hear about my friend's upbringing in Africa, which had been so different to my own, and it felt good to have a mate who understood what it was like to have been bullied.

When Curved Air released their first album *Air Conditioning*, it was one of the first ever vinyl picture discs and I thought it looked really cool, so I bought a copy. The sound quality was appalling but there were a couple of good songs on the record, which made it worth the price. I loved Sonja Kristina's voice on *It Happened Today* as it sounded so passionate and thought Darryl Way's electric violin playing on *Vivaldi* was exceptional, which was obviously down to his classical training but it was the simple idea of installing pick-ups under his strings, which enabled him to create such unique sounds with his instrument.

At Christmas, I bought *Led Zeppelin 111.* Apart from the full-on opening track *Immigrant Song,* it was much more acoustically driven than their previous albums, so it took me a few plays to appreciate it properly. *Friends, Gallows Pole* and *That's the Way* remain favourites to this day.

Mike and I, donning our Army trench coats, went to see heavy rock band Black Sabbath at the Guild Hall in Southampton on the 11th of January and got front-row seats. Ozzy Osborne sang and sweated on stage like a man possessed and Tony Iommi played some superb solos.

Geezer Butler supplied some throbbing bass lines but Bill Ward's drum fills were far too loud, which I found a bit irritating after a while. The songs we liked the best were *Paranoid, Iron Man and War Pigs*. Singing along with Ozzy as he yelled 'Generals gathered in their masses, just like witches at black masses' was great fun and this was the moment I tried head banging for the very first time standing right in front of the mighty Terence Michael Joseph 'Geezer' Butler who was doing the same violent moves as us only a couple of feet away and covering us with his sweat. Sabbath may have been considered satanic and in league with the devil by some overly concerned parents but at the time we felt we were in heavy rock heaven.

The support act was Curved Air and it was good to see them play some of the songs I had heard on their album. Sonja Kristina owned the room the moment she stepped onto the stage. I was mesmerised by her beautiful voice and her sultry stage presence. It was a lethal combination and the release of dopamine into my teenage brain would soon become evident but a little lower in my anatomy. I hadn't connected music and sex before but from now on the two would forever be entwined. The ticket for the double bill cost me ten shillings, or ten bob as we used to call it.

On the 15th of February 1971, Britain went decimal. Under the old system, we had 12 pence in a shilling and 20 shillings in a pound. With decimalisation, the pound kept its value but was now subdivided into 100 new pence and the shilling was abolished forever.

Jethro Tull released *Aqualung* on the 19th of March, which I thought was their best album yet. It cost me £2 and 40 pence. The powerful title track, *My God* and *Locomotive Breath* were my initial favourites but the more I played the record the more I liked the acoustic songs *Cheap Day Return, Mother Goose and Wond'ring Aloud*. I also loved the watercolour portrait of the bearded tramp in shabby clothes by Burton Silverman which he did for the album cover. I was so impressed with it I copied it as precisely as I could and was rewarded with an A by my previously unimpressed art teacher.

In April, Caravan released *In the Land of Grey and Pink*, which had the almost 23-minute track *Nine Feet Underground* on it, which is where some of my less musically inclined friends thought the album should be buried.

We were lucky enough to have Supertramp perform at our school the following month and we also saw Emerson Lake and Palmer, Yes, Iron Butterfly, Jethro Tull and Steeleye Span in Bournemouth and Tangerine Dream at Southampton University.

To pay for all the concert tickets, which cost between £1 and £2 depending on the popularity of the band, I did a variety of part-time jobs. I worked as a barman at The Forest Park Hotel in Brockenhurst, as a kitchen slave at The South Lawn Hotel in Milford on Sea and as a petrol pump attendant in Pennington. I only got paid 20p an hour in those days, so it took me ages to save any money but at each place I made some new friends.

On the 3rd of July, another great rock music hero, Jim Morrison died of a heart attack from using heroin. Like Brian Jones, Jimi Hendrix and Janis Joplin, he was also only 27 when he passed away.

In August, The Who released *Who's Next*, which I thought was their best album yet and particularly liked *Won't Get Fooled Again* and the song with 'teenage wasteland' in the chorus, *Baba O'Reilly*, which featured Dave Arbus from the band East of Eden on violin.

I went to a free concert at Hyde Park on the 4th of September, which Jack Bruce the bass player with Cream was headlining. His band was all exceptional musicians. He had Chris Spedding on guitar, Graham Bond on Keyboards, Art Themen on Saxophone and John Marshall on drums. The support acts were Formerly Fat Harry, Roy Harper and King Crimson. I still played their first album *In the Court of the Crimson King* a lot, so finally being able to see them perform *21st Century Schizoid Man* live was a real treat.

A week or so after this memorable gig, my friend Bruce invited me to watch the Morris troupe he had recently joined, perform some old English folk dances at a pub in the New Forest. Their rhythmic stepping was very impressive, so I challenged them to do their next dance to *21st Century Schizoid Man*. They absolutely nailed it and I think even the master of musical timing, Robert Fripp, would have given his approval.

My love for twin lead guitar harmonies began when my stepbrother John played me *Pilgrimage* by Wishbone Ash. I thought Andy Powell and Ted Turner's interplay on *The Pilgrim* was quite extraordinary but my favourite track was *Jailbait,* as I was impressed by the way the two guitarists left space for each other to allow their counterpart to do their own thing during their solos. I was still struggling with the few chords I had learned so far and couldn't imagine how I would ever be able to play solos as good as these talented guitarists so put the unreachable dream out of my mind… for now.

On the 18th of September, I went to The Concert for Bangladesh at The Oval Cricket Ground in London, which was billed as *Goodbye to Summer.* This time the headline act was The Who so it was what we termed a 'no brainer'. We arrived just as Lindisfarne went on stage to a huge cheer from the crowd. Quintessence were a bit too psychedelic for us and we sat down and chatted throughout their set but Mott the Hoople soon got us all on our feet again. I don't remember much about America except for their hit song *Horse With No Name.* They were followed by some poor chap on acoustic guitar who wasn't very good and subsequently got totally ignored. If we'd known his name was Eugene we would most probably have told him to be *careful with that axe,* so perhaps it's just as well we didn't and simply referred to him as the *'Artist With No Name'.* Atomic Rooster with Vincent Crane on organ played *Tomorrow Night* and *The Devil's Answer,* which got our attention and if it hadn't, Rod Stewart's leopard skin suit certainly would have. The Faces looked like they were having fun and as I looked around me, everyone was smiling. *Maybe I'm Amazed, Stay With Me, Maggie May* and *Had Me A Real Good Time* were their best songs. The last was how most of us were feeling long after they left the stage.

The Who started their set with *Summertime Blues,* so I was a happy camper, as were about 40,000 others who had made the journey to south-east London. At one point Keith Moon used a cricket bat to play the drums before throwing it into the crowd. Well, it was home to the Surrey Cricket Club after all. After performing a medley of songs from *Tommy* they then turned the spotlights on the audience and we all sang along as loudly as we could. Hearing *Won't Get Fooled Again* live for the first time was an experience I would never forget. Listening to them, I got the music. When The Who finally left the stage it looked like a right mess. Keith Moon had pushed his drum kit over and pieces of it were strewn everywhere and Pete Townshend had smashed his guitar before throwing what was left of it into the darkness, making an encore impossible, as the host Jeff Dexter said stating the bleeding obvious over the loudspeaker.

On the 21st of September, BBC 2 aired *The Old Grey Whistle Test* for the very first time. It was on quite late at night so I had to watch it with the volume really low so I didn't wake my parents. I loved the title music *Stone Fox Chase* by Area Code 615. This ground-breaking show exposed me to all kinds of music I hadn't heard of before, including songs by *Loudon Wainwright 111* and *Alice Cooper,* whose real name was Vincent Furnier. I also saw a young Englishman called Reginald Dwight sing one of his own songs called *Tiny Dancer*. He had recently changed his name to *Elton John.*

I'm told he has done quite well since then.

On the 29th of October Duane Allman of the Allman Brothers Band died in a motorcycle accident in Macon, Georgia. He was only 24.

I bought two new albums the following month, which couldn't have been more different from each other. Pink Floyd's *Meddle* which starts with *One of These Days (I'm Going to Cut You Into Little Pieces),* one of the most extraordinary opening tracks you will ever hear, and ends with the 23-minute epic *Echoes,* which I found entrancing. The other record was John Lennon's *Imagine*. The title track was so powerful that I doubted that any of the other tracks would be nearly as good… until I heard *Jealous Guy.* The melodic piano, played by renowned session musician Nicky Hopkins, was simply beautiful and brought a tear to my eye.

Yes released *Fragile* in November, which was the first of their records to feature Rick Wakeman on keyboards and the first of their covers to be designed by Roger Dean whose artwork I really admired. *Roundabout* and *Heart of the Sunrise* were the standout tracks for me on this LP. Led Zeppelin released their fourth album the same month. Apparently, they came up with the title of their song *Black Dog* after a large nameless black Labrador Retriever walked into the Headley Grange studio while they were recording. I liked every track but *Stairway to Heaven* stood out from the rest. The day after I heard this amazing song for the first time, I desperately tried to learn the chords, so I could impress the girls in the hope they would 'go out' with me. It did, and they did.

The first Genesis album I ever heard was *Nursery Cryme*. *The Musical Box* and *The Return of the Giant Hogweed* conjured up such wonderful imagery for me I became a huge fan of the band. Anyone who can write a song about a girl called Cynthia who knocks the head off someone called Henry with a croquet mallet was obviously a genius in my book. When I discovered Peter Gabriel, Tony Banks and Mike Rutherford had been to Charterhouse, a public school similar to the one I had attended, it explained their rather serious and repressed manner and I could immediately relate to them.

Before the end of term, my old art teacher left and was replaced by a much younger man and from day one he was an inspiration to the whole class. Mr Jones gave me the freedom to express myself instinctively, which up until now I had been told to suppress. He took me aside one day to tell me he liked the way I used my imagination but if I wanted to become a better artist I would need to hone and sharpen my skills and become more intuitive. He taught me about Henri Matisse who believed intuition and instinct were the best guides to be a true artist. This was music to my ears and I spent the rest of the term studying everything I could about this marvellous Modernist artist who had died on the same day I was born. In his later years, Matisse used scissors to cut out shapes and create collages, so I decided to try this intricate art form next and found I had a knack for it, which our new teacher seemed quite impressed with. Mr Jones asked me why I was doing them as a triptych. After seeing the blank expression on my face, he explained the name was what they called a series of three different pieces, which combine to tell a story. He then asked me a simple question but one which would change the course of my life forever, 'Do you want to tell stories with your art Jamie?'

'Yes…that's exactly what I want to do.' I replied, surprised at my answer.

'Then you should think about learning photography.'

Mr Jones kindly lent me his 35mm camera, so the following weekend I took some black and white photos of the yachts moored on the Keyhaven River and after having them developed, he told me he didn't think they were too bad considering it was my first attempt. The next weekend I took some more photos but this time they were of the abstract reflections made by the yachts, which he thought were much better and far more interesting. I liked the fact each reflection was something only I would ever witness first-hand but which I could then share with others. And this was when and how I became interested in becoming a photographer. I will always be grateful to Colin Jones for his insight and encouragement.

My end-of-year report by the headmaster wasn't quite as kind. He simply wrote four words. 'Contributes little, but thoughtfully.'

I wasn't quite sure how to take those words, or even what they really meant, but at the time they made me feel worthless, anxious and depressed. The feelings of isolation and fear of failure were never far away either, although this may have been some of the long-lasting effects of having gone to a boarding school.

Thankfully music was the remedy yet again and this time came in the form of an album by David Bowie called *Hunky Dory*, which I bought with the money my mother gave me for Christmas. I really liked the ballad *Life on Mars?* and after I had heard *Oh You Pretty Little Things!* I couldn't get the catchy song out of my head. However, *Changes* was the stand-out track for me as I felt it had a real sense of optimism and hope, which was just what I needed at the time, so thank you and Merry Christmas, Mr Bowie.

Morecambe & Wise outdid themselves on their 1971 Christmas TV special. The fabulous Shirley Bassey had to sing *Smoke Gets in Your Eyes* while the comedy duo re-arranged the scenery around her and then André Previn was forced to conduct an achingly funny rendition of Grieg's piano concerto. The hilarious sketch had the best punchline of all time when Eric says to the maestro, 'I'm playing all the right notes, but not necessarily in the right order!'

On the 22nd of January 1972, Mike and I went to see Pink Floyd play at the Bournemouth Winter Gardens on what was called the *Eclipse of the Darkside* tour. The first ten songs they played would eventually feature on their best-selling album *Dark Side of the Moon* but with a few title changes such as *The Travel Sequence* now known as *On The Run* and *The Mortality Sequence* which was re-named *The Great Gig in the Sky*. The live performance of this wonderful song was quite different to how we know and love it today. Richard Wright played an organ instrumental while a recording of journalist Malcolm Muggeridge reading verses from the Bible was heard over the top. It wasn't until a couple of weeks before the album was finished the band had the idea of adding female vocals over the end section. Their engineer Alan Parsons suggested a young session singer called Clare Torry who agreed to come to the studio on a Sunday evening and improvise some vocals for them with no idea she had just created musical history.

The following month, Mike and I went to see Jethro Tull at the Winter Gardens. After we had taken our seats, we noticed the cleaners were still sweeping the floor right in front of us, which we thought was a bit odd. It was only when they went on to the stage, hung their brown coats and caps on a hat stand and picked up their instruments we realised the cleaners were actually members of the band. They performed *Thick as a Brick* in its entirety and their musicianship was truly superb. The band were tight and managed the complex time signatures with consummate ease, although I read an article many years later where guitarist Martin Barre admitted they were petrified playing it live. As soon as the LP was on sale, I bought it and played it endlessly. The album cover was designed to look like a spoof local newspaper complete with nonsensical articles and mock adverts. It took me a week to read it.

The other record I played non-stop was *Grave New World* by The Strawbs. I thought Dave Cousins had a unique voice and also wrote some wonderful lyrics. The whole record was great but *Benedictus* and *New World* were the two songs I liked the most. Blue Weaver from Amen Corner had just replaced Rick Wakeman on keyboards, which was a hard act to follow, but he did himself proud.

At the end of April, Wishbone Ash released *Argus.* Their twin lead guitar harmonies were better than ever and the songs were memorable, especially *The King Will Come, Warrior* and *Throw Down the Sword.*

Alice Cooper released a single the same month called *School's Out,* which became a huge hit in England and with only a couple of months before the end of term, it felt like an appropriate anthem for me, but first I had to take my dreaded A Levels.

I completed my last exam on the 16th of June, which was the same day David Bowie released *The Rise and Fall of Ziggy Stardust and the Spiders from Mars.* I loved the whole album but my favourite songs were *Five Years, Moonage Daydream, Starman* and *Suffragette City.*

At the end of the month, my school days were officially over and my education could finally begin

On the 29th of July, Mark, Kipper, John and I went to the Crystal Palace Garden Party. We arrived just as Roxy Music started their set. They had recently released their first album, so we were excited to see them play some of the songs live, especially *Ladytron* featuring a haunting oboe solo by Andy MacKay, and *Re-Make/Re-Model* where every band member did a short instrumental solo during the end section. Bryan Ferry had an incredible voice, which I liked but it was the experimental sounds Brian Eno made on his VCS3 synthesiser, which I was truly impressed with. I had never heard anything quite like it. Inside the concert programme, there was a quote from one of my heroes, DJ John Peel, who said. 'Roxy are going to take the world by storm.' He was right.

Stone the Crows were up next featuring Jimmy McCullough on guitar who had recently replaced Les Harvey after he had been fatally electrocuted earlier in the year. They were followed by Edgar Winter's White Trash. When they played their most well-known song *Frankenstein* the crowd roared their approval. Osibisa were on next and their rhythm section was sensational. Halfway through their energetic set, a couple of girls of a similar age to us threw a blanket onto the ground next to us and started talking to us about the concert. This was the moment I met the first girl who I really fell for. Her name was Julie and we got on so well I didn't take much notice of the rest of Osibisa's set but when American folk singer Arlo Guthrie began singing we finally stopped chatting to listen. His satirical song *Alice's Restaurant* made us all laugh and I had no idea it was a protest song against the Vietnam War until Julie told me. When it was time to go home, she wrote down her name and number on the back of my concert program and I promised to call her the following day.

A week later Julie took the train from Maidenhead where she lived to come and stay with me. As it was the summer holidays, we were able to go to the beach at Milford-on-Sea and on the second night, after getting very drunk, we went for a swim in the sea in our undies, which sobered us up pretty quickly. On the last day of her visit, Julie told me she was about to move to Guildford to train as a nurse, which would make it hard to have any kind of meaningful relationship so we agreed to be just good friends. And after all, we were still only seventeen.

My best mate Mike moved to New Zealand with his family at the end of the month and we wouldn't get to see each other for the next three years but promised to stay in touch by mail.

To earn some money, I did all kinds of odd jobs over the summer, including working as a gardener for an elderly and rather reclusive couple. The house had been in the family for over a century and it had an enormous garden with ornate statues and a beautifully manicured lawn, which had stripes in perfect alignment in two different shades of green. I started work at 7 am three days a week and at 10 am a bell rang, which meant I was to go to the back door and wait. A hatch would then slide open and a mug of coffee and a piece of fruit cake would magically appear before the hatch closed again. This ritual continued each day until on one dreadful day I made an unforgivable mistake. I had no knowledge of the skills required to cut grass at two different lengths so moved their lawn just as I had done everyone else's on previous jobs. The result was the lawn was now all at one level. I was sacked on the spot.

There was at least one party every weekend. The unwritten rule was to bring your own booze but whoever the host was usually provided bowls of peanuts and Twiglets. There was always music playing in the background and in August there was rather a strange mix in the top ten hits from *School's Out* by Alice Cooper to *Run to Me* by The Bee Gees. You could always tell who was standing by the record player. If you heard *Silver Machine* by Hawkwind then it was one of the boys but if it was *Sylvia's Mother* by Dr. Hook if it was one of the girls.

John and I made some lovely new friends over the summer, Nick, Andy, James, Alexa, Catriona, Ros, Tricia and Vicki who we would remain close to for the rest of our lives.

After one particularly boozy bash, I stayed at Jon G's house after getting rather pissed with his younger brother Nick. We must have been far more drunk than we had realised at the time, as neither of us actually made it to bed. When Mrs G came down for breakfast in the morning, she discovered her wayward son asleep in the downstairs loo with his head bent over the toilet bowl and then found me snoring away in the dog basket in the kitchen. As for Gris, their Boxer, I must have let him out for a pee when we got home in the middle of the night and passed out on his bed, leaving the poor hound outside all night.

The sound of the telephone ringing woke me up with a start and I heard Mrs G talking to a woman at the other end of the phone who said she was from Brockenhurst College and had called to tell Nick his A-Level results.

'Yes. Yes, that's right. I see. Really? Oh Dear!' Mrs G said in a tone which suggested the results were not what she hoped for but had rather expected. She then explained to the woman I was currently staying with them so wondered if she could tell her my results as well, so she could let me know, 'Yes. That's right. Really? I see. Oh Dear!' As Mrs G placed the phone back on the receiver, she looked down at me in the dog basket and said with a resigned sigh, 'Well, you might as well stay there!'

Thankfully, although my exam results weren't as good as they should have been, I still managed get a place at Bournemouth & Poole College of Art to study Film and Photography for the next three years. But before then I had the rest of the summer holidays to enjoy.

I went to see Roxy Music again on the 6$^{th}$ of August when my friend Nick and I drove to Bournemouth to see them perform at Chelsea Village. They sang *Virginia Plain* twice by popular demand. The support act was The Mick Abrahams Band. Having been too young to see him when he was the original guitarist with Jethro Tull, it felt good to finally get to see him now. He was an exceptional blues player.

My stepbrother John and I went to the 1972 Reading Festival for three days in mid-August with my friend Mark. We tried to find somewhere to sit equal distance between the two stages and near the front but of course everyone else had thought of the same thing, so we ended up a bit further away than we had hoped but we still had a good view.

Friday's line-up included Good Habit, Cottonwood, Steamhammer, Jackson Heights and Genesis, who included *Twilight Alehouse* and *The Musical Box* in their set. Mungo Jerry were much better than we thought they would be and their one-off hit *In the Summertime* went down very well. Curved Air were the headliners and played *It Happened Today* and *Backstreet Luv*. When we went back to our tents at the camp site and I crawled into my sleeping bag, I was still thinking about the lovely Sonja Kristina, as I suspect were most of the other red-blooded makes trying to get some kip at Little John's Farm that night.

Saturday started with a short set by Jonathan Kelly. The underrated Irish singer-songwriter sang *Sligo Fair, Madeleine* and *The Ballad of Cursed Anna*. Welsh band Man played *Spunk Rock* as they always did, but now they had Deke Leonard as well as Micky Jones on guitars, their extra-long solos made the song seem to go on forever. I don't remember seeing Linda Lewis, so perhaps she came on when I went back to the tent to get a jumper, as it was a bit cooler than the previous day.

Focus blew us all away after playing *Focus, Focus 11* and *Focus 111*, making it unlikely we would ever forget their name. Jan Akkerman did some dazzling guitar solos and Thijs van Leer was a triple threat by being a keyboard virtuoso, a flautist extraordinaire and a charismatic vocalist, which was highlighted on their last song *Hocus Pocus*. After their set finished, a man who was sitting right behind us and smoking dope told us Jan Akkerman's guitar was a solid-state Fender and he created his unique sound using a Colorsound Power Boost, one of the very first overdrive pedals ever produced. We had no idea what he was talking about of course but not wanting to appear ignorant nodded our heads knowingly and accepted the joint he offered us with immense pleasure.

During Edgar Broughton's set he got everyone shouting *Out Demons Out*! which was a bit of a laugh, but it went on for far too long. I missed Jericho and a band called If, when I went for a wander to get a drink, but I was back with the others in time to see The Johnny Otis Show, featuring the aptly named backing singers, The Three Tons of Joy, and his son Shuggie Otis who was a bit of a wizard on guitar. The Electric Light Orchestra were up next and performed *From the Sun to the World* and the *10538 Overture*. Roy Wood had only left the band in July so all the singing duties were now down to Jeff Lynne and he didn't disappoint.

The Faces were on last, meaning it was party time with Rod Stewart, Ian McLagan, Kenny Jones and 'The Two Ronnies', Wood and Lane. *Miss Judy's Farm, Stay with Me* and *I'd Rather Go Blind* were the highlights plus the encore of *Twistin' The Night Away, Every Picture Tells A Story* and they closed their fun-filled set with *Maggie May*.

On Sunday we saw The Sutherland Brothers, Gillian McPherson,

String Driven Thing and Matching Mole with Robert Wyatt on drums. Stackridge were outstanding and as they were one of Mark's favourite bands we tried to get as close to the stage as we could. When they played *Do The Stanley*. we did the silly dance which the band had invented but it was the epic *Slark* we all wanted to hear and whistle to when Mutter Slater played the catchy melody on his flute. At one point when there was a break between band changes, we heard someone call out 'Wally!', presumably searching for a lost friend in the huge crowd. After hearing this man yell his mate's name a few more times other people around us started calling out 'Wally!' as well and before long hundreds of people had joined in creating a chorus of 'Wally! Wally!'

Vinegar Joe with Robert Palmer and Elkie Brooks got us back in the mood and then Status Quo proved they were still the best boogie band around. Someone near us said their new album was going to be called *In Search of a Fourth Chord*, which made us hoot with laughter. Quo were followed by Stray, Roy Wood's Wizard, Mahatma Kane Jeeves and finally by Ten Years After who gave a mighty performance with Alvin Lee playing guitar licks to die for.

We never discovered whether Wally was ever found or if he was even there. As we made our way to the car park one of the stewards told us it was more likely just someone copying what had happened at the Isle of Wight Festival in 1970 when the original call for Wally amongst the massive throng was alleged to have been made.

On the drive home we discussed which band we had enjoyed the most. John had loved the Johnny Otis version of *Willie and the Hand Jive* but for Mark and I, it was Genesis with Peter Gabriel which had ticked all our musical boxes, especially with *The Return of the Giant Hogweed.* The crowd must have agreed with us, as the applause went on for a good four or five minutes after they left the stage.

The best gig of 1972 for me was David Bowie and The Spiders From Mars at Starkers Royal Ballroom in Boscombe on the 31st of August, and the ticket only cost one pound. Bowie had dyed his hair bright orange, put on heavy eye shadow and was wearing his Ziggy Stardust outfit and a pair of silver platform boots, which made him look like an alien. Mick Ronson was on guitar (and boy, could he play it), Trevor Bolder was on bass and Mick Woodmansey on drums. They performed all my favourites from *The Rise and Fall of Ziggy Stardust and the Spiders from Mars* album plus a few older songs, which everyone seemed to enjoy. It was a truly magical musical night and one I would treasure forever. As we were leaving the venue, I overheard one of the other fans say, 'Well, that was the best quid I've ever spent in my life!'

Truer words were never spoken.

*Filmmaking, whatever the window dressing or the scale of a film may be, is eventually about telling a story.*

Farhan Akhtar

## CHAPTER 6: AND YOU AND I

Although part of me was really excited to be going to film school in Bournemouth, another part was a bit reluctant to go, as it would mean leaving the comfort of home and moving into unfamiliar surroundings again. However, my hesitation was only temporary and a couple of weeks later I moved into a tiny bedsit in Boscombe.

As I would now have to get myself to and from college each day, I upgraded my means of transport from my old Honda 50cc moped to a second-hand BSA Bantam 175cc, a two-stroke unit construction motorcycle with slightly raised handlebars. Even though I didn't look nearly as cool as Dennis Hopper in *Easy Rider,* I thought I was the cat's whiskers, especially when I 'head out on the highway'… or the A31 as it is more commonly called.

The film school was flexible about what hours we studied, which allowed me to make my own timetable, so I would often get up early and take myself on mini-adventures on my motorbike within a ten-mile radius of Bournemouth to take photos, study in the afternoon and then go to concerts in the evenings. Over the next three years, my relationship with music, photography and filmmaking would become almost inseparable with a barely visible line between the different forms of artistic expression.

For the first few weeks, I felt like an outsider looking in, which was most probably because the others were all older than me and I thought they might not want me to be part of their group. I was also painfully aware how much better they all were at photography than I was and how little I knew about the subject but I needn't have worried, as unlike the cowardly bullies at my public school who preyed on my vulnerability, these more mature students were all exceptionally kind, had an interest in film-making and a similar passion for music, so at last I had a sense of inclusion, which really helped with my self-confidence.

Richard was Polish and quite a bit older than me, so when I first met him, I thought he might be my lecturer. He had a huge walrus moustache, which he twiddled with constantly when he was in deep thought. Alan was Scottish and had a very strong Glaswegian accent, which made him sound like a tough guy but he wasn't and we got on like a house on fire. Jean-Pierre was French, good looking and very confident, or arrogant as the English call anyone who dares to look happy with their lot. I once saw him walk up to two pretty girls and tell them he was going to have a party in his bed in the afternoon and then ask them if they would care to join him. To my surprise and with more than a little envy, I watched as the girls giggled and calmly walked off with him, one on either arm. Bulent was Turkish and not only taught me how to play Backgammon but also got me stoned for the first time in my life.

Despite my enthusiasm for trying something new and illicit, I was a little nervous as to how the weed would affect me. I watched as my new friend from Istanbul rolled a huge joint and after taking a couple of puffs handed it to his girlfriend who did the same. When it was my turn, I must have taken too big a drag and suddenly had a coughing fit, which made them double up with laughter. After I had recovered, I took another puff and this time managed to inhale without coughing. I had been warned I might not get high after the first time but nobody told me I might just get a headache. I was a bit disappointed, but the following morning I had to admit I had never slept better.

As I now had some older friends to discuss what was considered 'good' music, their slightly more sophisticated tastes began to influence what I listened to and I was exposed to bands like King Crimson, Camel, Caravan, Gnidrolog and Renaissance who were all experimenting with their own styles, which a few years later would collectively be labelled as progressive rock. I was lucky enough to see them all perform while I was in Bournemouth as well as Wishbone Ash and Wild Turkey, who had recently been formed by Jethro Tull's original bassist Glenn Cornick.

Although I loved going to gigs and listening to records, the radio was my main source for discovering new music at the time. There are three DJs I owe a huge debt to for my musical education and who have all had a major influence on my musical taste. The first was Alan Freeman, whose nickname was 'Fluff' because of a fluffy jumper he often wore. He was an Australian who had lived in England for many years and he was best-known for presenting a weekly show called *Pick of the Pops*. This Sunday show featured all the latest songs topping the charts but on Saturday afternoons he presented *Rock Show* on BBC Radio 1 and played heavy rock and progressive rock music. It was because of Alan's show, I became a fan of bands like Gentle Giant and Caravan. The second was BBC DJ John Peel who was famous for promoting new artists and many of the bands he introduced me to on his show are still amongst my favourites today like Be Bop Deluxe, Focus and Streetwalkers, to name just three. 'Whispering' Bob Harris was the third. He was the host of *The Old Grey Whistle Test*, which featured non-chart music and influenced me even more than the radio shows as on this programme we could see them perform live. It was on this program, I first saw Lynyrd Skynyrd, Little Feat, The Allman Brothers and Peter Frampton. Believe it or not, the show was commissioned by Sir David Attenborough when he was controller at the BBC. He was also responsible for *Monty Python's Flying Circus* and *Match of the Day,* which showed highlights from the day's top football matches.

During his final term at boarding school in Sherborne, my stepbrother John invited our parents and I to a special concert by classical guitar maestro Julian Bream. The hall was so full; John and I had to sit on fold up seats on the stage only a few feet from the great musician himself. The whole audience was surprised when Julian began his show playing the lute rather than a guitar but within seconds, we were all transfixed as the music was so beautiful. In the second half, he played guitar music by composers who I had never heard of like Villa-Lobos-a Parita and Granados but I loved it all and to witness such virtuosity at such close quarters will always be a special musical memory.

When Yes released *Close to the Edge* in September, it took me a while to appreciate the album, as I wasn't keen on the first 4 minutes of the 18-minute title track but thought the rest was musically inventive and original and by the time they reached the climax I was fully on board. I also loved the lyrics, which one of my friends told me were partly inspired by Herman Hesse's novel *Siddhartha,* which inspired me to get the book out of the library. Steve Howe's acoustic guitar intro and outro on *And You and I* as well as his slide guitar and Rick Wakeman's keyboard solo near the end made this song the standout track for me. *Siberian Khatru* was a real rocker by comparison and I loved the fusion of rock, jazz and classical influences, as it sounded so fresh and original.

On the way home from the gig, I was wondering whether music and photography might have anything in common, and then I suddenly made a connection. Musicians always know exactly when the next beat is and they know instinctively when to make a change that could alter the mood of the piece of music they are playing. Photographers need the same sense of perfect timing. They also have to use their instincts and know exactly when to press the shutter to create the best image possible at that decisive moment.

I slept rather well after that epiphany… although it might have also been something to do with the four pints of Newcastle Brown Ale, which I had downed earlier that night.

A month later, Genesis released *Foxtrot* and outdid Yes time-wise by creating a 23-minute epic called *Supper's Ready,* which conjured up many whimsical images for me including Narcissus turning into a flower, going to Willow Farm to look for butterflies, flutterbyes *and* gutterflies and the most memorable image of all, Winston Churchill dressed in drag. I enjoyed hearing both songs but some of my friends thought they went on and on… for far too long. Perhaps Igor Stravinsky got it right when he said. 'Too many pieces of music finish too long after the end.'

In October, Santana released *Caravanserai,* which was a great example of jazz-salsa-rock fusion and despite not being in the prog rock stable was certainly progressive, at least from my point of view. I played this album non-stop for days and the two instrumentals, which attracted my attention the most were *Song of the Wind,* which had a really tasteful guitar solo on it and *La Fuente del Ritmo,* which not only had some great guitar licks but also had some great percussion. The combination of drums, timbales, congas and bongos might best be described as disciplined improvisation.

Despite the numerous concerts I had been to and the records I had bought, my life wasn't all about music. I still had to learn as much as I could about filmmaking and photography, which meant attending lectures, watching movies and reading books about portrait, still life, fashion and street photography. Finding the right balance between my love of music and visual storytelling was a constant battle to start with but once I began to appreciate how each of my interests was heightened by the other, I started to relax and accept my life would always be a melting-pot of passions.

As a few of the other students were now taking photographs on medium format cameras and getting some amazing results, I thought perhaps I should do the same thing, so I sold my 35mm camera and bought a second-hand Mamiya C330 Twin lens reflex camera to replace it. This camera had a waist-level viewfinder which took a while to get used to and the images were square so I had to compose my shots very differently to how I had done up to now. The C330 was used by professionals to shoot portraits, so I decided I have a go, as soon as I could find someone to model for me. My first attempts weren't very good but when one of my school friend's sisters, agreed to pose for me I soon got the hang of it.

Rafaela was very photogenic so it was hard to take a bad picture of her and as a thank you I took her to the cinema to see *The Adventures of Barry McKenzie.* The Australian comedy told the story of an Aussie lager-lout, played by Barry Crocker, who is sent to Pommyland with his Aunt Edna Everage, played by the comic genius Barry Humphries. Such is the power of product placement, Bazza had a can of Fosters in his hand for the majority of the film, which we thought was hysterical and started drinking the Aussie lager from then on. Although I discovered later, Fosters wanted nothing to do with the odious Crocker character at the time and only agreed to support the film when the producers threatened to go to a rival brand.

While booking some tickets for an upcoming concert the next day, the girl who answered the phone said she liked my voice and asked me if I had been to a Public school. After I told her I had, she then asked me if I would like to meet her for a drink, so I said yes and we agreed to meet at a bar we both knew the following evening. I waited at the pre-designated spot and ten minutes after the agreed time, a very pretty young woman came up to me and asked if I was the man she had spoken to on the phone. I told her I was but before I could ask her if she would like a drink, she said rather unkindly, 'Oh, you don't look anything like your voice.' I took her disappointed tone as a strong indication our date would most probably be a one off. It was an accurate assessment.

I then met an attractive girl called Anne who had long red hair, a huge smile and a laugh that could wake the dead. When I asked her if she would model for me, she agreed without hesitation. I enjoyed taking portraits of this beautiful girl and decided to ask her out on a date. We agreed to meet at the steps of the library and then walk to the cabaret restaurant Maison Royale together for a couple of drinks. I decided to take the bus rather than my motorbike so I could have a few drinks and in a last-minute moment of vanity decided not to wear my glasses as I had been told I was better looking without them.

This would prove to be short-sighted of me.

Although I was blind as a bat, I could still see well enough if I squinted really hard when I needed to focus and managed to get off at the correct stop near where we had arranged to meet. I waited for ten minutes and when there was still no sign of her, I thought she must have decided not to come, but just as I was about to give up, I felt a tap on my shoulder and when I turned around it was Anne. She looked furious.

'Who are you waiting for?' she demanded.

'You of course! Who else?' I replied, somewhat confused.

'Well, I just wondered if you were meeting someone else, as you were sitting on the same bus as me for the whole trip and didn't even bother to say hello!'

Once I had explained my lack of 20:20 vision she saw the funny side of it and joked she could now officially say she had been on a blind date, although it was pretty clear from now on, we were going to be 'just good friends'. We had an enjoyable evening at Maison Royale and while we were there one of Anne's friends came up to our table and told her to stay clear of a man who was working as a consultant for the club, as he was a bit 'touchy-feely'. When I asked what his name was, she replied. 'Jimmy Savile'.

In the morning, one of my photography lecturers told me that he was pleased with my progress with both my 35mm and medium format photographic work, but now it was time for me to learn how to take large format photos on a 4x5 camera. This proved to be far more complicated as the image appeared upside down on the focusing screen as well as reversed from right to left. I never quite got the hang of it but it did give me my first opportunity to work in colour using transparency film. My first attempt was to take a photo of a porcelain bowl full of colourful fruit and vegetables. The focus was sharp and the exposure was correct, but it had taken me so long to get everything positioned just as I wanted, the sticks of celery had drooped under the heat of the lights and ruined the photo. In my second attempt the celery looked much fresher and the exposure was correct but the image was slightly out of focus, so I must have knocked the tripod a fraction before pressing the remote shutter trigger. After a few more frustrating attempts, I realised I just didn't have enough patience to do large format photography to a good enough level to turn professional, so reverted back to 35mm.

My photography and filmmaking studies were now becoming just as important to me as music, so in an attempt to find the perfect balance between them, I limited myself to only listening to albums after dinner and only going to concerts once or twice a month.

In November, I heard Lou Reed's *Walk on the Wild Side* on the radio so often I bought the double A-side single and was glad I had as *Perfect Day* was the other track. Both songs were produced by David Bowie and Mick Ronson. I considered buying *Transformer* as both those tracks were on the album, but I couldn't afford to buy it as well as *Framed* by The Sensational Alex Harvey Band, so the two-track single was a happy compromise. I loved the title track *Framed* on the SAHB album, which was a cover of the Willie Dixon song *I Just Want to Make Love to You. There's No Lights on the Christmas Tree, Mother. They're Burning Big Louie Tonight* was also included on the album, and I had the catchy chorus ringing in my ears all through the festive season.

On the 10<sup>th</sup> of December, Nick, a mate of mine from Milford on Sea, and I went to see Family at the Bournemouth Winter Gardens. Roger Chapman was in fine form and I particularly enjoyed *My Friend the Sun, Holding The Compass* and *The Weaver's Answer*.

Three days before Christmas, Nick and I then went to see The Strawbs at Chelsea Village. I enjoyed hearing Dave Cousins sing some of the songs from their *Grave New World* album live but *The Hangman and the Papist* stood out for me, as it was such a powerful story and still gives me the chills today. Imagine being a hangman and discovering your next victim is no other than your brother, who has been just sentenced to death for his religious beliefs.

After lunch with my parents on Christmas Day, we put on the TV to watch the Queen's speech and as the Top of the Pops Christmas Special was on before Her Majesty, we watched the end of it. One of the DJs was Jimmy Savile and I remember my mother saying, 'I don't like the look of that man. There's something a bit creepy about him.'

The last song was Hawkwind's *Silver Machine,* which had come out in the summer and been a surprise hit. I had bought the single as I liked it so much. The bass player was a skinny lad from Stoke called Ian Fraser Kilmister whose nickname was Lemmy.

The first gig of 1973 was The Sensational Alex Harvey Band at Chelsea Village. Apart from performing songs off their album

*Framed*, they also did a cover of *Dance to the Music* by Sly & The Family Stone. The support band was Gnidrolog, which being dyslexic was a nightmare to attempt to write down correctly in the new diary I had bought as my annual Christmas gift to myself. *I Could Never Be A Soldier* was their best song but I may have been slightly influenced by the Jethro Tull-esque flute playing on it.

During the next term we had an American guest lecturer come to our Film School called Maurice Binder whose talk had a huge influence on me. Maurice was considered one of the best Film title sequence designers in the world. He had created the opening title sequences for 14 of the James Bond films up to then including the famous gun barrel sequence for *Dr. No*. He also created the titles for *The Battle of Britain* and *Barbarella,* which featured Jane Fonda peeling off her space suit in zero gravity. Maurice told us he achieved the shot by getting the beautiful actress to lie on a large piece of plexiglass, placing an image of a spaceship beneath her and filming the action from above creating the optical illusion she was doing her striptease in outer space. In-camera effects fascinated me and I hoped I would get the chance to do something like this in the future.

Our film theory tutor was a rather serious looking man who only ever wore black clothes. Although he didn't appear to have much of a sense of humour, he certainly knew a lot about all the famous film directors. Each week we would watch a film by a different director like Alfred Hitchcock, David Lean, Federico Fellini or Claude Chabrol. He would then tell us about how the films were made and discuss the content, style and execution. We also watched a few old classics, which I always looked forward to with child-like enthusiasm.

This is when I first saw *The Third Man* (1949) starring Orson Welles as Harry Lime. I loved the harsh lighting cinematographer Robert Krasker had used in this black and white movie to set the dark tone of the story and I thought his use of dynamic angles really added something to the film's dramatic atmosphere by suggesting everything was just a little off, which of course it was. The theme music by zither player Anton Karas, is one of the most recognised pieces of film music of all time and puts a smile on my face every time I hear it. The other brilliant example of film-noir, which inspired me was *A Touch of Evil* (1958) written and directed by the great Orson Welles. The movie starts with one of the longest opening shots of all time. We see a time-bomb being set and placed in the boot of a car...or 'the trunk' as my American friends would say...and then we follow the car's progress for a total of 3 minutes and 20 seconds until the bomb explodes. Cinematographer, Russell Metty, went on to win an Oscar for Best Cinematography for *Spartacus* at the 1961awards.

Apart from old classics, we also watched some more recent films which had been made in Europe and the one I love most to this day was an Italian movie called *Investigation of a Citizen Above Suspicion* (1970), which was directed by Elio Petri. The story is about a chief of police who kills his mistress and manipulates the murder investigation by planting obvious clues, which get ignored by the police under his command. Is he so powerful he is really above suspicion? I have always been a fan of black-humour but this movie also had plenty of suspense and was beautifully filmed by Luigi Kuveiller, which helped it win the Oscar for Best Foreign Language Film in 1970.

When we asked our lecturer what his favourite genre was, he told us he loved Westerns so over the following weeks we were treated to *Rio Bravo* by Howard Hawks, *The Searchers* by John Ford and *Once Upon A Time in the West* by Sergio Leone. Watching the lengthy opening scene where the bad guys are waiting for the train taught me how to block a scene, how to get the timing exactly right in an edit and how to maximise your sound effects. It was a master class in film making.

We also screened *The Magnificent Seven* by John Sturges, which was really a re-make based on a Japanese film called *Seven Samurai* by Akira Kurosawa. Our lecturer showed us the film so we could compare the two side by side. I became an instant fan of Kurosawa and wanted to find out more about this brilliant director.

During my research I came across the name Ishiro Honda, which sounded a little familiar so I looked him up and discovered he had directed *Godzilla* the film which had premiered on the same day I was born. This was the first film with large-scale special effects which had ever been produced in Japan and as I was now interested in visual effects I decided to find out as much as I could. I found out the head of the special effects team was a man called Eiji Tsuburaya and discovered how the sequences involving the destruction of the miniature sets was achieved by using powerful lighting and high-speed filming to make the action slower. I was also interested to note Ishiro Honda, whose father had been a Buddhist monk, had said he had found the best way to get good performances from his actors was without having to raise his voice. I told myself if I ever got the opportunity to direct actors, I would try to remember this advice.

Meanwhile Bulent, decided my knowledge of Marijuana needed updating. He had already taught how to roll my own 'doobie' to perfection but now he wanted to teach me how to make hash brownies. While I was being 'educated' he put on *The Captain and Me* by The Doobie Brothers. The opening guitar riff on Tom Johnston's *China Grove* still makes me feel high today, even without smoking a Naughty African Woodbine.

After Pink Floyd released *The Dark Side of the Moon*, the intake of spliffs increased considerably with each listen. It was a remarkable album, which starts with a heartbeat and then explores the themes of time, death and mental illness. Roger Water's lyrics were infused with pain and made me think about my mental health for the first time. The confusion and despair I had felt when I was still at boarding school were gradually dissipating but I still had moments of intense insecurity and the question I was now asking the resident lunatic in my head was, 'What do I want in life?' I had no desire for fame but hadn't yet worked out what I really wanted except for drugs, rock'n'roll and sex, but 'not necessarily in that order'. The track I liked the most was *The Great Gig in the Sky*, written by keyboard player Richard Wright with session singer Clare Torry providing some truly emotive vocals despite being totally wordless. I still get a lump in my throat whenever I hear her incredible contribution to what would become one of the most played records in my ever-growing collection.

On the 24th March, I went to see King Crimson perform songs from their *Lark's Tongues in Aspic* album at the Bournemouth Winter Gardens. Robert Fripp was on guitar, John Wetton on bass and vocals, David Cross on violin and Bill Bruford on drums plus an extra percussionist called Jamie Muir, which made their powerful set very entertaining to watch.

On the 13th of April, David Bowie released *Aladdin Sane*, a pun on 'A Lad Insane', which included a rather camp cover version of the Rolling Stones *Let's Spend the Night Together.* The best track in my mind was *Drive-In Saturday.* Bowie initially wrote the song for Mott the Hoople but they rejected it, which was a bit of a surprise considering the last song he had given them, *All the Young Dudes,* proved to be their biggest ever hit and apparently had originally been intended to go on the *Ziggy Stardust* album.

When Nick and I went to see Roxy Music at the Winter Gardens, they started their set with *Do the Strand* followed by *Beauty Queen* and *Editions of You.* At a specific point during *In Every Dream Home a Heartache,* Bryan Ferry sang the words, 'I blew up your body,' and the whole audience joined in with, 'but you blew my mind!'

It was a fabulous moment of unadulterated joy shared with total strangers, which made me feel at one with them and share a common sense of belonging to something bigger than ourselves. The encore was *Virginia Plain.* We didn't know it at the time but it would be the last tour Roxy ever did with Eno.

Having managed to get my interests in music, photography and film into a respectable as well as acceptable routine, I now had time to indulge in my other passion. Travel.

A week before Easter, Nicci invited me to stay with her in Mallorca over the break, which would not only give me an opportunity to spend time with my sister but also give me the chance to go to the beach and get some sun on my pale skin. Unfortunately, this idyllic scenario had to be put on hold when it started to rain about an hour after landing at the airport in Palma. I took the unexpected opportunity to read one of the books I had brought with me. The choice was between *The Inimitable Jeeves* by P.G. Wodehouse and *Hallowe'en Party* by Agatha Christie, which featured her Belgian detective Hercule Poirot. I chose the latter and had to smile when I read Christie's dedication at the front, as it was to P.G. Wodehouse - 'whose books and stories have brightened my life for many years. Also, to show my pleasure in his having been kind enough to tell me he enjoyed my books.'

While we were sunbathing one day, Nicci asked me if I had had a proper girlfriend yet. When I admitted I hadn't, she told me not to worry and gave me some sisterly advice. 'Be patient little brother. If a girl is interested in you, she will let you know.'

After I'd had the chance to relax for a couple of days, Nicci said she had organised a ticket for me to go to another bullfight. I told her I had mixed feelings about bullfights after seeing my first one the last time I was there but she told me this one would be different as it would all be done on horseback with beautiful Andalusian horses which were originally used in dressage. Bullfighters on horseback are known as Rejoneadors and the ones on display today were considered the very best. Angel and Rafael Peralta. As soon as the brothers entered the ring, it was clear their horsemanship was exceptional but I was concerned for the horse's safety as they had no padding. I let out a gasp every time the bull got anywhere near them but the rider's timing and skill was so perfect the bull never managed to get close enough to harm them. The man sitting next to me explained to me the reason the rejoneador was making the bull chase the horse so close to its backside was to find out how it was likely to attack once the fight started. As Angel placed a pair of barbed darts, called banderillas, into the shoulders of the first bull, I winced and wished I hadn't come but I had been fascinated by the balletic way he had done it considering both his hands were occupied and therefore had to control the horse's movements with his knees. The Peralta brothers were experienced showmen and made their horses do intricate dressage-like movements which the crowd loved but after the third bull had been killed, I'd had enough and left.

When I got back to college, one of my photography lecturers looked at the bullfight photos and told me he thought I had 'caught the drama of the struggle between man and beast perfectly' but quickly followed this high praise with a slightly more honest appraisal of my work, which roughly translated to 'and it's about time your damn photos were all in focus and exposed properly!'

On the 25th of May, Mike Oldfield's Tubular Bells was released. The first album on Richard Branson's Virgin label. I heard it 4 days later when DJ John Peel played it on his BBC radio show Top Gear (BBC, 29th May 1973). He said it was 'one of the most impressive LPs I've ever had the chance to play on the radio, really a remarkable record.'

When I took my driving test, I was a bit nervous initially but then I remembered my mother's advice. 'Treat everybody on the road as idiots, including yourself, and then you will be alright.' Her words made me smile and from then on I felt completely comfortable behind the wheel. The examiner must have thought so too, because when we were only half way through the test he told me to pullover near the shops and got out of the car. I asked him if he wanted me to wait for him but he said there was no need and I could drive anywhere I wanted from now on as I had passed. My budget was only £100 but luckily it was all I needed to buy my first ever car. A blue two-door Mark 11 Mini.

The following Saturday, the first episode of *The Ascent of Man* aired on Television. (BBC, 1973) The series was written and presented by Dr. Jacob Bronowski who travels the world investigating man's scientific achievements and technical discoveries up to modern day. It was the first programme I had ever seen which made me stop in my tracks and really pay attention to what was being said. I didn't understand everything by any means but the stunning visuals made me continue watching and want to at least try to understand this clever man's wise words. 'There is no absolute knowledge. And those who claim it, whether they are scientists or dogmatists, open the door to tragedy. All knowledge is imperfect. We have to treat it with humility.'

I loved the way the series had been filmed, so wrote down the two cameramen's names in the hope I might meet them one day and tell them how much I had enjoyed their camerawork. My mother wrote a letter addressed to both of them care of the BBC and after explaining her son was a film student in Bournemouth she asked if it was possible for me to spend a day on location with them if they were ever filming in the area. I never expected a reply, but two weeks later I received a call from the main cameraman, Nat Crosby, telling me he was about to start shooting a Drama series called *Vienna 1900* and some of it was to be shot in Warminster, which was only an hour's drive North of Bournemouth. He then added I would be welcome to visit the set if I could make it the following week and he would be happy to talk to me and give me some encouragement.

I immediately accepted his kind offer, as I knew if I was to have any chance of following my childhood dream of working in Hollywood one day, I would have to make the most of every opportunity because they don't come along very often. I would also have to get used to making quick decisions but thankfully this was reasonably easy for me as I had never been one to plan my spontaneity too far ahead.

After filling my Mini with petrol, I drove to the location the night before I was expected. I had already decided to sleep in the back of the car to save on paying for a B&B and although it would be rather uncomfortable, it would only be for one night and also be the best way to make sure I wasn't late for my meeting with the cameraman the next day. After driving for just over an hour I saw a sign letting me know I was almost at Warminster so started to look for somewhere to spend the night. After taking the next left turn I found myself in a small car park right by a pretty lake. There was only one other vehicle parked there. An old Ford Transit campervan. As I couldn't see anyone around, I had a quick pee against the nearest tree and decided to then take a stroll by the lake to stretch my legs before it got dark, I got back to the car park just as a middle-aged man wearing a baggy hat and some even baggier clothes was setting up a fold-up chair next to his campervan. The man had a small but friendly looking dog with him which ran up to me and rolled on its back, hoping I would rub its tummy, which I duly did. The dog's owner asked me if I would like a cup of tea and I gratefully accepted. As he poured boiling water from a thermos flask into a teapot, he asked me why I had stopped at this particular spot, so I told him I was planning to sleep in my car as I didn't want to be late for a meeting in the morning with one of the best cameramen in the country.

'One of the best, eh? What's this cameraman's name?' the man asked.

'Nat Crosby,' I replied.

'Is your name Jamie by any chance?'

I was totally taken aback for a moment wondering how on earth he could have known my name and then it clicked. This man must be Nat Crosby.

Nat told me he always took his campervan on location so his dog could come with him. We then talked about *Vienna 1900,* the miniseries he had come to shoot and he promised he would try to get permission for me to take photos as long as I was willing to let the producer's use them for publicity. He then took himself off to bed in his comfy campervan and I did my best to get some rest in the back of the Mini.

In the morning, Nat introduced me to the director Herbert Wise who shook my hand and told me to call him Herbie. He was more than happy for me to take photos as long as I stood well behind Nat's camera and didn't talk during a take. I couldn't believe my luck when after an exciting day watching them film, I was then invited to stay for the rest of the week and told they would cover the expense of a room in their hotel in exchange for copies of my photographs. I was over the moon. It was fascinating to watch the Austrian director at work and during a break, Herbie said he would show me how he 'blocked a scene'. When he saw the confusion on my face, he kindly explained what this meant, 'It's really just working out where the actors should stand and move in relation to the camera. A bit like choreography in a ballet.'

Over the next few days, I watched how the actors performed and moved in front of the camera including Roberts Stephens as Dr Graesler, who was one of England's most respected actors and married to a brilliant young actress called Maggie Smith. I also got to meet Dorothy Tutin, who had starred in the classic 1952 film adaption of Oscar Wilde's play *The Importance of Being Ernest.* I took a photo of her young daughter Amanda who was one of the extras, dressed in period costume and holding two balloons. It was the best photo I took on the set all week. I was also befriended by a charming up-and-coming actor called Norman Eshley who made sure I was given food and drink every time the actors had their breaks. It was a great experience to watch such professional cast and crew at work and for a few days be a small part of their 'film family'.

The photographs I took on the film set plus the bullfight on horseback photos I had taken in Mallorca became part of my first-year exhibition at the college and students doing other courses were invited to see our work. I noticed two pretty girls standing in front of my photos so decided to ask them what they thought of my images but it soon became apparent they weren't interested in my photography at all. They were studying fashion so were far more interested in looking at the period costumes the actresses had worn during the filming of *Vienna 1900.*

One of the girls told me her name was Rowena and said she liked what I was wearing, which was a collarless white shirt bought from the Army & Navy Stores, an old-fashioned multi-coloured waistcoat found at a charity shop and a pair of knee-length boots. My friends had teased me about my rather Bohemian choice of clothes and given me the nickname 'Byron' saying the combination of my old-fashioned clothes and my shoulder-length long wavy hair made me look more like a poet from the English Romantic movement than an up-and-coming photographer. Luckily for me, this look must have been what my new admirer found attractive and a couple of days later we went out on our first date. Rowena had prepared a lovely picnic, which we ate sitting on a rug in a secluded field in the Dorset countryside. It was a very romantic setting but being inexperienced in the art of love making I wasn't quite sure how to make the next move, but I need not have worried as she took the initiative and began to kiss me passionately. My sister had been right. This young woman was definitely interested in me and was now letting me know in no uncertain terms. After much fumbling, undoing of buttons and removing of our clothes we made love and I finally lost my virginity.

'About bloody time Byron!' one of my mates teased after I had admitted my recent amorous activity over a couple of beers to him the following weekend.

On the 23$^{rd}$ of June, I drove to London to see Jethro Tull perform their upcoming album *Passion Play* live at the Empire Pool, Wembley. Robin Trower was the support act and warmed the audience up perfectly with his amazing guitarwork. When Tull eventually came on after a rather long gap between acts there was a huge cheer. The new music took a bit of getting used to and was a bit heavy going at times, as instead of playing the flute, Ian Anderson played a soprano saxophone, which gave the band a very different sound and wasn't what most us were expecting or had come to hear. The new album comprised of a number of short songs, which had been arranged into one continuous piece of music lasting about 45 minutes. On their previous album *Thick as a Brick,* it had worked brilliantly but this time didn't have quite the same instant satisfaction musically, at least not for me.

I went out with Rowena a couple more times and as it seemed to be going well, I asked her if she would like to be my girlfriend, but she told me she wasn't interested and split up with me. I was very upset at being rejected and became quite depressed for a while.

Listening to music had helped relieve feelings of depression for me before, so I felt it was worth discovering whether it would help with heartbreak too. Thankfully, it did and I made a reasonably quick recovery after buying Joe Walsh's latest album *The Smoker You Drink, the Player You Get*, which included the uplifting song *Rocky Mountain*

*Way.* I loved Joe's talk box, which allowed him to modify his guitar sound using his mouth as a filter to shape the sounds via a plastic tube right next to his microphone. Every time I hear the song it takes me right back to when I first heard it and how it helped me get over being dumped.

On the 3$^{rd}$ of August, Lynyrd Skynyrd released *Pronounced 'Lĕh-'nérd 'Skin-'nérd.* My favourite song on their debut album was *Freebird.* Allen Collins blistering guitar solo, which he played on a 1964 Gibson Explorer, was the best I'd ever heard. The other song I liked was *Simple Man.* The lyrics 'Forget your lust for the rich man's gold. All that you need is in your soul,' spoke directly to me and would become a big influence on how I chose to live the rest of my life.

*The beautiful thing about learning is that nobody can take it away from you.*

B.B. King

## CHAPTER 7: THE CINEMA SHOW

Being obsessed with music is one thing, but understanding it is another. For me, it was a way of relaxing and de-stressing but I also had a genuine appreciation for original music, which made me actively seek out new bands who strived to be different, which was one of the reasons I was on my way to Reading to attend the 1973 National Jazz Blues Rock Festival in late August. My stepbrother John came with me plus our mutual friends Mark, Kipper and Andy. We arrived just in time to see Commander Cody and the Lost Planet Airmen but it was Rory Gallagher who we had really come to see as we had enjoyed his performance with Taste at the Ilse of Wight so much three years earlier. I lapped up every moment the Irish blues guitarist was on stage, right from his energetic first song *Messin' With The Kid* to his last *In Your Town,* which featured some sublime slide work.

It felt great to be with my good mates who were all into the same music as me but part of the joy of going to festivals is talking to the people sitting, standing or camped next to you who are complete strangers on the first day but who soon become friends even if only for the duration of the festival.

This was the case on Saturday when Lindisfarne had us all singling along to the chorus of *Fog on the Tyne* and *We Can Swing Together* before The Sensational Alex Harvey Band got us shouting along to the chorus of Alice Cooper's *School's Out.* The Faces set included a superb cover of *The Stealer* by Free but it was Rod Stewart's version of Jimi Hendrix's *Angel,* which was still playing in my head by the time we all head back to our tents.

Sunday started with Scottish singer-songwriter John Martyn playing a few songs from *Solid Air,* followed by a French group called Ange whose atmospheric music conjured up all kinds of *bizarre* images for my over-active imagination, especially *Le Cimetière Des Arlequins,* which if there had been an annual award for the most expressive use of a mellotron, would have won *le grand prix.* Ange were exactly the kind of band I was hoping to discover at the festival as they were totally unique and their songs completely original. Stackridge were on next and they soon got us all on our feet with the jaunty instrumental *Lummy Days* and ended their amusing set with *Let There Be Lids* using dustbin lids as percussive instruments, which wasn't as rubbish as it sounds.

One of the best things about attending a festival is being exposed to new artists and bands you have never heard of before. The experience widens your knowledge and tests your musical boundaries. This is exactly what happened when the ever-so-slightly eccentric George Melly came on stage with the Feet Warmers. Their take of trad jazz and sense of fun went down surprisingly well with the mainly hippie crowd and my friends and I loved every minute of their set. Tempest came on stage next but I was really only interested to see them because the band was the brainchild of ex-Colosseum drummer Jon Hiseman, who I greatly admired, but when he did his inevitable drum solo, it went on far too long and a few bored members of the audience started to build a tower using all the empty beer cans they could muster. There was a huge cheer when the tall can-tower eventually collapsed, which marked the end of the fun but unfortunately not the drum solo. The Spencer Davis Group were on next and they soon made us all feel happy again playing old hits like *Keep on Running* and *Gimme Some Loving.*

The headline act was Genesis and their faithful followers were rewarded with theatrical interpretations of *Watcher of the Skies*, *The Musical Box*, *Supper's Ready* and *The Return of the Giant Hogweed* before ending with *The Knife*, which sent us all home happy.

Although my main obsession was still music it now had stiff competition because of my passion for film and photography and they would constantly fight for top billing for the rest of my life. Initially, you might think there aren't many similarities but there are. For example, beautifully composed music creates visuals in my head in a different but just as pleasing way as taking well-composed images with one of my cameras. Both music and photography have 'rhythm' and to be good at either you need to have it in spades. The next time I took some fashion photos at the studio at college, I played *Superstition* off Stevie Wonder's great album *Talking Book* and got the model to dance with me as I took the photos. It was great fun and completely daft as an experiment but it worked and my 'choreographed' images were my best yet. Even the lecturer was impressed with the results and told me they were 'full of positive emotion', which was high praise indeed from a man who only ever wore black.

In October, I went to see Genesis again but this time at the Gaumont Theatre in Southampton. The band performed a few songs from *Selling England by the Pound*, including *Firth of Fifth* and my favourite *The Cinema Show* with a really long keyboard solo played by Tony Banks on the ARP Pro Soloist, one of the first pre-set synthesizers. At the start of the second verse 'Romeo locks his basement flat. And scurries up the stair', so as I was about to move into a basement flat myself the song really resonated with me. Mine was in Bournemouth and the building had originally been an old hotel before it had been badly damaged by a fire. My parents had decided to buy it and convert the building into 18 holiday flats to give them a regular income. When they offered me free accommodation in exchange for helping them out with odd-jobs from time to time, I gratefully accepted.

Although I attended lectures every day, I also had to study at home quite a bit, which involved reading numerous library books about the technical aspects of photography. While I studied, I listened to Tangerine Dream's album *Zeit*, which I found soothing rather than distracting, as the electronic music drowned out all the other extraneous sounds allowing me to focus all my attention on the complicated content and more importantly remember enough of it a week later during a practical class at my college. This musical experiment may well have been the first time I ever got my left and right brain to work in harmony. Who knows? I'm still in two minds about it.

After telling my lecturer about how Tangerine Dream had helped me to fully concentrate, he asked me if I had tried listening to classical music while I studied, 'If not, give it a go, as I think it might help you come up with abstract solutions to logical problems.'

I didn't really understand what he meant at the time, so I relayed the comment to my friends the next day. Richard attempted to explain how music helps improve your cognitive skills, so I turned to Alan to ask him what cognitive meant but thankfully he seemed just as baffled as I was. After Richard had finished laughing *at* us, not *with* us take note, he explained, 'Cognitive skill is the ability to recall specific events and details. In other words, it means memory.'

'Oh, is that right?' said Alan now in full Glaswegian sarcastic tone, 'In that case, I'll try to fucking remember!'

When The Who released *Quadrophenia*, Charles Shaar Murray said he thought it was the 'most rewarding experience of the year.' It was hard to disagree with the respected New Musical Express journalist whose reviews I always read with great interest and often agreed with. *Love, Reign o'er Me* is one of the best songs Pete Townshend ever wrote and Roger Daltrey's vocals on this track are truly impressive.

In November, I went to see Yes perform at the Bournemouth Winter Gardens. They played all three tracks from *Close to the Edge* but in reverse order followed by all four sides of their upcoming album *Tales from Topographic Oceans.* Alan White had replaced Bill Bruford on drums, who was a hard act to follow, but he did a splendid job and his skills really shone on *Ritual (Nous Sommes du Soleil)* and on the encore *Roundabout.*

The Groundhogs played at the same venue shortly afterwards. The songs from their upcoming album *Solid* got a rather lukewarm reception, as the fans weren't familiar with the new material but as soon as they played a few tracks off *Split* and *Thank Christ for the Bomb,* I suspect everyone thought 'Thank Christ for that.'

I spent Christmas Day with my parents and watched Noel Edmunds and fellow BBC DJ Tony Blackburn present a special edition of *Top of the Pops,* which included *Cum On Feel* the Noize by Slade, *Can the Can* by Suzi Quatro and *See My Baby Jive* by Roy Wood's Wizzard, who also had a huge hit with *I Wish It Could Be Christmas Every Day*.

The first lecture in 1974 was by Saul Bass, who had designed the title sequences for many films including Alfred Hitchcock's *Vertigo*, *North by North West* and *Psycho* as well as Billy Wilder's *The Seven Year Itch*. He had also designed some of the world's most iconic posters such as *Anatomy of a Murder* for Otto Preminger and many corporate logos. I was really impressed by his designs and his work was a big influence to me later in my career.

We were also given a lecture about the power of music which had been specifically written for films. I loved Bernard Herrmann's suspenseful music for Hitchcock's *North by North West,* Maurice Jarre's score for David Lean's *Lawrence of Arabia* and Ennio Moriccone's unforgettable theme for Sergio Leone's *The Good, the Bad and the Ugly* but I hadn't really appreciated why I liked these particular pieces of music so much, or how the music had triggered my emotions, or how each score had influenced how I perceived the visuals. After this informative lecture I paid a lot more attention to the soundtracks of the movies I went to see and on what effect they had on my overall enjoyment of the film.

As part of our course each student got to spend a week with a film production company to see how the professionals produced their work. I was sent to London to get work experience with a TV Commercials company called Brooks Fulford Cramer. Bob Brooks and Len Fulford were two of the most successful advertising photographers in the business who both specialised in food and product photography. Ross Cramer had just joined them from Saatchi's and he was given the task to look after me, which he did, but in his own mischievous way.

On my first day of work experience, Len Fulford was shooting a beer commercial and it was my job to take away the 'stand in' glass of beer which had been sitting under the lights while he composed and lit the shot and then replace it with a fresh one when he was ready to take the shot. I wasn't sure what to do with the beer in the old glass, but didn't think they would want me to pour it down the sink and simply waste it. And as a student with very little money, this was an unthinkable action, so I asked Ross if I should drink it rather than waste it, he said, 'Why not, it's only a light beer. And it's free!'

Despite having been under the lights for quite some time and therefore a little warm, it was still very drinkable. Unknown to me, Len was fastidious and prone to take a lot of photos until he felt he had the best shot in the bag. After five takes of disposing of the liquid amber in the same way as the first glass, I realised I was now getting a wee bit pissed. When Ross came back on set, he took one look at me and burst into a fit of giggles but then took me to their office kitchen to make me some coffee. When he had finally stopped laughing, he told me it wasn't a light beer after all and it was actually the strongest beer on sale in the UK, and the advert claimed it was 'Strong as a double Scotch, less than half the price.' Needless to say, I couldn't do any more work for the rest of the day so Ross paid for a taxi to take me back to my digs where I promptly passed out.

To make up for his prank, Ross asked me to help 'set dress' the food products for his shoot the next day. He wanted me to arrange the food in the way I thought looked best from the angle where his camera was positioned. This was much more up my alley, as I seemed to have a knack when it came to anything to do with spatial awareness. When the client looked at the final composition on the monitor, he said he was happy and no changes were needed. Ross was very pleased with the outcome and invited me to join the crew for a celebratory drink after we had wrapped. I had an orange juice.

Although, I had only been a minor part of a film crew for a few days, it gave me a real taste of what my life might be like in the film industry, if I followed the same path I was currently heading. I had enjoyed witnessing the professionalism on set but most of all I had noticed the camaraderie between everyone in the crew. It felt like they were all one big family and if this was what my career might look and feel like in the future, then I couldn't wait to get started.

When I got back to Bournemouth, I took my trustworthy Mini to the local garage for a service but unfortunately discovered it was no longer roadworthy, so traded it in for a maroon-coloured Hillman Imp, which had the engine at the rear. This little car was fun to drive and the handling was excellent due to its low centre of gravity. It also had a car radio, which made driving to college each day a lot more interesting. The first song I ever heard on it featured the lyrics, 'This Town Ain't Big Enough For Both of Us,' which was taken from the 1932 movie *The Western Code.* The full line in the film was, 'I'm getting tired of your meddling. This town ain't big enough for the both of us and I'm going to give you 24 hours to get out. If I see you in Carabinas by this time tomorrow, it's you or me!' Forty-two years later, brothers Ron and Russel Mael were working on an idea for a pop song, which had a dialogue cliché after each verse but in the end, they decided the line they liked from the old cowboy film would be enough for their needs. Their band was called Sparks and the song *This Town Ain't Big Enough For Both of Us* was a huge hit for them.

At the end of April 1974, Steely Dan released *Pretzel Logic*. When I had heard the single *Rikki Don't Lose That Number* I thought the guitar solo by Jeff 'Skunk' Baxter was out of this world, so bought their album based purely on the one track and I wasn't disappointed.

On the 8th of May, I went to *The Summer of '74* at Charlton FC in London with Vicki and my friend John N, who we called Nicol to differentiate him from all the other 'Johns'. Nicol was well over six foot tall and ate Twiglets almost continuously except when he was talking about Grand Prix races, which he knew everything you could ever possibly want to know about as well as quite a lot you probably don't.

Bad Company were up first and got us in the right mood with a dazzling cover of Mott the Hoople's *Ready For Love* but *Can't Get Enough* off their self-titled album was the crowd's favourite, along with a stimulating cover of Free's *The Stealer*.

When Lindisfarne came on stage, everyone joined in the choruses to *Fog on the Tyne* and *We Can Swing Together* and when it was Lou Reed's turn to shine, we all sang along to *Vicious* and *Walk on the Wild Side*, so by the time Humble Pie, with the sensational and soulful Steve Marriott on vocals, began their set, we were already in high spirits. They ended with *I Don't Need No Doctor,* by which time there was a bit of fisticuffs going on in front of the stage, so ironically it's quite likely some of them did.

After an unusually long wait, The Who eventually appeared on stage and started their set with *I Can't Explain* followed by *Summertime Blue* and *Young Man Blues,* which all went down well but the best song of the night by far was *Baba O'Reilly.*

Pete Townshend did his famous windmill arm-swinging while strumming his guitar and Roger Daltrey swung his microphone in the air on a long lead before catching it every time. John Entwistle on bass was as laid-back as ever and Keith Moon went bonkers on drums, so no change there either. His kit seemed to have sprouted a dozen tom toms and two gongs since I had last seen him play.

After *Won't Get Fooled Again, Pinball Wizard* and *See Me, Feel Me* their fans went mental but there was still more to come. *Magic Bus, My Generation, Naked Eye, Let's See Action* and finally *My Generation Blues.* What a band, what a night.

Having been to so many concerts already this year, my happy jar was full but I still had room for more so when Dire Straits released their first album in June, I added it to my collection. Although *Sultans of Swing* got a lot of air play on the radio, I preferred the opening track *Down to the Waterline.* Be Bop Deluxe also released their first album the same month. *Axe Victim* really made me sit up and take notice because Bill Nelson's sensational guitar solos were unique, especially on the title track, *Adventures of a Yorkshire Landscape, Jets at Dawn* and *No Trains to Heaven.* The LP cover also grabbed my attention because it featured a guitar made from a human skull on it, which was rather eye-catching.

The first time I ever heard *Sweet Home Alabama* was on my car radio in July. The song was off Lynyrd Skynyrd's album *Second Helping* and as it only had three chords, C, G and D, it was relatively easy to play along to but the tracks I liked jamming to the most after listening to the whole album were *Workin' for MCA* and *Call Me The Breeze* because their three lead guitarists played some blistering solos, which blew me away and made me want to join in. However, having the desire and having the skill are two entirely different things.

I now had a fairly impressive vinyl collection all stacked in alphabetical order using the artist's first name or band name but, as my beloved rock albums were now interspersed with blues, jazz, folk, electronic and classical records, I started to question my decision and after a sleepless night got up early the next morning to re-arrange my LPs by last name and band name. I had never felt so satisfied in my life.

The 1974 Reading Festival in August promised to be even better than the year before so my step brother John and I along with our mutual friends Mark and Andy decided to go for the second year in a row. The Friday line-up included 10cc, who were much better than we had anticipated with *Rubber Bullets* proving to be a hit with the crowd and The Sensational Alex Harvey Band, who were as entertaining as ever and demanded our participation on the chorus of *School's Out*, so we did. Well, it would have been rude not to.

There is something truly primal about being part of a huge crowd at a festival creating spontaneous order together out of seeming chaos like a flock of birds or a school of fish using swarm intelligence to decide which direction to go next. The sense of being 'at one with everyone' stays with you forever.

On Saturday we saw Procol Harum with Gary Brooker, Thin Lizzy with Phil Lynott and Traffic with Stevie Winwood, so it was a pretty special day and on Sunday we saw Barclay James Harvest, Chapman and Whitney's Streetwalkers and Focus. When the Dutch band played *Hocus Pocus* we tried our best to keep up with Thijs Van Leer, as he yodelled, whistled and did a comedic scat, which wouldn't have been out of place on *The Goon Show*. The two DJs for the weekend were my musical mentor John Peel and Jerry Floyd...no relation to Pink. Despite many calls for 'Wally!' from the crowd, he didn't make an appearance this year... as far as we know.

Over the summer, I met and dated a lovely local girl but as she put too many demands on our budding relationship, it didn't reach full bloom, so I returned to my one true love, music, which unlike human relationships, is unconditional.

On the 13th of September Supertramp had released *Crime of the Century* in September. I first heard it at my old kindergarten friend Phil's house with a group of our mutual friends. We all thought it was one of the best albums we had ever heard because it felt like the band had somehow found the perfect fusion of progressive and pop music. I still think *School* is one of the most exciting opening tracks of all time. The melancholy harmonica intro gave me goosebumps and by the time Rick Davies electric piano joined in, I was wondering where these impressive musicians would take us next. It was a thrilling ride. *Bloody Well Right* had a great chorus, which I thought would be popular with audiences when played live but the two tracks I liked the most were *Asylum* and *Crime of the Century*.

In November, I saw Queen at the Bournemouth Winter Gardens on their *Sheer Heart Attack* tour. Freddie Mercury had an extremely powerful stage presence and Brian May's riffs and solos were something to behold, although his guitar solo was a bit self-indulgent. *Killer Queen* and *Seven Seas of Rye* were the two stand-out songs for me and they ended their rousing set with the well-known stand-up song *God Save The Queen*.

When Pink Floyd performed at Wembley, they started their set with *Shine On You Crazy Diamond* from their upcoming record *Wish You Were Here* and then did two new songs called *Raving and Drooling* and *You've Got to Be Crazy*, which were later renamed as *Sheep* and *Dogs* and appeared on their album *Animals*. After performing the whole of *Dark Side of the Moon* they then played *Echoes*. It was a truly epic night.

At the end of the month, Jethro Tull came to Southampton to promote *Warchild* and in December Supertramp came to Bournemouth to do the same for *Crime of the Century*. 1974 had provided some magnificent musical memories.

On New Year's Eve, I went to our favourite watering hole, The Chequers, to meet some of my old friends for a drink. Kipper was already at the bar waiting to get served and standing next to him was a very attractive woman with long blonde hair. Having discretely ensured my friend wasn't after her himself, I introduced myself and discovered her name was Sara. We hit off straight away and I asked her out for a drink the following weekend. One date was enough to realise we had had both fallen in lust at first sight and we became an item. Sara stayed with me in Bournemouth two nights each week and we would also catch up in Lymington at the weekends as well. We had a great time 'going out' together and apart from the strong physical attraction, I also really enjoyed her company. But as all play and no work makes Jack a mere toy, I made a new year's resolution to focus less on my sex life and more on my studies. My good intentions lasted a week.

During the first term of 1975, our film lecturer told us to split up into groups of three and come up with an idea for a film and as there was only one old wind-up 16mm Bolex camera at the Film School, we would have to share it between us. I teamed up with my Polish friend Richard and Scottish friend Alan. Richard wanted to make a film about the myth of a group of Polish cavalrymen who had allegedly charged German tanks in the battle of Krojanty on the 1st of September 1939. We thought it was a cool idea so we agreed Richard should be the director. The Bolex was the perfect camera for us to learn filmmaking techniques. We all had a go with it with varying degrees of success but as Alan was obviously the best out of the three of us, he became the cameraman, which meant I would be the editor. Our lecturer told us the project was too ambitious and it would be impossible to do in the time we had. Well of course, this was a gauntlet we simply had to pick up.

Our first problem was to find some tanks to film so the next day we drove to the Tank Museum located in Bovington Camp, in Dorset. After chatting to a kind woman on reception we managed to get the name and phone number of Major Meredith who was currently in charge of the base of the Royal Armoured Corps.

As Richard mumbled under his huge moustache and Alan had a

strong Glaswegian accent, it was decided I should be the spokesman for the group, so putting on my poshest public-school voice I made the call. To my surprise the Major picked up the phone himself, so with the thought of nothing ventured nothing gained firmly in the back of my mind I said exactly as I had rehearsed in the car with my friends, 'Excuse me Major but do you believe in the word Impossible?'

'Certainly not young man.'

'Good. In which case, I am hoping you will want to help us sir.'

'Go on.'

'My friends and I are making a film about the Polish cavalry who charged German tanks on the first day of the Second World War for our student film and we have been told by our lecturer it is impossible. But if you were to allow us to film your tanks on manoeuvres, we could intercut those shots with those of the cavalrymen, which we will film separately. Are you willing and able to help us do the impossible sir?' There was such a long pause I thought the line had gone dead but then I realised the Major was laughing.

'Be at the front gate tomorrow morning at seven am sharp and I will see what we can do.'

We arrived bang on time and to our amazement Major Meredith was there to meet us personally. After he briefed us as to where we could stand safely to avoid being run over by one of the Chieftain Mk.5 tanks doing their training exercises, we were taken to the military firing ranges in Lulworth in a six-wheeled FV603 Saracen armoured personnel carrier where we were allowed to film the tanks going through their paces. Although they weren't the kind used by the Germans in WW2, they were perfect for our purposes.

A few days later we went to the New Forest to film the Polish cavalry, who were actually three fellow film students wearing uniforms created by girls from the fashion department at our college and riding horses we had hired from a local stable. After we had all the footage processed and printed, I then intercut the shots to create the impression the tanks and horses were at the same location and after adding suitable sound effects we were all pleased with the result. The examiners must have thought the same as both Alan and I passed our design diplomas with credit and Richard got a distinction.

I rewarded myself with Jeff Beck's latest release *Blow by Blow*. The legendary George Martin produced the album, which may have been the reason for the inclusion of the cover version of the Beatles song *She's a Woman,* but my favourite track *'Cause We've Ended as Lovers* was written by Stevie Wonder and dedicated to the great Roy Buchanan.

At the end of April, I drove up to Heathrow to pick up by old friend Mike, who was finally returning from his sojourn in New Zealand. He was full of stories about his adventures and I couldn't wait to go there myself one day.

To celebrate Mike's return, we went to Chelsea Village to see a Welsh band called Man who were best known for their extended jams especially on their cult classic *Spunk Rock*!

Deke Leonard had recently disbanded Iceberg and re-joined Man, so it was a real treat to finally get to see him trading meandering marathon solos with fellow axeman Micky Jones.

And on the 25th of May, Mike and I and a couple of our mutual friends to see Led Zeppelin at Earls Court, which was the last of their five shows at the venue. Seeing them play live was inspiring. They played for almost four hours and their long set included all the songs we loved like *Kashmir, Trampled Underfoot, Stairway to Heaven* and *Black Dog.* As we drove home we thought we had just witnessed Robert Plant, Jimmy Page, John Paul Jones and John Bonham at their peak but of course, only time would tell.

I had a huge party to celebrate passing my exams and leaving film school. It was held at the Red House in Barton-on-Sea and all my friends turned up including Mark, Kipper, Mike, Andy, Jon G and his brother Nick. I drank far too much whiskey and eventually passed out. My step-brother drove me home but stuck my head out of the window and wound the window up under my chin so if I was sick, I wouldn't throw up in his car.

On the 11th July, Fleetwood Mac brought out a self-titled album. It was the first to feature guitarist Lindsey Buckingham and vocalist Stevie Nicks whose haunting song *Rhiannon* had an infectious melody, which stuck in my head for ages.

As well as a certificate from my film school to prove I had a brain of some sort, I had also managed to find a way of giving all three of my obsessions, music, photography and filmmaking equal top billing in the said same brain, so I felt pretty good about the direction my life was heading. All I needed to do now was to find a job, which allowed me to indulge my passions, so rather than look for a normal job with a regular income, I decided to find a way of doing what I loved for a living while also getting paid 'enough' to maintain my chosen life-style. It didn't take as long as I feared.

I wrote to more than a dozen companies trying to get a job in the film industry and only got three replies. Two of them to kindly inform me I needed experience to work with them but unfortunately not how to get the much-needed experience. Thankfully, the other letter was more promising and informed me their company was looking for a runner, which is also known as a gofer, as in 'go for this' and 'go for that', and so I accepted the interview with great excitement. I took the train to Waterloo and a tube to Leicester Square before walking up to Soho. Walking through Wardour Street for the first time was quite exciting for me as this was the centre of the film industry in London and where a number of production companies were based all working out of tiny offices along this street and the ones either side of it. By the time I got to Oxford Street, I was in great need of relieving myself. If you are caught short, the nearest pub is the most natural location to proceed to but it is considered polite to purchase a beverage at the bar first before making use of the amenities, so I ordered a pint before rushing to the loo. Unfortunately, I discovered to my horror the Gents was temporarily closed while the plumbing was being fixed. My own plumbing was in dire need of fixing too, so I downed the pint and went to look for another pub. Having been assured their lavatory was in perfect working order before buying another pint, I then went in search of it at speed. I was just about to unzip myself at the urinal, when a person of rather dubious hygiene approached me and made a somewhat indecent suggestion. Needless to say, I declined his kind offer and after necking my pint as quickly as I could I went in search of another loo.

Apart from still being desperate for a pee, I was now also in danger of being late, so I decided to go straight to Fitzroy Square. As soon as I arrived, I explained to the receptionist I urgently needed to use their facilities, and she kindly pointed me to their toilet. It felt so good to finally have a pee I let out a loud moan of relief. I heard the sound of a lavatory being flushed behind me and as I turned around to look, I saw an elderly and rather dishevelled man, who I thought was most probably the janitor, come out of a cubicle. He asked me if I was feeling alright so I told him my about my ordeal and how I had been worried about being late as I really wanted the job. He must have found my tale amusing as I could still hear him laughing after he had left me alone in the toilet to wash my hands.

While I waited in reception, I talked to Jenny, the Australian receptionist, and gratefully accepted the extra strong mint she offered to stop me smelling like a brewery. Eventually I heard my name being called out and I made my way to the managing director's office.

Imagine my surprise when I realised, I was about to be interviewed by the janitor! His name was Jack Shepherd and realising how keen I was, he kindly offered me the job there and then.

I started my first job in the Film industry on the 24th of July 1975. I was hired by United Motion Pictures as a tea boy and runner, which meant making endless cuppas for the editors, so they didn't have to leave their cutting rooms, and carrying heavy 16mm film cans between our offices to the film laboratory in Soho Square.

Not exactly my dream of working in Hollywood… but I had to start somewhere.

*When you are asked if you can do a job, tell them, 'Certainly I can!'*
*Then get busy and find out how to do it.*

Theodore Roosevelt

## CHAPTER 8: SHOW ME THE WAY

Now I was working in London, I had to find somewhere to live but as my wages were only £17 a week, I couldn't afford anything too flash. After viewing five filthy flats in a row, all with sepia-stained toilets with matching odious odours and occupiers, I eventually found a tiny room in a shared flat in Avonmore Gardens, West Kensington. I agreed to rent it, partly because the loo had been cleaned relatively recently, partly because my new flatmates were into music, but mainly because it was only £5 a week.

Apart from the single bed, which took up the majority of the space, my bedroom was so small I could only fit one rickety old kitchen chair in the corner but it was the ideal piece of furniture for my second-hand Dansette Tempo 4-speed portable record player to sit on, and there was enough room to place a handful of LPs underneath. My room was right above the Kensington railway line but I was so exhausted by the time I got home each night, I soon got used to the noise and rumble of passing trains. The only heating was from a coin-operated gas fire in the hallway. On one particularly chilly night the coin box was so full we couldn't add anymore coins or get hold of the landlord to unlock and empty the meter, so we had to come up with an alternative way to stay warm. One of my flatmates suggested we put crumpled newspapers between our sheets and blankets as an insulator, which worked surprisingly well and we didn't freeze to death, so didn't end up in the headlines the following morning.

Over the new few months, I had very little spare time, or money, to go to concerts or out for drinks with friends, as I now needed to focus all my energies on my film career.

To make a few extra quid, I worked between 7pm and midnight three nights a week selling hamburgers cooked on a portable hotplate from a stand in Leicester Square. There were always two of us at the stand, one cooking the meat and onions and the other handling the money and handing the rolls to hungry customers who had just come out of the nearby cinemas. We did quite well as there wasn't much competition back then. Although McDonalds had opened their first restaurant in Woolwich in November 1974, it would take another ten years before the American company would become profitable in the UK. When we got mugged by a gang of skinheads one night who stole all our hard-earned cash, I decided it might be a good time to quit and find an easier way to increase my income.

Although I couldn't afford to buy any new LPs for the time being, the ones I had brought with me were more than enough to keep me company. *Crime of the Century* by Supertramp and *Moving Waves* by Focus both had such a positive energy about them they helped me to relax and de-stress at the end of a long day.

Jack Shepherd, the owner of the company, was a kind man who always gave me a smile when we passed in the corridor, but the executive producer, who was in charge of all the productions, was a malevolent little man who had a rather high-pitched voice with a faux cockney accent and thin shoulder length wispy hair, which he blow-dried in his office each morning. He never even bothered to learn my name and just shouted 'Boy!' whenever he wanted me to do something for him, expecting me to stop whatever I was doing and immediately come to his aid, which, wanting to keep my job, I always did. His unreasonable behaviour and verbal bullying reminded me of my sadistic teacher at boarding school and for a few weeks he made my life a misery.

One day, I heard one of the editors call him a megalomaniac but not really knowing what the word meant, I decided to look it up in the dictionary but being slightly dyslexic I misread the word 'megalomaniac' and looked up the definition for 'melomaniac' instead. Although the two words are spelt almost identically, they have very different meanings. A megalomaniac is 'a person who has an obsessive desire for power' and a melomaniac is 'one with an abnormal fondness of music; a person who loves music.'

'That's me!' I thought. It was a defining moment, as the word described me perfectly and still does to this day. My compulsive and constant need to hear new and original music is as strong now as it was back then, I love to change the music genre to suit whatever mood I am in and I feel immense joy whenever I hear or see a new artist. When I was having such a hard time being bullied at boarding school, music had been my saviour and got me through the worst, but I was now a different person to who I had been when I was a timid schoolboy and didn't have to take any crap from anyone anymore, so from the next day onwards, I decided to simply ignore the producer's constant demands, offensive language and belittling remarks and just get on with whatever menial task he thought suited my low status each day. As a result, by not letting myself be intimidated by his megalomaniac tendencies and need to be master over others, I took the power away from him and empowered myself in the process.

Making never ending cups of tea for the editors allowed me to watch them while they worked and ask them questions when they had a break. I got on particularly well with the owner's son Barry, who was an experienced film editor, so one day I asked him if I could be his assistant, as I was keen to learn everything I could from him. He thought about it for a day or two and then persuaded his father to not only promote me from runner to assistant editor but also increase my wage to £25 a week. This was when my career really started.

Over the next few weeks Barry taught me how to log the rushes and how to synchronise the sound with the pictures by using a contraption called a synchroniser. The sound was recorded on location on a portable stereo reel-to-reel tape machine called a Nagra IV-S, which was considered the workhorse of the film industry because of its reliability. The audio was then transferred from the ¼' on to a 16mm perforated magnetic film to make it the same size as the rushes, or dailies as they were also called. I then had to do 'rubber numbering' which involved printing matching numbers using a latex-based solution on the edges of sound and picture so the editor could match the edge numbers and find correct audio which synced with the image.

The films were all edited on a 16mm Steenbeck, which was a flat table-based machine where I laid the synced-up film and sound rushes on their sides on rotating plates on the left-hand side and attached the head of each reel to a take up plate on the right-hand side. The film could be seen on a screen above the plates after passing in-front of a backlit multi-sided rotating prism. To play forwards, backwards or pause, the machine had a built-in control at the front of the table. Barry would make the decisions were to cut by marking both the film and sound with a chino-graph pencil and would then either cut out or add in more frames to the scene. He cut the film selecting shots I had hung from pins on a rack next to him, which were all in a specific order and would join them together with a tape splicer. I also learned how to track lay the sound and how to compile a cue sheet, so when it was time to do the audio dubbing the engineer could see what sounds he had to work with before he heard them which made his job much easier. I coloured my cue sheets to make it clear which tracks were sync voices and which ones were sound effects.

After each film was completed and approved, we had to get the film neg cut and graded at either Humphries Film Labs or Kays Laboratories. This allowed me to spend a lot of time at both places talking to the technicians and trying to learn everything I could about their craft. They showed me how to cut the neg while wearing white cotton gloves so I didn't leave fingerprints on the frames and how they created double-exposures, fade-outs and dissolves at the Lab and also taught me the basics on how to do back projections, matte paintings and blue screen shoots, which would all come in use later in my career.

I loved attending the sound mixes at John Wood Studios in Soho. John was a legendary dubbing mixer, so I had to ensure my cue sheets were always spot on. They also recorded narrations there so as UMP used well-known actors and TV personalities to do their voice-overs, I got to meet a few including BBC news reader Angela Rippon, Blue Peter's John Noakes and Lesley Judd, and the actors Patrick Allen and Richard Briers.

In September, Pink Floyd released *Wish You Were Here*, a tribute to their former band member Syd Barrett, whose mental illness and drug abuse had finally got the better of him. As I now had a little extra income, I was able to afford the album and found it quite moving, especially all nine parts of *Shine On You Crazy Diamond*. I was surprised to discover Roy Harper had sung vocals on *Have a Cigar* but it worked quite well and I had to laugh when I heard the lyric, 'Oh, by the way, which one's Pink?'

The following week, I bought two more albums. The first was *Voyage of the Acolyte* by ex-Genesis guitarist Steve Hackett. The opening track *Ace of Wands* and last track *Shadow of the Hierophant* were the two stand out tracks in my opinion but Steve's distinctive guitar style was there for all to hear on every track. The other album was *Minstrel in the Gallery* by Jethro Tull. I really liked *Cold Wind to Valhalla* and *Black Satin Dancer* but it was the almost 17-minute epic *Baker Street Muse* I enjoyed hearing the most, partly because of whimsical lyrics like 'Indian restaurants that curry my brain', partly because of Ian Anderson's exquisite acoustic guitar and expressive flute playing, but mainly for the overall professional quality of musicianship from the entire band.

As I seemed to have found a balance between my 'abnormal fondness of music' and learning about the film industry, my love of photography would have to take a back seat for a while. I wasn't too concerned, as it felt more like a hobby anyway… at least for now.

On the 19th of September *A Touch of Class,* the first episode of *Fawlty Towers* was shown on BBC Two. The date is etched in my mind as it was the day, I laughed so hard I nearly peed myself. John Cleese was to blame.

I shared my 21st Birthday party in November at the Angel Hotel in Lymington with my Australian friend Hugh, who was two days younger than me. We invited all our mutual friends. There were a hundred of us drinking non-stop and dancing to a local rock band we had hired for £30 called Spider, who played covers of all our favourite songs.

My Hillman Imp was now too old and rusty to drive as far as

London on a regular basis, so I bought a green Renault 5 for £500. It was a three-door hatchback with a stick-shift on the dashboard to change gears. It also had a built-in cassette player so my next purchase was to buy a tape to listen to on the journey back to London. The choice was easy as Queen had recently released *A Night At The Opera,* which included the magnificent *Bohemian Rhapsody,* which we all loved to sing along to especially 'Scaramouch, Scaramouch, will you do the Fandango!' and a few Galileo's at different pitches before the compulsory head-banging section began.

Jenny, the Australian receptionist at UMP, stayed with us for Christmas and then flew home to Australia two weeks later. She had been really supportive to me when I had first started to work as a runner, so I would miss her a lot. Before she left, I asked Jenny if she had minded being so far away from her own family, she just shrugged and said she wouldn't have become the person she now was if she hadn't decided to travel overseas. Her words gave me food for thought and made me wonder whether I could also find the courage to do what she did and live on the other side of the world for a while.

On the 6th of January 1976, Peter Frampton released *Frampton Comes Alive!* This incredible double album by the ex-Humble Pie guitarist soon became a firm favourite especially the songs *Show Me the Way* and the final track *Do You Feel Like We Do.* Frampton's use of the talk box really got the crowd going nuts. They couldn't get enough of it. I knew exactly how they felt.

In February, Genesis released *Trick of the Tail* with Phil Collins taking over vocal duties from Peter Gabriel for the first time. The opening track *Dance on a Volcano* proved the band still had a future but the best track was the last, an instrumental called *Los Endos,* which would become a fan favourite for years to come.

*Rebel* by John Miles came out the same month. The opening track *Music* is one of the best rock ballads of all time. I could really identify with the lyrics, 'Music was my first love. And it will be my last.' And the second verse said it all for me. 'To live without my music would be impossible to do. In this world of troubles my music pulls me through.'

John's words really resonated with me, as music had pulled me through when I was getting bullied at school, and since then had helped shaped my identity into a much more self-assured young man, one who was finally comfortable with himself.

On the 19th of March Paul Kossoff of Free, died of heart failure in his sleep during a flight to America. He was 26.

Having a Union card to work in the British film industry was compulsory at the time, so when The Association of Cinematograph, Television and Allied Technicians (ACTT) told me I would either have to stay with the same company for another year to get my card or I could go overseas for a year to find work elsewhere with the guarantee I would be given a card as soon as I returned. I had gained a lot of technical know-how in the reasonably short time I had been working at UMP, but if I stayed with them for another year I was unlikely to learn much more and by having to stay at the same level would mean not earning any more than I was already being paid, so the decision to stay put or travel overseas to look for work was starting to swing in favour of the latter, at least in my head. It would obviously be a risk to go to somewhere like Australia and I didn't want to end up looking a complete fool, but perhaps remaining in the UK would prove to be a bigger risk.

On the 1st of April I was given a small pay rise, so I was now able to afford to go to a few concerts, including The Fabulous Poodles at The Marquee, as well as Be Bop Deluxe and Ange, who I had first seen at the Reading Festival. I also got to see Memphis Slim at Ronnie Scott's and Brand X, with Phil Collins of Genesis fame on drums, at The Nashville Rooms at the Famous Three Kings Pub. The rest of my spare time was spent in record shops expanding my knowledge of the American Blues by listening to LPs by the other famous three kings. Freddie, Albert and B.B.

It felt good to be able to attend live gigs again, so working in London definitely had its upside. The down side was the constant threat of being blown up the IRA. On the 29th of January a dozen bombs had exploded in the West End but luckily only one person was injured. On the 21st of February a bomb had gone off at Selfridges. This time five people were injured. And on the 27th of March a bomb exploded in a litter bin at an exhibition hall in Olympia which was very close to my flat. This time 70 people were hurt.

At the end of April, my buddy Hugh told me he was going back to Australia. I didn't blame him as the UK was a very scary place to live at the moment. Before he left Hugh told me I would be welcome to stay with him if I ever got myself to Adelaide. I thought it was highly unlikely at the time but the idea did sound quite appealing I must admit.

I was still following every match played by Southampton FC, so when the Saints got to the FA Cup Final, I was really excited. On the 1st of May 1976, I invited my friends, Mike, Harry and Jon G to watch the match on TV at my parent's house. My mother made us a red and white striped cake, the team's shirt colours, and we demolished it during the game, which Saints won 1-0 with a goal by Bobby Stokes.

On the 19th of May 1976, Gordo, who had been my mentor when I was at my prep school, passed away of old age. He had been a teacher for over sixty years first at Lancing and then at Walhampton, so must have inspired many other young boys like me along the way. I could still remember him saying, 'kindness is the greatest virtue' and as I bade him a silent farewell, I vowed to try my best to be kind to everyone I met for as long as I lived.

A few days later Mike, Harry, Philip and I went to see The Rolling Stones at Earls Court. The band opened with *Honky Tonk Women* and ended with *Sympathy for the Devil*, which were our two favourite Stones' songs. Who says you can't always get what you want?

On the 31st of May, I went to see The Who at Charlton FC again with Nicol and Vicki and about 80,000 others, so there was very little room to move.

The event was called *The Who Put the Boot In*. The first support act we saw were Streetwalkers who I was keen to hear as the band included singer Roger Chapman and guitarist Charlie Whitney both ex-members of Family. The highlight for me was a great rendition of *Burlesque*. The Outlaws came on next and completely blew me away. Hughie Thomasson and Billy Jones exchanged some awe-inspiring guitar solos and by the time the band had finished playing *High Tides and Green Grass,* I had become a huge fan. When Little Feat came on they were so laid back a few members of the crowd didn't really take to them and a number of empty beer cans were thrown at the stage. I wasn't impressed by their actions and the band clearly weren't either as they didn't come back on for an encore, which was a pity as I had really enjoyed *Dixie Chicken* and *Triple Face Boogie.* The Sensational Alex Harvey Band were up next and lived up to their name. Alex was in fine form and soon got the crowd going with brilliant versions of *Framed* and *Faith Healer.* They did come back on for an encore. A cover of *Delilah* the Barry Mason/Les Reed song made famous by Tom Jones but now re-invented and re-invigorated by the infamous Alexander James Harvey.

By the time The Who took to the stage, it had started to rain heavily and we were absolutely drenched. When Roger Daltrey appeared, he slipped and slid from one end of the stage to the other before getting up and introducing the band as 'The Who on Ice!'

They opened with *I Can't Explain* followed by a couple of other old songs before performing a few from *Quadrophenia* and *Tommy*. They finished their set with *Won't Get Fooled Again* and despite the crowd chanting for more the show was over.

My next job at UMP was to add the sound effects to a very popular BBC children's television show called *Captain Pugwash,* which was created by John Ryan. Cardboard cut-outs of his characters were filmed in live-action using levers to move them. The story was about a group of pirates who sailed the high seas on a ship called the *Black Pig*. A very funny man called Peter Hawkins provided the voices and kindly allowed me to watch as he recorded them in our sound studio. Captain Pugwash was known for his exclamations such as 'Suffering Seagulls!' and 'Blistering Barnacles!'. His pirate crew consisted of Willy, Barnabas and Master Mate as well as a cabin boy called Tom.

One of the Sunday newspapers at the time had re-named them as Master Bates, Seaman Staines and Roger (have sex with) the cabin boy, which we all thought was terribly funny at the time but apparently John Ryan was mortified his beloved innocent characters had been given such sexually suggestive names.

Adding sound effects to sync to pictures was fun but creating them was even more so. The technique is called Foley, named after its originator Jack Foley, and this allowed me to spend time in the recording studio and play around to recreate and record the right sounds or in the case of my next job the more absurd the better.

*The Goodies* was a comedy sketch show on the BBC starring Tim Brooke-Taylor, Graeme Garden and Bill Oddie. Bill wrote and performed their songs and he was the one who told me what he thought would work best for the silly sound effects. He was right every time.

To get the correct sound for footsteps on a gravel surface a Foley artist would normally walk on gravel in a small pit in the studio in similar shoes to those the actor on screen was wearing but Bill had another, and better idea. Walking barefoot on a well-known breakfast cereal. We used my hands in a bowl of flour to create walking on snow and coconut halves for the sound of horse's hooves. To imitate the sound of birds flying overhead we used an umbrella being opened and closed quickly, moving closer to and further away from the microphone. As I said, it was fun.

The music for the films we edited came from a company called the KPM Music Group. Their extensive library consisted of a variety of stock tracks composed and recorded exclusively for film and television purposes. One of my favourite jobs was to find the right track for the editors to use on whatever film they were currently working on. This task was perfect for me as it allowed me to combine my passions for both music and filmmaking.

On the 22nd of June, I went to the Globe Theatre to see Barry Humphries in *Edna Everage Housewife Superstar* with some mates. She was brilliant but from the moment she said, 'Hello Possums!', I couldn't stop thinking about going to Australia and by the time Edna was throwing her 'gladdies' to the audience at the end, I had made a decision.

Although, the sporadic IRA bombs were a source of daily concern, I made my decision based solely on the need to further my career sooner rather than later. UMP had been a great place to learn the basics of filmmaking but it was unlikely I would learn much more with them even if I gave them another year. What I really needed was to go somewhere I would be given new opportunities and learn new skills, which according to my friends Jenny and Hugh who I had kept in touch with, was Australia, so I handed in my notice the very next day and applied for a working holiday visa.

Three days later, I bought *Tales of Mystery and Imagination,* the debut album by The Alan Parsons Project. I was enchanted by the musical retelling of some of Edgar Alan Poe's stories. The record was produced by Alan Parsons, who had been the engineer on Pink Floyd's *The Dark Side of the Moon,* so it was no surprise the production values on his own album were equally superb. I was interested to discover at a later date, the second track, *The Raven,* was the first ever rock song to use a digital vocoder.

To save enough money for my upcoming antipodean adventure, I mowed lawns, filled cars with petrol at the local garage and served drinks at the pub. In my spare time I went to parties and took a number of different girls out on dates. I then met a very pretty girl called Val who was a hairdresser and we hit it off straight away. Her working hours were flexible so we were able to go sailing together and take long walks in the New Forest to find secluded spots to… be romantic.

In the summer of '76 we had a heat wave, the second hottest summer average temperature since records began. It was so dry water supplies reached critical low levels. We weren't allowed to use hosepipes and we were told to pour our washing up water down the loo rather than flush it. Val and I made the most of the weather and swam in the sea and sunbathed on the beach nearly every day and slept together as often as we could. The ideal acclimatization before heading down under or so I thought, until we sunbathed nude one day and got very, very sunburnt. I immersed myself in a cold bath to lower my body temperature and drank plenty of water but even after a week's rest, I was still far too sore in my nether regions to do any more lovemaking. Val must have recovered quicker, as one of my friends rang to tell me she now had a new boyfriend. To cheer me up, I bought myself Lynyrd Skynyrd's album *One More from the Road,* which included an extended version of *Free Bird* with one of the best live guitar solos of all time. Allen Collins was a real force of nature and one of my all-time musical heroes.

According to Joseph Campbell, the author of *The Hero with a Thousand Faces,* the hero's journey always begins with a Call to Adventure. My call came in the form of a letter letting me know my Australian working holiday visa had been approved, so I sold my car and then used the proceeds to buy a ticket to Melbourne. The cost was £327.50.

It was really sad saying goodbye to my Mum, but the call to adventure was far too strong and I knew in my heart if I didn't take this calculated risk and try to further my career in Australia, I would regret it forever. The time had come to cut the umbilical cord and fly to the other side of the world to begin a new adventure… one where anything could happen.

*Follow your bliss. The heroic life is living the individual adventure.*

Joseph Campbell

## CHAPTER 9: IT'S A LONG WAY TO THE TOP

There was movement at the airport, for the word had passed around. Yet another young backpacker from old blighty had just landed in Melbourne, Victoria. It was mid-morning on the 13th of October 1976 and I was totally knackered after the long-haul flight but excited to finally be in Australia. I had hoped to stay for a year but at immigration they only gave me a six-month temporary visa, which was a bit disappointing.

After I retrieved my heavy backpack and went outside to search for the taxi rank it immediately started raining. I assumed, being summer in the southern hemisphere, it would be sunny and unbearably hot but my taxi driver informed me Melbourne had changeable and unpredictable weather conditions.

When I arrived at my destination in Toorak, I knocked on the front door and after a couple of minutes, a dishevelled young man with knotted hair and wearing a wrinkled T-shirt opened it and said, 'Who the Fuck are you?'

It was fairly obvious by his lack of happy demeanour and genial greeting, I had woken him up from a deep sleep, so I apologised for the early hour and explained how I had just arrived from the UK and had been invited to stay for a few days by his flatmate Clare.

'Ah, I see! In that case you'd better come on in mate, you look fucking bushed. I'll put the jug on and then you can tell me what the fuck's going on, okay?'

The first thing I noticed was, rather than a kettle, he used a ceramic jug, which heated the water using a bare-element, which he explained, after telling me his name was Dave, didn't electrocute the user as the containers didn't conduct electricity. After a brief conversation we worked out his flatmate was the younger sister of one of my female friends in the UK who must have made the kind offer on her sister's behalf without telling her, or had told her and she hadn't informed him, which Dave thought was the most likely scenario. Fortunately for me,

Clare was a travelling sales rep and away on business until the weekend so Dave suggested I use her room for the next couple of nights. I was relieved my immediate accommodation problem had been resolved but also realised I would have to find a job much sooner than I planned so I could rent my own place as soon as possible.

Still feeling jet-lagged, I went to the nearest phone box with a pocket full of unfamiliar looking coins I exchanged at the local corner shop for one of my brand new and rather colourful ten-dollar notes, which featured a portrait of poet Henry Lawson on one side and one of architect Francis Greenway on the other, who I discovered later had been transported to Australia as a convicted forger. If this was a typical example of the Aussie sense of humour then this was the place for me, I thought to myself as I started flicking through the phone book to look for the numbers of local post production companies.

After making a short list of potential employers in alphabetical order with their numbers next to them, I took a deep breath and made my first call. The first four companies told me they had no need for an assistant editor and unlikely to want one in the near future, which was a bit disheartening. However, on my fifth attempt, the woman who answered the phone told me she knew of an editor who was looking for an assistant and kindly gave me the number of a film editor called Mike Reed. I called him straight away but he was too busy to talk then and asked me to come to his office at lunchtime.

When I first met Mike, I could tell he was the type of man who doesn't suffer fools gladly so I didn't beat about the bush and just gave him a brief explanation of what experience I had gained in England and how I had come to Australia in the hope of furthering my career. He thought for a moment and then said, 'I'll give you three days trial next week and if you're any good I'll pay you 120 bucks and if you're not, you can fuck off! Sound fair to you?' Just what I needed. Incentive.

I had only been in Australia for two days and already had some work in the Australian film industry, so I was 'well-chuffed', as Aussies often say when feeling happy about something, and the following morning I found a one-bedroom flat to rent right next to the Kooyong tennis club. In the evening, I finally met the elusive Clare who had returned from her latest sales trip, who said I could stay another week at their house and sleep on the sofa until I got the keys to my rental home.

When I told Clare I was interested to hear some Australian rock music, she turned on the radio but all the local stations seemed to be playing nothing but ABBA's *Dancing Queen,* Rod Stewart's *Tonight's the Night* or and Bryan Ferry's *Let's Stick Together* on rotation so I then asked my host if she had any records by Aussie bands and was rewarded with a grin.

'You're going to like this!' she said as she put on AC/DC's *High Voltage.* She was right.

The first track was *It's A Long Way To The Top (If You Wanna Rock 'n' Roll).* The use of bagpipes in a hard rock song worked a lot better than I could ever have imagined. Clare told me when Aussies sang the chorus, they actually sang *It's a Long Way to the Shop (If You Want a Sausage Roll).* She then played me *Eagle Rock* by Daddy Cool, *Most People I Know (Think That I'm Crazy)* by Billy Thorpe and a few other great songs by The Ted Mulry Gang, Little River Band, Sherbert and Skyhooks. I had no idea there was so much talent in the Australian music industry. 'This must be what a pirate feels like when he discovers a map with an X on it to mark the spot where the treasure was buried.' I said to the girls. Julie told me the reason there were so many great bands in their country was because they'd paid their due' on the never-ending pub circuit where they not only gained experience playing nearly every night but also discovered what the Aussie crowds wanted to hear, which was a 'sound' unique to Australia and not just an imitation of American and British bands. If what I'd been hearing was a taste of things to come then they were well on their way, the amazing array of fresh and original music would get better every year and eventually become known collectively as 'Oz Rock'.

I started working for Mike Reed's Post Production (MRPP) on 19th October as Mike's assistant editor on a couple of TV commercials for

*Just Jeans* and *Export Cola*. My experience in London seemed to impress him and on the last day of the trial he offered me a job until Christmas and offered to pay me $300 a week. This was more than four times what I would have been earning in the UK, so it looked as though I had made the right decision to come to Australia.

Exactly ten days after arriving in the country, I moved into a flat in Selwyn Court near Kooyong Road in Toorak. A week later Clare's cousin and his partner arrived in Melbourne and as they needed somewhere to live they asked if they could rent my spare room, which immediately cut my rent in half and gave me a chance to save some money.

I sent my Mum an aerogramme to tell her my exciting news. Aerogrammes were lightweight postal forms and had an overseas stamp already printed on them. After writing a letter, you had to fold the form in a specific way and use your tongue to stick the flaps down before sending it. I can still remember the foul taste. It usually took ten days for Mum to receive one of my letters and another week or so to get her replies but it was much cheaper than using the phone, which would have cost a small fortune in those days.

Along with the sound of people playing tennis at the nearby courts, distant lawnmowers and kids splashing in pools, the most deafening sound was the cicadas that began their synchronized call at dusk every evening after I got home from work. I discovered it was the males who make these loud calls to attract females when they are ready to mate. These noisy insects hold the record for being the loudest in the world and peak around November, so unbelievably there was worse to come.

In the mornings, I took a green and yellow tram to get to work, which I loved as it felt so different to being in London. The ticket collectors were always friendly and said 'G'day!'

One of my duties as an assistant editor was to splice pieces of film together with clear Scotch tape, which I did everyday with no problem until we ran out. When I told Mike he gave me some cash and asked me to buy him some Durex. I refused outright, telling him it was far too personal so he should do it himself. After a brief argument and after the understandable misunderstanding became apparent, there was much laughter and I agreed to his request. In England Durex is a brand of condom but in Australia it was a brand of splicing tape. Coincidentally, the job Mike was editing was for XXXX Beer (pronounced four-ex) but in the USA Fourex is a brand of condom, so the jingle made us all giggle out loud as the words were 'I can feel a four-ex comin' on!'

My friend Hugh, who I'd shared my 21$^{st}$ birthday with the previous year now lived in Adelaide, so flew down to Melbourne to share our 22$^{nd}$ together. As it was Mike Reed's birthday a few days before ours we decided to celebrate our combined birthdays over dinner at one of the best restaurants in South Melbourne. After getting totally sloshed and paying the enormous bill we clambered into Mike's little Volkswagen to get a lift home but just as Hugh and I had managed to squeeze ourselves into the back seat of the tiny vehicle Mike yelled, 'Fuck! The negatives have been stolen!' He then explained he had left the cans of negative of the latest TV commercial he had been editing on the backseat of his car to take to the laboratory later and as they were no longer there, it was potentially a major disaster.

'Fuck! If this gets out I'll be a laughing stock. What shall we do?' He asked his wife Fran.

'I've got an idea,' she said. 'Let's try the other beetle over there!'

In our drunken state we had got into an almost identical looking VW parked on the other side of the road. Neither vehicle had been locked, which was common practice back then. Luckily for Mike, all the cans of negative were still in his car, which was a huge relief.

While Hugh was staying with me, he introduced me to Vegemite. Unlike a lot of Poms, as the Aussies call us Brits, I absolutely loved it. In fact, so much so, I never went back to Marmite, as I preferred the flavour and have kept a jar in my cupboard ever since.

When I was back at work the following week, I worked on a radio commercial, which required the services one of an Australian legend. Barry Humphries, better known as *Dame Edna Everage*. Unfortunately, the voice over wasn't to be in the unforgettable voice of the infamous *Housewife Superstar!* but as her alter-ego, Barry himself. However, he did say 'Hello Possums!' as he arrived at the studio which was good enough for me.

Having focused on my film career since arriving in Australia, I felt it was now time to indulge in my passion for some live music again, so when I found out Status Quo would be performing in Melbourne, I rang the Paul Dainty Corporation, who were the tour promoters to cheekily ask if I could get a press pass to attend the concert. When the receptionist asked me where I was from, I told her I was from England. She replied, 'Oh No worries then,' and gave me the address of the office where I had to collect my pass. It was only after I had put the phone down, I realised she might have meant, what company was I from rather than country, but perhaps with my accent they simply presumed I was working for one of the English music papers.

When I picked up my pass in the morning, I met Michael Chugg, the company's tour manager. Deciding honesty was the best policy, I told him I wasn't from an English newspaper and was just in Australia on a working holiday. His reaction wasn't what I expected. He simply smiled, handed me a press pass and told me to enjoy the gig, which took place on the 2$^{nd}$ of December at the Sidney Myer Music Bowl. The Kevin Borich Express were the support act, so I was finally going to see an Australian rock band perform live for the first time, although I found out later Kevin himself was from New Zealand.

While the roadies set up for Status Quo, I got a tap on the shoulder from an Aussie girl with long blonde hair who held up her expensive camera with an even more expensive zoom lens attached to it and said rather cheekily, 'Mine's bigger than yours!' Her name was Di and her red-haired companion was called Julie, an equally lovely young woman. We became instant friends. When Quo finally came on stage they started their set with *Junior Wailing,* a cover version of a song by Steamhammer. I really enjoyed the whole show but thought they were at their best playing *Roadhouse Blues*, another cover, but this time by The Doors. In the morning, I sold one of my photos to the Melbourne based rock music magazine *Juke* for the grand sum of AUD$8 and they featured it in their next addition. It was my first ever sale. I then sent a 5x7 print of the photo by post to Michael Chugg, c/o the Paul Dainty Corporation with a thank you note.

Selling one of my photos was a big deal for me at the time, as although it wasn't much money, it allowed me to think of myself as a professional...of sorts, and the fact I was also being paid to work in the Australian film industry and could afford to attend live gigs meant I was now indulging in all of my passions at once and it felt good...really good.

Since I had been in Australia, I had learned to communicate with other people a lot better than I had when I was working in London and as a result I had managed to not only interact with complete strangers but also make a few new friends. My life was finally beginning to take shape and as a result my self-confidence was growing day by the day.

Over the next few weeks, Di and Julie took it upon themselves to further my education of the Australian music scene. We played records by AC/DC, Billy Thorpe & The Aztecs, The Angels and Daddy Cool whose song *Eagle Rock* was a true classic destined for immortality. The girls then introduced me to an Australian music TV show called *Countdown*, which was usually hosted by record producer and music critic Ian 'Molly' Meldrum but the first episode I ever saw had Daryl Braithwaite, the lead singer of Aussie rock band Sherbet, as guest host with Molly just doing an interview with the band later in the show. AC/DC performed their song *Dirty Deeds Done Dirt Cheap* in the ABC studio and there were a couple of Sherbet songs in the mix plus others by Ol'55, John Paul Young and the Ted Mulry Gang but the most memorable music video was of Fleetwood Mac with Stevie Nicks singing her own song *Rhiannon* about a celestial being.

The other TV show I watched with Di and Julie was *Hey Hey It's Saturday!* The variety entertainment program was co-hosted by Daryl Somers and a pink puppet called Ossie Ostrich performed and voiced by Ernie Carroll. But it was voice over artist John Blackman's ad-libbing and double entendre humour my friends seemed to enjoy the most.

It was while watching this show the girls taught me how to do a Tim Tam Slam, which involved having to nibble the ends off both corners of the heavenly chocolate biscuit and then use the rest like a straw to suck up my cup of tea.

The sensation is known as the Tim Tam Rush!

At the weekend, Di, Julie and I drove to the Healesville Sanctuary in the Yarra Valley. The Zoo was set in natural bushland, so we couldn't have had a better opportunity to see some Aussie wildlife in its natural habitat and we were able to get some good photos.

Australia has more deadly snakes than anywhere else in the world and a long list of other creatures which can kill you like saltwater crocodiles, sharks, box jellyfish and numerous venomous spiders, including the infamous funnel-web, which is considered the most dangerous anywhere on our planet. I would get to see all these fascinating if somewhat frightening animals in the future but my first encounter with any native species was with a harmless marsupial with large furry ears.

The koala was sitting halfway up a gum tree munching happily on a eucalyptus leaf. A little later we saw two brush-tailed rock wallabies who seemed completely unfazed by our presence, so we took some photos of them, and then just as we were leaving, we saw a small mob of kangaroos who were so tame we were able to hand feed them. On the drive home we listened to some Aussie rock on the radio and the girls knew all the words, so sang along to *Jump in my Car* by the Ted Mulry Gang, *Million Dollar Riff* by Skyhooks and *Slipping Away* by Max Merritt and The Meteors.

When my contract was up with Mike, I told him how grateful I was to him for giving me my first break in the Australian film industry. I had learned something new every day and was sure I wouldn't have been given the same responsibilities if I had stayed in the UK.

When Jenny, the receptionist who I had met when we were working together in London, invited me to spend Christmas Day with her 'relos' in Brisbane, I leapt at the chance and a few days later flew up to Sydney to meet her. She told me she was really happy the way things were turning out for me and it was good to hear how life had got better for her too since she had returned home. We drove up the east coast so I could see a bit of New South Wales on the way up to Queensland. On the way, she played a cassette of *Hotel California* by The Eagles, which was the first album featuring Joe Walsh on guitar and what a difference he made to the band's sound. I loved the whole album but the solo on the title track was mesmerising and I wanted to hear the song again and again. Looking back now, I can hear a voice in my head saying, 'Be careful what you wish for!'

After eating a huge roast turkey lunch, which her mother had cooked, I tasted my first ever passion fruit straight off the vine in their garden. It was sensational and my over-the-top reaction to it made everyone laugh. Jenny asked me if I would like to make a quick phone call to my Mum to wish her a Happy Christmas and when I got through to her, I got quite emotional hearing her voice again after being away for so long. As Jenny wanted to stay with her family for a few more days, I flew back to Sydney on my own.

Seeing Sydney Harbour Bridge from the air is something I will never forget. It was also fascinating to see the Sydney Opera House, designed by Danish architect Jørn Utzon, as it had only been completed three years earlier. Jenny said I could use her flat in McMahons Point as a base, so I took a taxi there to drop my bag off before taking a ferry to Circular Quay and a long bus ride to Bondi Beach where I had a quick swim in the Pacific Ocean. On New Year's Day 1977, I bought a ticket to see the play *The Magistrate* at the Opera House, which I thoroughly enjoyed and then caught the overnight train back to Melbourne.

When a group of rowdy drunks boarded the train, carrying enough 'grog' to drink all the way to Perth let alone Melbourne, sat right behind me, I realised any idea of getting some sleep was going to be impossible. Oh well, I thought, if you can't beat them join them so turned around to say 'G'day'. One of the lads then handed me a can of lager and I joined in the celebrations. After another beer or possibly three, I was in need of a pee so went in search of the loo. On the way back I saw there were plenty of empty seats well away from my drinking companions, so I sat down on one of them and closed my eyes in the hope of finally getting some kip.

I had just started to doze off when I felt someone brush past and sit down next to me. When I opened my eyes to see who it was, a pretty young woman was smiling at me. After apologising for waking me up she introduced herself. Her name was Mia, she was Italian and had just had Christmas with her parents in Sydney. We continued chatting until midnight when the lights in the carriage suddenly dimmed, which was the cue to get some sleep. As it was getting cold, I took off my jacket and put it around Mia's shoulders to keep her warm. She then leant on my shoulder and we both dozed off. Well, she dozed off and I began to have naughty thoughts about her. When she woke up, she must have noticed the effect of my nocturnal fantasies, as she took my jacket off her shoulders and placed it over my jeans. I was just about to say something in way of an apology when she started to kiss me. At the exact same moment, the train went through a tunnel, just like in the old silent movies when they wanted to suggest sex was about to take place. The grin on my face remained until we arrived.

Sadly, I never saw my Italian belladonna again, as I only had a few months left on my visa, so decided to leave Melbourne and stay with Hugh in South Australia until I had to go back to the UK. Fortunately for me, my buddy had a spare room in a house in Aldgate, so I had somewhere to sleep as soon as I arrived. I really liked the Adelaide Hills but it was evident if I wanted to find any work in the film industry then I would have to look for it in the city, so I sent a letter to every film company I could find in the Adelaide phone book. While waiting for replies, I did any work I could to pay my way, including being a waiter, a barman, a washer-upper and installing sprinkler systems.

After discovering the Hendrix-inspired guitarist Robin Trower was going to be performing at the Festival Theatre in February, I decided to go and see him. And as the gig was being promoted by the same organisation had given me the press pass to see Status Quo, I decided to give them a call to ask if I could get another one for this concert.

'Loved the Quo photo mate!' Michael Chugg, the tour manager said once I had got through to him and asked me how he could help. I was very glad I had made the effort to send him a photograph of the band in way of a thank you as now asking for another press pass didn't seem quite as cheeky. Not only did he agree but told me what time to be at the band's hotel the next day to get it off him personally. When I met him in the foyer of the Park Royal, he introduced me to one of the roadies who was called Scrooge, and as he handed me my pass he said, 'This is the cheeky Pommy bastard I told you about!'

'Talking of cheek,' I replied in a rare moment of over-confidence, 'Any chance I could have two, so my mate Hugh can come with me?' To my surprise he said. 'No worries!'

Australian group Blackfeather were the support act but it was Robin Trower we had come to see and he didn't disappoint. *Bridge of Sighs* and *Too Rolling Stoned* being the stand out songs for me. Hugh and I both took photos of the gig. We had bought one roll of Tri-X 400 each and pushed it to 1600 which would allow us to take handheld shots rather than have to take a tripod. We had decided to only shoot in Black & White, so we could develop the negatives in Hugh's homemade darkroom when we got home. After the final song we went backstage to meet Robin and asked him if he remembered playing at our school in Brockenhurst in 1971. To our surprise he did. After I had developed my film, I sent a copy of the best shot to the Paul Dainty Corporation to say thank you again and was rewarded with yet another press pass by return of post to see Rod Stewart on the *Foot Loose & Fancy-Free* tour at Memorial Drive on the 11th February. Hugh didn't seem to mind it was only me who got the pass this time as he was going to take a girlfriend to the gig anyway.

The Australian soft rock band Air Supply were the support act. They were fronted by singers Graham Russell and Russell Hitchcock who both had splendid voices. Their song *Love and Other Bruises* was their best by far. In the break I saw Scrooge, the roadie I had met recently, helping the band take their gear off stage so gave him a wave. When he had finished, he came over to where I was standing in the photographer's pit and grabbing my arm helped me climb onto the stage. He then beckoned me to follow him to the wing and told me to sit there as I'd get much better shots. Being allowed to sit on the edge of the stage, I was not only able to get a good shot of Rod strutting his stuff but also some close-up images of his brilliant guitarist Jim Cregan and energetic drummer Carmine Appice. *Juke* magazine used one of my photos of Rod but I don't remember what I got paid or even if I did this time. Rod's set was an interesting mix of his own songs like *Maggie May* and *The Killing of Georgie (Part 1 and 11)* plus The Faces' *Stay With Me* and covers of The Beatles' *Get Back* and The Sutherland Brothers *Sailing*.

Two of my all-time favourite albums were released later in the month. *Rumours* by Fleetwood Mac and *Songs From The Wood* by Jethro Tull.

Although *Rumours* was essentially a pop record, which as a fan of the blues era of the band wasn't up my alley, the quality of the song writing and the impressive production values were so good I was won over and played it endlessly. Lindsey Buckingham's *Go Your Own Way,* Stevie Nicks' *Dreams* and Christine McVie's *Don't Stop* were pure gold but it was *The Chain,* credited to all five members of the band, which was my favourite. I loved the bass solo and it has since become one of the most recognizable in music history.

*Songs From the Wood* was very different to anything Tull had done before and I thought it was their best album since *Thick as a Brick.* Interestingly, they had also started as a blues band but this time out they had decided to combine English folk melodies with heavy rock music and it was marvellous. The musicianship was exceptional and the lyrics by singer-songwriter and occasional-one-legged flute player Ian Anderson were playful and pithy. I particularly liked the image of 'galliards and lute songs served in chilling ale'.

Now I had such a positive balance in my musical memory bank account, it was time to focus all my energies on my film career. I had been very fortunate to have been given the opportunity to work in both advertising and factual entertainment since my arrival but if I was to have any real chance of achieving my end goal of working in Hollywood, I needed to keep following my dream, and finding a job working on an Australian feature film would definitely be step in the right direction.

I had no idea how to make this momentous leap but one of the things I had learned since I had been in Australia was not to be afraid to ask for help, so I rang Mike Reed in Melbourne to ask his advice. As usual, he was blunt and straight to the point, 'Just get on the fucking phone! Call every post-house editing a feature film, which you can find a list of in the latest edition of Australian Cinema Magazine, and let them know you are available. That's how you got the job with me, so just rinse and repeat!' He then added with a more sympathetic tone, 'you're a good assistant editor Jamie...and I'd be happy to give you a reference if you that will help? Good luck mate!'

I felt a lot better after talking to my old boss, and really appreciated his belief in me.

Now it was my turn.

*Luck is nothing more than opportunity and preparedness being in the same place at the same time. You make your own luck.*

Michael ONeill

## CHAPTER 10: SOLSBURY HILL

The South Australian Film Commission (SAFC) had only been operating since 1972, so was still in its infancy as a production company when they rang to ask if I would be interested in being the assistant editor on a feature film called *Storm Boy.* The idea of working on a 'fillum', as some of the older Aussies used to call movies 'back in the day', was very appealing and would be a real stepping-stone in my career, so I told them I would be very interested in deed. They promised to get back to me the next day to discuss the job further.

Unfortunately, I didn't get the gig in the end as they wanted someone with previous feature film experience, which I didn't have yet. Three days later I received another call from the SAFC, asking me if I would like to apply for the assistant editor role on a movie called *The Last Wave* being shot in Sydney by legendary film director Peter Weir of *Picnic at Hanging Rock* fame. I asked them if I would have the same problem as I had no prior feature experience but apparently there were no other assistants available, so they thought they might give me a go. I got very excited at the prospect of working with such an eminent director but my hopes were dashed overnight when they eventually found someone with more experience.

Although I should have felt flattered to be even be considered for these jobs, self-doubt started to creep in and I began to wonder if my Hollywood dream was in reality just a pipe dream. Ever since I was a small boy, I had lacked self-confidence and self-belief in my own abilities. This was most probably because of the fear of making mistakes when I was at boarding school and the resulting punishment as a consequence to my failures. However, I was a grown man now and knew making mistakes was the best way to improve and grow, so I was determined to find a way to overcome my fears whatever the outcome.

In an attempt to cheer me up, Hugh bought me Peter Gabriel's first solo album. The second track *Solsbury Hill* was so uplifting I couldn't help but smile. The positive energy this song evoked was like being given an instant happiness pill.

Having played some fairly heavy guitar riffs on Alice Cooper's *Welcome to my Nightmare*, it must have been quite a change of speed for Steve Hunter strumming his Martin D28 acoustic guitar on this superb track. In fact, this is exactly what happened, as I discovered a few years later, they had recorded three tracks in the studio using a variable speed oscillator chorusing effect, slowing one track down and another sped up, creating a triple track of exquisite and everlasting beauty.

After singing the words, 'My heart going boom, boom, boom...' with Mr. Gabriel for the umpteenth time, I was feeling much more optimistic about life.

I had the music turned up so loud, I nearly missed hearing the phone going ring, ring, ring.

The call was from a film company called Scope Films who said they were interested in me working for them... but there was a catch. The job was based in a small town called Gumeracha, which was only about an hour's drive from where I lived in Aldgate, but as there were no buses from one destination to the other, I would need to work another way of getting there and back each day. I told them I was really interested and would get back to them as soon as I had found a way of resolving my transport issue.

When I arrived at the café, where I was washing dishes three nights a week, the other members of staff were talking about ABBA who were very popular in Australia at the time. The letters in the name ABBA stood for the band member's first names: Agnetha, Benny, Bjorn and Anni-Frida. One of the waitresses asked me if I would like to go to the concert with her the following evening and the ticket was only $9 but, as I was so low on cash, 1 turned her kind offer down. Ironically, when I explained my pitiful financial situation to her, ABBA's song 'Money, Money, Money' was being played on the radio.

'It's a sign!' she said as a joke. 'ABBA are the answer to all your money problems!' We both laughed and then I went back to washing dirty dishes. Lots and lots of them. As I stood at the sink, the afternoon sun shone through a crack in the window and made a beautiful pattern on the wall. I wished I had my camera with me as it would have made a great shot and was the eureka moment when I knew ABBA really could be the answer to my prayers. If I could find a way of going to the concert for free then I could take some photos of the band and try to sell them to the local paper. I now had a plan so after my shift was over, I plucked up courage and made a call to the local paper to see if they would be interested in buying some photos of Australia's current favourite band. They told me their staff photographer was already going to the concert so they wouldn't need any but then suggested I contact the promoters for the ABBA tour and gave me a number to call. After I had told the receptionist I was a photographer from England and wanted to know if I could get a press pass to see ABBA, she put me straight through to the tour manager. By pure coincidence it was Michael Chugg.

'You again!' he said with a chuckle. After telling me the name of ABBA's manager and the name of the hotel where the band were staying, he added. 'Tell him Chuggi sent you!'

On Tuesday the 8th of March, I borrowed Hugh's Yamaha RD 350cc to get myself to the Park Royal Motor Inn, where I collected my pass and then rode to the Westlakes Football Stadium. Once I got to the venue, I made my way to the photographer's pit in front of the stage where there were at least a dozen other photographers already in place, and behind us were around 20,000 fans all screaming 'We want ABBA!'

All I had to do now was get some good photos but just before the concert was about to begin one of the security stewards, a huge man with muscles like Popeye on steroids, pointed at my camera and told me I wasn't allowed to use flash because it distracted the musicians. I didn't feel inclined to argue with a man of his stature, so just thanked him for letting me know and then desperately tried to remember what I had been taught at film school about shooting in low light conditions and changed the aperture and shutter speed settings on my camera accordingly. Moments later Agnetha, Frida, Bjorn and Benny took to the stage and hundreds of flashes all went off around me at the same time. Still partially blinded by the lights, I suddenly felt a strong pair of hands lift me up onto the edge of the stage. When I looked down to see who had just given me a better view of the band, I saw the same security steward who now had a huge grin on his face, so I gave him a thumbs up with my left hand and then put my right index finger on the camera shutter. It was showtime!

ABBA started with *Tiger* and then played a number of other songs I had heard on the radio including *Waterloo, SOS, Money, Money, Money, Mama Mia* and *Fernando*. The encore was *Dancing Queen* followed by a reprise of *Thank You for the Music*. It was a magical evening and I felt very lucky to be there…on stage with them.

After the entertaining show was over, I rode Hugh's motorbike straight to Group Colour, a local film Laboratory, to put my roll of film in for overnight processing. When I told the elderly man at the counter, I had just come from the ABBA concert but hadn't been able to use any flash, he asked what settings I had used, nodded to himself, and then took the roll of film out of the camera and quickly disappeared through a set of swing doors without a word.

I went back to the Lab as soon as it opened the next morning and was relieved to discover my images had come out better than I had dared hope. I took them to another company specialised in creating posters and after I had shown the photos to the owner, he bought four of them on the spot for $50 each.

With the proceeds, I bought a 1964 EH Holden off Hugh's brother-in-law Don for $200, got the 'rego' sorted, filled the tank up with petrol at the nearest 'servo' and then rang Scope Films to say I could start work as soon as they wanted me to. It was a huge turning point in my life. I had been able to make money using my photographic skills which would now help me further my film career. Plus, I had achieved this minor miracle by attending a live gig.

'It doesn't get much better than this', I thought as I drove my car up to Gumeracha, and then to voice my true feelings, wound down the window and yelled at the top of my voice, 'Cooee! I love this fucking country!'

The owner of Scope Films was a man called Edwin Scragg who looked like a cross between Harpo Marx and Dr. Who (the one with the scarf!), and was one of the most interesting people I had ever met. (For interesting read, eccentric, enthusiastic and entertaining.)

'The Scraggs' consisted of Edwin and his wife, Jane, and their two young daughters Emma and Sarah, who were just as much fun as their parents and soon made me feel like part of their family or perhaps menagerie would be a more apt word as they also had a Labrador called Kali, a cow named Sleek, two donkeys called Abraham and Rimsky, and a dozen chickens, who thankfully weren't individually named and went under the collective title 'The Chooks.'

The animals weren't the only ones with 'interesting' names. Edwin's neighbour was a lovely man called Devon Ambrose and the local policeman's name was Peter Panic! (I'm not joking.)

Scope Films produced high-end corporate films and as Edwin had hired me to not only work as his assistant editor but also as his assistant cameraman, I learned a number of new skills from him over the coming weeks and as his home was a working farm, he also taught me how to milk a cow by hand, ride a donkey and collect eggs from the chooks. He also showed me how to mark, dock and castrate lambs and how to spread fertiliser, trim lawns on a tractor mower as well as erect wire fences around the property. It was hard work but fascinating, fun and had the bonus side-effect of also keeping me fit.

I usually got home quite late during weekdays, so apart from hearing the latest pop and rock songs on my car radio, I had to wait until the weekend to listen to my own music. I still had the same cassettes I had brought with me from the UK but Hugh had a fairly decent and diverse collection of LPs, so when we were both at home we would play one of his records on his rather impressive hi-fi system.

On my commute between my home and Scragg End, I passed hundreds of eucalyptus trees, so I always kept my eye open for a koala sitting in one of them and had my camera sitting next to me on the passenger seat just in case I saw one and wanted to grab a quick snap of it. The iconic marsupial relies on eucalyptus leaves for food, so it was just a matter of being patient and when I did eventually see my first koala in the wild, I was absolutely 'stoked', as the Aussies say when they are excited about something.

Before I left work for the day, Emma and Sarah would sometimes ask me to stay longer and read them bedtime stories and when we inevitably finished reading all of their old children's books, they asked me to make if I could make one up, so I wrote a story specifically for the two girls called *Zamel the Camel.* The reason I chose *(camelus dromedarius)* as the hero in my story was because the logo for Scope Films was an image of a man wearing a pith helmet on his head, holding a telescope to his eye, and sitting astride a dromedary camel. To make the story more appealing to the girls, I drew detailed illustrations of all the native animals in the story, which included a cockatoo, a kangaroo, a wombat, a koala and a male and female camel. It took me absolutely ages to complete the drawings but seeing the smiles on the girl's faces when I read the story to them made all my hard effort worthwhile.

In April, Edwin got the green-light from a mining company to make a film called 'Weipa Greenies', which had to tell the story about the regeneration programme they were doing at the bauxite mine. As this meant we had to fly to Far North Queensland to shoot it, my dream of seeing other parts of Australia was about to come true.

On the first day of the production, Edwin and I flew a 727 to Townsville where we then took another flight to Cairns in an old DC9 before meeting up with Wayne, our soundman and Malcolm, our grip, who had both flown up from Sydney earlier in the day, and then we all flew together in a small Fokker Friendship to Weipa on the Cape York Peninsula.

Edwin had brought a Super 16mm Aaton camera with him to do the filming and while we were in Weipa, he taught me how to use it and also how to use his home-made time-lapse system, so we could film sunrises and sunsets every day. One of the bonuses on the shoot was being allowed to drive a Ford Falcon, which was the first time I had driven an automatic. One of the minuses was being bitten by what felt like a million mozzies.

After the shoot was over, Edwin suggested I take a few days off when we were in transit in Cairns before coming back to Adelaide, just in case I never had another opportunity to come back to Queensland, so I did. I booked myself into a cheap motel for the night and in the morning took a 45-minute ferry ride to Green Island. On board I met a lovely nurse called Val who must have taken a shine to me, as she took me under her wing until sunset and then took me under her doona until sunrise.

The next day, I hired a 4WD Mini Moke and drove it up the coast to Port Douglas to see Four Mile Beach, followed by a wonderful walk in the oldest surviving tropical rainforest at Mossman Gorge, and then took a scenic rail from Kuranda to see Barron Falls before heading to the Atherton Tableland where I saw the magnificent Milla Falls, which cascaded into a pristine waterhole surrounded by lush rainforest.

Travelling on my own was fun. I felt totally free and at peace with myself, and as I took a quick dip in the clear cool water and looked at the mini-paradise around me, I suddenly came to the realisation I was enjoying my own company and didn't need anyone else in my life to share the moment with. Solitude by choice would become a way of life for the rest of my life.

My next destination was Lake Tinaroo, where I saw a middle-aged man wearing a pair of bright pink sunglasses catch an enormous Barramundi just as the sun was setting, so I took a couple of photos of him. While he de-gutted the fish he adopted the Aussie salute, which is what Australians call the action of constantly flicking away flies.

'They belong to my missus!' he said smiling and pointing to his brightly coloured sunnies. After he had finished filleting the fish he carefully put the sliced pieces into a plastic bag and then put them into an Esky. He then pulled a couple of cold beers out of the same ice box and kindly handed me one, introducing himself at the same time, 'I'm

Cocky!' and then explained how his nickname was quite common for small-scale farmers like him.

As it was now getting quite dark, I told Cocky I needed to head off fairly soon as I hadn't organised anywhere to stay the night yet. He said 'No worries!' and then as an afterthought said I could stay on his farm in Tinaburra for the night in exchange for helping him milk the cows in the morning. After following his Ute back to his house in my rental, Cocky invited me inside and introduced me to his wife, 'Meet the missus!'

'G'day I'm Debbie,' she said shaking my hand firmly, 'If you don't mind me saying, you look completely done in!' It was true, I was exhausted. After barbecuing the Barra and drinking a few more tinnies, I crashed out on their sofa for the night but was roused at 6am sharp to pay my dues or more precisely to milk the cows.

Thankfully no hand milking was required at this farm, as they had suckers, and after I had attached them all, my host handed me an ice cold tinny.

'It's a bit early, isn't it?' I questioned, as I took the cold can of beer from him.

'Yeh, Nah,' was his reply, which translated into English meant 'I understand what you are saying old chap but I don't agree with your comment so you can either fuck off...or you can have a beer with me...it's your choice.' I chose the second option and after we had both taken a swig, he held his tinny up to his face for closer inspection and then said almost reverently, 'Ah, breakfast of champions!'

Not long after I had got back to South Australia, Edwin took me to Mannum on the Murray River to film an old steamboat at sunrise but it wasn't quite as beautiful a week later as we got caught in a dust storm while filming in Gawler. When we got back to the farm, we had to completely dismantle the camera to remove the red sand, which was a lengthy and painstaking task. On the next shoot we had to film in an abattoir in Adelaide at the crack of dawn. This is where I saw one of the lambs escape the clutches of the slaughterer and run amok covered in blood before eventually being caught and meeting a grisly end.

When we were putting the camera gear back into the van, I told Edwin how the experience had put me off eating meat for a while, but he wasn't going to let me get away with being a wimp and when we stopped at a café for breakfast on the way home, he ordered egg, bacon, sausages and a lamp chop for both of us. I surprised him, as well as myself, by scoffing down the lot without a hint of remorse or regret.

'A year ago, I was struggling to make ends meet,' I told Edwin as we left the café, 'and here I am today filming at an abattoir where they make meats end!'

'Don't give up your daytime job!', he replied with the tiniest hint of a smile on his face.

The following weekend, I flew to Melbourne for a few days to catch up with my friends Di and Julie who played me AC/DC's latest album *Let There Be Rock* as soon as we got to Julie's house. Hearing *Whole Lotta Rosie* for the first time blew me away and remains my favourite Acca Dacca song to this day. The song is about a woman of generous proportions who the band's singer Bon Scott had supposedly had carnal knowledge with at an earlier date.

While I was in town, I also caught up with my old boss Mike Reed who seemed genuinely pleased I had managed to get so much location experience since I had last seen him, as he thought by understanding some of the problems faced on a shoot, I would become a better and more understanding editor.

As soon as I got back to the Adelaide Hills, Hugh and I went to the Aldgate Pump Hotel for a debriefing session over a few cold beers, as it had been a while since we had caught up. Later in the evening I met a very attractive nurse called Carmel and ended up back at her place for a further de-briefing… so to speak.

As my working holiday visa was about to expire soon, I went into Adelaide to renew it but was turned down by a rather officious and odious immigration officer, which was a huge disappointment as I everything was just beginning to go well in every department of my life.

Hugh's stepfather Keith ended up being the hero of the hour by not only arranging for me to meet Donald Cameron, who was the current Senator for South Australia, so I could ask plead my case for an extension to my visa, but by also coming with me for support. It was because of his timely intervention the decision was eventually overturned and I was allowed to stay in Australia until October.

When I told Edwin told the good news, he said he was really happy for me but sadly didn't have any more work for me for the time being, so suggested I call the South Australian Film Commission to let them know I was available and promised he would give me a good reference.

I wasn't too worried, as having extended my visa meant I now had more time to listen to music and take photos. In a stroke of serendipity, an opportunity to combine both my interests presented itself a few days later when I was given a backstage pass from publicist Patti Mostyn in exchange for some Black & White photos of Dr. Hook and the Medicine Show at the Festival Theatre in Adelaide.

My passion for photography and music were now in perfect harmony, which was more than could be said for the band's opening number but once they had got the sound levels sorted the rest of the gig was excellent. I had heard *Sylvia's Mother* on the radio but was unfamiliar with their other songs. Their blend of country and rock wasn't normally my cup of tea but I have to admit, I enjoyed the gig far more than I had anticipated and while they were on stage, I was able to get some fairly respectable shots of their vocalist and percussionist, Ray Sawyer, who wore an eyepatch and cowboy hat, which made for quite an iconic image ...or so Patti told me after she had seen my photographs, which was very kind of her.

Ten days later, Mike Chugg gave me a press pass to see Bryan Ferry at the Apollo Stadium on his first world tour since leaving Roxy Music. Jon English was the support act and warmed the crowd up beautifully. When Mr. Ferry started his set with *Let's Stick Together*, I was pleased to see he had done exactly as the song requested by retaining two of his old Roxy Music pals, Phil Manzanera on guitar and Paul Thompson on drums. Chris Spedding was on guitar and ex-King Crimson singer John Wetton on bass.

It felt good to be able to combine my love of photography and music but as I had come to Australia to further my film career, it was time to focus on my long-term goal.

In another stroke of good fortune, I got a call out if the blue one day from a well-respected production manager called Ross Matthews. Apparently, I had been recommended to him by the South Australian Film Commission, who had informed him of my lack of previous experience working on feature films but had also told him they thought I had 'potential'. Ross then asked me if I would be interested to come to Sydney to be the assistant editor on his next movie, which was called *The Irishman,* set in the 1920s, and told the story of a hard-drinking Irish teamster, played by actor Michael Craig, who is reluctant to admit his Clydesdale horses are being made redundant by the new timber trucks run by actor Bryan Brown's character.

The director was Donald Crombie and the producer was Anthony Buckley, who I had heard of as he was the editor on one of the best films ever made in Australia called *Wake in Fright,*

Ross then told me I would be paid $270 a week and be put up in a hotel in Chatswood for the duration of the edit, 'So are you interested mate?'

After, a moment's pause I said, 'Yes please... and thank you.'

Hugh was really pleased for me and told me not to worry about leaving him to rent the house on his own, as he wanted to move soon anyway and then his brother-in-law offered to buy my car for exactly the same amount of money I had paid for it, so all I had to do was re-pack my backpack, leaving a few items with Hugh for safekeeping until I returned and then fly to Sydney.

The morning I arrived at Spectrum Films in Willoughby on the city's North Shore, I was met by the two owners of the post-production company, Hans Pomeranz and Nick Beauman, who I soon discovered were both friends of Edwin, who had called them in advance and sung my praises, which was kind and considerate of him. Hans then introduced me to the editor I would be working with, Tim Wellburn, who was absolutely charming and immediately put me at ease.

My main job was to sync the rushes, matching the picture to the sound of all the previous day's takes. After I had finished the syncing process, I had to do edge numbering on both the image and sound reels before putting the synced rushes into a tea chest and sending them to Charters Towers in Queensland where the director would view them and decide the takes he wanted us to use in the edit. The town was so remote it took two flights and a long drive to get them there each day.

The widescreen images of twenty Clydesdale draught horses pulling timber across the Burdekin River were absolutely glorious. Heath Harris had done an incredible job wrangling the horses and getting them all to work as a team, and Peter James, the Director of Photography, had filmed the crossing beautifully. 'PJ' had made the decision to use a film stock called Gevacolor Type 680, a high-speed double-masked original negative film, which gave him an extra dimension as it was rich in greens and browns and was also good with flesh tones, so really added to the look of the movie. But unfortunately, this film stock was extremely brittle and would often break while the rushes were being viewed on location, so I would then have to order re-prints and re-sync everything again from scratch, which was as time-consuming as it was exhausting. To entertain the camera crew on location, I wrote down an Irish joke on a piece of paper every day and persuaded a wonderful animator called Peter Luschvitz, who was working in the adjoining office, to illustrate them for me. We attached the cartoon to the inside of the box-lid, so the crew would get a laugh every time they opened it. I spent nearly all my breaks talking to Peter about the movies we both loved. He was a very talented animator and taught me about all the techniques he used, which I found fascinating.

The production company had promised to put me up in a hotel but what I hadn't appreciated until I got there was the Hotel Charles was actually a pub just happened to have a few tiny bedrooms above its bottle shop. It was a really noisy pub, which meant I usually wouldn't get to bed until after midnight but as I was working between 72-80 hours every week eventually the exhaustion caught up with me and I was able to fall sleep as soon as my head hit the pillow.

It wasn't all work and no play. I got every Sunday off and when we did get a free night off during the week, I made the most of it. I was able to get a much-needed dose of live music when I went to see the traditional Irish folk band The Chieftans at the Regent Theatre, although having to buy my own ticket and not get a free pass was a bit of a novelty I must admit. Most of their songs were instrumentals and had unpronounceable names but the one I will never forget was *O'Keefe's Slide/Round the House and Mind the Dresser*!

I also discovered a family run cinema in North Sydney run by two movie-buffs called Bill Glass and Bill Pitt who by happy coincidence often put on a double bill. I had many a long chat with them about old classic movies and sometimes they would tell me little-known facts, such as the movie *Casablanca* was based on a play called *Everybody Comes to Rick's*. It was at this tiny venue I first saw *The Rocky Horror Picture Show* written by Richard O'Brien and directed by Jim Sharman. Tim Curry was perfect as Dr. Frank-N-Furter and I thought Susan Sarandon was wonderful as Janet. This was also the first time I saw Meatloaf, albeit on screen.

As I spent so much of my time at work standing next to an editing bench, I wasn't at my physical best, so when one of the other assistant editors at Spectrum suggested I learn to surf to get fitter, I initially thought it was a great idea, 'I think it may even be compulsory, if you stay in Australia for more than six months!' he said laughing at his own joke. Well, I think it was a joke; I hadn't actually read the small print on my visa extension.

The following weekend, a few of us went to Palm Beach on the Northern Beaches to give surfing a go but trying to get up and then stand up on a surfboard was much harder than I thought it would be and my first attempt was woeful. I did manage... once... sort of... but only got up on my knees and never managed to actually stand up. When a massive wave broke on top of me and pushed me under and then swept me around, I made the mistake of taking a big breath at just the wrong time and swallowed a mouthful of Pacific Ocean. It felt like I was being squeezed to death but thankfully the intense pressure only lasted a few seconds and when I had got my head above the surface again, I was able to swim back to the shore where I was greeted sympathetically by some local surfers.

'Bro, you're a kook!'

'You got well and truly rag dolled!' which after being translated, I discovered meant I was completely clueless as far as surfing was concerned. I reluctantly agreed with their accurate assessment and decided I would stick to boogie boarding from now on and risk the inevitable ribbing from my mates who duly obliged.

I had forgotten all about my failed surfing attempt by the following evening, as I was expecting a visit from Charles Marawood, the man who had been hired to write the film score for *The Irishman,* who was coming to our edit suite to see the sequences we had cut so far to get a feel for the music he was going to write for them. As he was only available after-hours, I was asked if I would mind sitting with him and showing him whatever he wanted to view on the Steenbeck. When I met Charles, he told me he had been in the Australian Imperial Force (AIF) during the war and in 1968 had written a song for Marlene Deitrich called *Boomerang Baby.* As we watched the film sequences together, he made some rather strange humming noises and then scribbled a few notes on a pad at the same time. He then asked me to play everything again but without any soundtrack. This time, as the 'silent movie' played in front of us, he hummed quite loudly into a small tape recorder he had brought with him, and this is how he composed his music. It was incredible to be a fly on the wall to their unique creative process and a real privilege as well.

On the way to work one day, I walked past a firm of Marine Architects, so went in to ask if they would be interested to meet my friend Hugh, as he had all the right training to work for them but there were no opportunities in his chosen field in Adelaide. Rather surprisingly they told me they would love to meet him, so Hugh spoke to them on the phone and shortly afterwards they offered him a fulltime job, which meant he would have to move to Sydney.

A week later I went to two concerts two nights running with Wayne, the soundman from the shoot in Weipa and his lovely wife Roe, who I had become good friends with while I was in Sydney. The first gig was a rather quirky double bill with Supercharge from England and Mother Goose from New Zealand at the Elizabethan Theatre. The second was another double bill but this time with two lads from Glasgow at the Town Hall. John Martyn and Bert Jansch who was ex-Pentangle. I had bought John's album *Solid Air* a few years previously so new some of his songs already but seeing him play *I'd Rather Be The Devil* and *May You Never* live gave me a whole new respect for his musicianship.

On my last day working on *The Irishman,* Hugh started his new job as a marine architect in Sydney. To celebrate, we went to see Jethro Tull at the Hordern Pavilion. I had managed to arrange for two stage passes this time, which allowed us to sit close to the stage in the wings, so we were both able to get some fairly good photos that night. Tull's set included *Songs from the Wood*, as well as old favourites like *Thick as a Brick, Minstrel in the Gallery* and *Aqualung.* The shared experience of attending this excellent concert was a great way for us to say goodbye and go our separate ways.

Two days later, I heard on the news Marc Bolan from T-Rex had been killed in a car crash in Barnes. He was only 29. The pioneer of glam rock had once written the lyrics 'Life's a gas... I hope it's going to last.' Unfortunately for him it didn't and it made me appreciate life doesn't last forever, so I should make the most of every day.

It felt very sad to be leaving Australia, as I had made some lovely friends, attended a few memorable gigs, discovered some exciting new Aussie bands, taken loads of photographs while traveling this immense country, and had opportunities in the Australian film industry I would never have been given in England, but my visa was about to expire and it was time to go home. However, having satisfied my passions for music, photography and filmmaking over the course of the year, I now had another one to add to the list. Travel. To this end, I decided to return to the UK 'the pretty way', and travel home overland 'the pretty long way' via the infamous Hippie Trail from Kathmandu to London. I had never been so excited in my life.

*If you travel far enough, you'll eventually meet yourself.*

Joseph Campbell

## CHAPTER 11: FREE BIRD

Life is a journey not a destination, or so the saying goes, but an hour into my flight to Bali, the turbulence became so severe, the odds for arriving at my first destination in one piece weren't looking in my favour. However, when the man sitting next to me, a retired commercial pilot, calmly explained, 'Turbulence isn't as dangerous as most people think… and don't worry, *most* planes are built to handle the worst!' I decided to relax, close my eyes and listen to some peaceful music rather than look through the plane's window for any signs of induced drag, which according to my fellow passenger 'might increase the downwash on the trailing edge of the wing. Now *that* could be a concern as it would reduce the effectiveness of the…'

I missed his last and possibly most important words because I had placed my headphones on and was being distracted by Paul Rodgers distinctive raspy voice singing *Live for the Music* off Bad Company's third album *Run with the Pack,* one of only ten cassettes I had managed to make room for in my tightly packed backpack. While I listened to the 'supergroup' made from ex-members of Free, Mott the Hoople and King Crimson, I decided to go through the travel itinerary I had made before leaving Australia.

My journey back to the UK was going to start with a few days R&R in Indonesia before flying up to Singapore and then on to Malaysia. From there I planned to fly to Thailand to meet a group of other travellers who I would take an overland coach trip with starting in Kathmandu on the 13th of October and ending in London in the last week of November. This meant I had the next two weeks to myself and was free to do exactly what I wanted, when and where, which not being one to plan my spontaneity too far ahead was the ideal scenario for me.

After surviving the bumpy flight and arriving in Denpasar more or less in one piece, I walked out of the airport into the blistering sun and hailed a 'bemo' to take me to Kuta Beach. The vehicle wasn't like any other taxi I had ever seen, it was a small open-air minibus with all its seats removed and then replaced with benches either side, so the passengers had to look at each other, or as in my case an old woman holding a chicken, presumably on the way to or from a market.

Finding a Losmen to rent was relatively easy, as there were signs everywhere offering accommodation. It wasn't exactly the Hilton but suited my needs and only cost 600 rupiah a night, which was ridiculously cheap. The tiny room only had a wooden camp bed with a thin mattress, a sheet and a pillow but all incredibly clean. In the courtyard there was a head height tap poking out of the wall with a small saucepan hanging on a nail next to it, so you could pour water over your body while you stood under the tap. Behind the wall I found a deep hole in the ground which acted as a loo. Apparently, this was one of the upmarket ones as it had concrete footrests to help you squat more easily. Goodness knows what the downmarket ones were like. I tried not to dwell on it. An elderly lady placed a mosquito coil outside my room at night and replaced it with a thermos of steaming hot tea and two fresh bananas in the morning. As tap water wasn't considered safe to drink in those days and bottled water wasn't an option yet, I had to put special tablets in the water to disinfect it before drinking it, which tasted foul, so the fresh tea was always welcome.

In the 1970s Kuta was a tiny fishing village and totally unspoilt. The Indonesians were very open and friendly and all the children looked happy as they smiled and waved to me. I only saw a few other western tourists on the almost empty beaches, so it was absolute bliss to swim in the sea and then sunbathe for a couple of hours.

As I lay in the sun getting a tan, I thought about the benefits of travelling on my own and how having to make decisions for myself had already helped improve my self-confidence. What I needed next was to work out what I wanted to gain from my upcoming adventure on a personal level. The one thing I was certain about was to put my film career on hold for the next two months, get out of my comfort zone by attempting things I had never done before, even if it meant making mistakes, and hopefully overcome any remaining self-doubt in the process.

To this end, I hired a motorbike for a few days to explore the island and was soon inspired by everything I saw. The temples were beautiful and each one was a little different to the other, the markets only sold local products and the lush paddy fields were a photographer's dream come true. I wanted to take dozens of photos at every opportunity but as I only had room for one dozen rolls of film in my backpack, I had to limit the amount I took in each country. This was also the first time I used 35mm Kodachrome slide film, which was much more expensive than using colour negative film, so I had to be as frugal as possible.

Witnessing a cockfight for the first time in Ubud was quite distressing. Two cocks with blades attached to their feet were released and pecked and scratched each other until one of them bled to death. It seemed extremely cruel to me but in an attempt to be curious rather than judgemental I asked one of the locals, who spoke a little English, to tell me why they did this ritual. He explained how cockfighting was part of a religious ceremony and temple cleansing and the spilled blood was to ward off evil spirits.

At the end of the day, I watched the sun set behind the shrine at Tanah Lot while eating chicken satay on bamboo sticks, which was much more to my liking, although, on my way back to Kuta Beach, I did wonder whether I might have just eaten one of the losers.

From Bali I flew to Singapore, which was quite a change as it was so built up and The Miramar Hotel was extremely expensive compared to my last accommodation so I could only afford to stay for two nights. The main reason for stopping off there was to purchase some cheap contact lenses. My eyes were bright red for days but it felt amazing to finally be able to see without continually pushing my heavy coke bottle thick lenses up my nose every five seconds. I celebrated my new acquisition with a Singapore Sling in the Long Bar at the Raffles Hotel, which was indulgent but delicious.

Singapore to Kuala Lumpur was quite a short flight but long enough to enjoy listening to Peter Gabriel's first album on my headphones. The opening track *Moribund the Burgermeister* was about St. Vitus dance, a nervous disorder where the sufferer has involuntary and irregular body movements, which coincidentally were the same symptoms the man sitting in the seat next to me was currently displaying. Thankfully, after asking him if I could be of assistance, I discovered the man was simply trying to get a set of keys out of his trouser pocket, which had been causing him discomfort ever since we had taken off. Once the offending objects were safely in his hand, my fellow passenger told me he was American but lived and worked in Kuala Lumpur because his wife was Malaysian. I explained how I was only passing through KL, as I was slowly making my way to Nepal where I had organised to join an overland coach tour to London. My new friend Gene then kindly invited me to stay at his house for the night and his lovely wife Maureen cooked a wonderful Indonesian meal me. I had struck gold, which in Malaysia is about 99.5% purity, so I felt very fortunate indeed.

Before going to work the flowing morning, Gene dropped me off at the Batu Caves. While I was walking up the steps to the entrance, a group of young Malaysian men asked me to take some photos of them with their camera. I duly obliged and we exchanged pleasantries and handshakes.

Once I was inside the caves, I initially stuck close to a tour group who had entered at the same time but soon lagged behind because I wanted to take photos of the impressive stalactites and stalagmites without any of the other tourists in the background.

After a while, it dawned on me I was being followed by two rather unsavoury looking characters, so I started to walk a bit faster to catch up with the tour group. The two men then picked up speed to keep up with me, so I ducked under a railing in an attempt to take a short cut but when they did the same thing, I realised I was in trouble so started to run but they ran faster and eventually caught up with me. One of the men began hitting me while the other one tried to snatch my camera off me. Luckily for me, one of the young Malaysian men in the group I had taken photos of outside the caves must have seen what was going on and after getting the attention of his mates, they all came to my rescue. What followed was straight out of a Bruce Lee movie. They kickboxed my two assailants into submission, I retrieved my camera, said a quick thank you to my saviours and then left the caves as soon as my wobbly legs would allow.

The attempted mugging put me off staying in KL for longer than necessary, so after one more night with Gene and his wife, I decided to fly to Georgetown, on the island of Penang, a day earlier than I had originally planned.

I booked a room at Hotel New China, which only cost seven Malaysian dollars a night. It proved to be a good decision as a fascinating Frenchman was also staying there while he was making a film about the Penang Chinese Opera. Over a couple of beers at Fagin's Kitchen, Norbert told me it was an ancient art form which combined iron-rod puppets with musical performances. In the morning, he drove me around the island so I could see a couple of the Teochew Puppet shows for myself. On the way back to the hotel, Norbert told me I should visit the morning markets before I left the island, so I got up early and took a rickety old bus to get to the market shortly after it had opened.

As I was the only westerner sitting on the bus, unsurprisingly all the other passengers who were locals, were staring at me or to be more precise they were staring and pointing at my long curly hair, which was now shoulder-length and had become quite fair after so much exposure to the sun. One of the children seemed to be particularly fascinated by my forearms and unashamedly rubbed their fingers through the hairs on them. Perhaps this was because they don't have body hair in the way we smelly foreigners do. I thought I should politely ignore them and just look out of the window, which is exactly what I did until the next stop when I felt the body of someone sit down right next to me. When I turned in my seat to nod an unspoken 'good morning' to whoever it was, I was confronted by two beautiful brown eyes staring directly into my pale blue ones. The brown ones belonged to a rather pretty Malaysian girl who then gave me one of the biggest smiles I had ever seen. A few minutes later, I felt her leg rub against mine. Surely not, I thought. Nice well-brought up young girls do not rub their legs suggestively against complete strangers on a crowded bus, especially in Malaysia, so I pretended not to notice. But then it happened again and this time it continued for much longer. Was this really happening? Was I being seduced on a bus on the way to the market? The very thought made me somewhat excited but embarrassed at the same time. What was I to do? What was the correct thing to do in this situation? I had no idea, never having been in one like this before, so did what any other English gentleman would have done in similar circumstances. Absolutely nothing.

When I felt my leg being rubbed yet again, it appeared the girl really did want me to respond which is when I began to have some slightly erotic fantasies. But what was I supposed to do? What was considered the right etiquette? Should I ask her to come back to my hotel? When she rubbed my leg vigorously once more, I realised I had to respond right away or never know what delights might be in store for me, so I rubbed my leg against hers as hard as I could to let her know of my growing interest and to give her the sign I was ready, willing and able to perform whatever the Malaysian equivalent of horizontal folk dancing was.

Suddenly, I heard a 'Quack, quack, quack!' from a basket placed on the floor of the bus between both our legs. To my horror, I realised my amorous advances had not been bestowed on me by this beautiful local girl at all but by the bill of an overly tactile and possibly terrified duck the girl was taking to the market to sell.

When I arrived in Bangkok, the traffic was a complete nightmare and it took forever to get to the Prince Hotel. After I had checked in, I made my way to the bar where I had arranged to meet up with Sid, the Sundowners representative. Over a cold beer, he told me how he had travelled the same route numerous times before, so I was in safe hands.

I had really enjoyed travelling solo for the last two weeks, so I wasn't a hundred percent sure about travelling in a group but after Sid explained some of the benefits, it made good sense. Apart from having the company of like-minded people, I would only have the one form of transport to get on and off, as well as it being somewhere to leave my luggage when I wanted to go wander off on my own. It would also be much more cost-effective.

When I met my fellow 'Sundowners' an hour later, 8 of them were from the UK, 6 of them from the USA, 2 each from Canada, Holland and New Zealand and the rest from Australia. There were 38 of us in total, so the coach would be 'fair dinkum chockers' as Ruth, one of the 18 women in our group, told me when we first met.

The first couple I met were Steve and Honor, who were from Surrey and both of them had a great sense of humour, so when we went to Damnoen Saduak, Thailand's oldest floating market, I tagged along with them. The smells, sounds and sights were sensational. As I took photos of the colourfully dressed women selling fruit and vegetables from their long-tail narrow boats in the canals, Sid told the group this was just one of a number of floating markets and due to there being so many canals in Bangkok it had the nickname 'Venice of the East'.

Later we were taken to the Grand Palace and Wat Phra Kaew, which is also known as the Temple of the Emerald Buddha and afterwards to Wat Pho, also known as the Temple of the Reclining Buddha. It was getting hard enough to remember one name let alone two for each temple so when we were told there were four hundred temples in the city, we decided perhaps one more would suffice for our needs and made our way to Wat Arun or alternatively the Temple of Dawn, which ironically looked at its best at sunset.

There are only so many buddhas you can appreciate in one day, so I was quietly relieved and quite exhausted by the time we finally made our way back to the hotel to freshen up before being taken to a Thai boxing match in the evening. When I discovered it also had an alternative name, Muay Thai, I knew it was time to leave... depart...or fuck off.

The flight to Nepal was an experience in itself. Looking down at Mt. Everest was truly spectacular. The Himalayas had only been a name on an atlas for me until now but here I was flying over the snow-capped mountain range. When we arrived in Kathmandu, we booked into the Blue Star Hotel and I had to share a room with one of my fellow travellers, an Irishman called Patrick. What were the chances?

In the morning, my Irish friend and I decided to hire a couple of bicycles and ride to Swayambhunath, the Monkey Temple. After crossing a rather rickety bridge we then had to abandon our bikes while we climbed up some steep steps to get the temple, which was decorated with gold and had many colourful prayer flags hanging on wires from the top of the stupa. We saw a troupe of monkeys and as some of them looked quite vicious we kept our distance. According to legend, as Manjushree, the bodhisattva of wisdom was creating the temple hill, the lice in his hair turned into monkeys. Not long after leaving the hilltop temple, I saw a man having his head shaved bald in the street, so perhaps he wanted to get rid his head lice before they did the same transformation.

The smell of incense sticks in Durbar Square was so over-powering we stopped for a quick pow-wow and decided we might as well continue riding our bikes south in search of some hash. We concluded the smell of a joint wouldn't make much difference to our immediate surroundings and we were at the start of the Hippie Trail after all. No trip to Kathmandu, pun intended, would be complete without going to Freak Street, where flower children from all over the world had been drawn to since the 1960s to purchase legal weed. Patrick rolled a huge spliff and we got very stoned, very quickly, which made us giggle. I then had a very bad case of the munchies.

As we entered the shop, the owner told us The Beatles had eaten there once, so we ordered two slices of cake from him, which looked like they were full of 'yellow matter custard.' We then popped into the nearby pie and chi shop for some sweet tea. An hour later, our hunger pangs had been sated and we started to return from wherever our subconscious minds had taken us and went back to our hotel.

We were woken up 4 am the following morning and then driven to a spot about an hour's drive away, which had an absolutely stunning view of the snow-capped Himalayas. The dawn light over the vast mountain range looked majestic, which made the strenuous climb up the ridiculously steep hill to see them worth the effort.

As we were walking to a restaurant for dinner, my left contact lens fell out. Using mime, I persuaded a small group of children to look for the lens on their hands and knees, promising whoever found it would get a small reward. Trying to make the children understand what I was actually looking for was very funny, as they had no idea what contact lenses were and thought, by my hand gestures, my eye must have fallen out. When one of the boys found my 'left eye' he was duly given his prize and I became an instant celebrity. The children followed me everywhere for the rest of the night.

My 'right eye' fell out the very next day when we took on some local Nepalese men in an impromptu football match. As we were 0-1 down within ten minutes, we had to become a bit more aggressive, so the next time the ball floated above me, I leapt up as high as I could and headed it with such force my right contact lens went flying towards the goal with the ball. I need not have worried, as my loyal young fans were way ahead of the game and were already fighting over who would find my 'right eye' first.

We left Khatmandu on the morning of the 13$^{th}$ of October. Our plan was to travel along the Hippie Trail all the way to London. It had been more common in the 60's to drive the route from West to East but travelling in both directions had now become quite well-established. This was the first time any of us had seen the Sundowners coach we would be travelling around 4,500 miles on over the next few weeks. It looked a bit dilapidated and didn't fill us with much confidence, so it wasn't too much of a surprise when after only ten minutes into our journey, the coach broke down. Not a great start.

Our driver, Ecka, was totally unconcerned and after lifting the hood and making an adjustment or two, he had the engine going again and we were finally on our way.

Although Pokhara's spellbinding beauty always get a mention in travel reviews and is certainly memorable for its backdrop of pristine snow-capped mountains, my own memories of the place are a little tainted by two incidents happened in quick succession. The first took place just as we sat down at our table for dinner. An enormous rat dashed across the dining room floor towards us, which made the girls shriek, although it could possibly have been me. I then looked down and saw the rat was now sitting right on top of my left hiking boot, so I shook my foot vigorously and it eventually ran off. The cheeky rodent then ran towards the kitchen door, presumably to join its mates who were already tucking into our starters. The other incident took place only moments later. As I had a dirty fork, I asked the waiter if I could have a clean one. After he took my fork off me, he inspected it, turned his back to me, coughed up some phlegm and spat on the utensil before rubbing it on the bottom of his shirt and handing the now 'clean' fork back to me. After which, I rather lost my appetite.

We drove to the Indian border without incident despite Ecka having to navigate our coach around some rather sharp hairpin turns carved into side of the steep mountains. When we arrived at the rather run-down looking Hotel Lumbini, we were told we had to share rooms again, which was fine until we discovered it was not just sharing with each other but with hundreds of tiny insects, which were crawling all over the beds. A good rule of thumb if you are ever planning to stay in cheap accommodation. If it looks like a flea pit it, then it most probably is a flea pit.

Crossing the border into India took us four hours, so I had plenty of time to listen to music on my cassette player. Lynyrd Skynyrd's *One More from the Road* was still my favourite and every time I heard *Free Bird* it made me smile like a Cheshire cat, as it was exactly how I saw myself at the time. I had also brought Peter Frampton's *Frampton Comes Alive*, Fleetwood Mac's *Rumours* and Supertramp's *Even in the Quietest Moment*, so I had my musical mood swings well-covered.

On the way to our next stop, I saw a few elephants but mostly cows, lots of cows… and lots of cow poos. We continued driving for the rest of the day with what the Americans on our coach called 'comfort breaks' every couple of hours. This involved stopping in the middle of nowhere, getting off the coach with the men going to the side of the coach to do their business, facing the way we had come from, and the women going to the back of the bus where they could crouch and pee with some degree of privacy at least.

In Varanisi, or Benares as it is also called, we stayed at the Hotel de Paris, which had been used as an officer's mess in the past. I shared a room with the same people as the previous night.

We got up at 5 am to take a boat trip on the Ganges at sunrise, which was stunning. We saw hundreds of locals praying by and bathing in the river. The scent of joss sticks was everywhere as well as jasmine from the garlands being sold by young women near the river bank. While we were being told by our guide flowers are for both happy and sad occasions, I saw some garlands floating towards me from the direction of where a cremation had just been performed. I took a photo just as the ashes were being thrown into the river not far from where people were bathing.

I will remember the poignant scene and pungent smell forever.

On our way back to the coach, a beggar held out her hand asking me for money but Sid told me not to give her anything as if I did I would have to give something to all of them. As if on cue, the crowd now surrounded us, started to surge forward and I felt myself being pushed away from my travelling companions. Sid grabbed my arm and dragged me with him towards the coach just as a large group of beggars gathered around the entrance making it hard for us to board. When we were all back in our seats and heading back to the hotel, Sid explained he had noticed a sharp rise in inequality over the last few of years doing the same trip, with the richest people getting even richer while the poor struggled to survive on a minimum wage.

In 1971 India had experienced war against Pakistan, followed by inflation and protests by students. Indira Gandhi, the prime minister at the time, had ordered a state of emergency from June 1975 to March 1977, so the combination of these events, along with extreme wealth being created for a few through capitalism and inheritance, had done little to help the plight of the poor. The only thing they shared with the wealthy was a love of cricket. This fact was made clear to us when the local staff challenged the Sundowners to a cricket match on the lawn in front of the Hotel de Paris. They were very competitive but we were equal to the task and I am proud to say I did hit one six but then was declared out on the very next ball when one of the hotel waiters, who was taking the match far too seriously in my opinion, stepped into the fountain, soaking his trousers up to the knees, just to catch the ball, which he did to great applause.

Having drunk a few well-earned beers and eaten a spicy Guinea-fowl curry, we were then entertained by some dancing monkeys, a contortionist and a snake charmer. Afterwards we took turns having our photo taken with a huge python hanging around our shoulders, which would have made Alice Cooper proud and hopefully 'worthy' in his mascara-lined eyes.

As the drive to Agra was going to take all day, I grabbed one of the seats at the back of the coach so I could listen to music through my headphones. *Go Your Own Way* by Fleetwood Mac was playing when our coach suddenly came to a stop. When I looked out of the window, I saw a dead body at the side of the road lying next to a mangled motorbike. It was a man or at least the bloody remains of one, and it was evident he had been run over by a large truck. An old man was placing a circle of stones around the victim's body but everyone else just walked past with total indifference. Sid told me later he thought their apparent apathy might have been down to police intimidation. He had heard a story about a man who stopped to help a road accident victim and then become a suspect, as the police assumed he was only helping because he had a guilty conscious.

Having had a proper night's sleep at Hotel Jaiswal in Agra, our group was now ready for action again and what a day we had ahead of us. The legendary Taj Mahal was first up on our itinerary. The huge ivory-white marble mausoleum sits right on the bank of the river Yamuna and is a photographer's delight. The Taj was built as an expression of love by the Mughal emperor Shah Jahan for his favourite third wife, Mumtaz Mahai, who bore him 14 children but tragically died after giving birth to the last one. It is a truly magnificent piece of architecture and when seeing it for the first time should be the one and only occasion you ever utter the word 'awesome' in public.

As Ruth, one of my fellow travellers also wanted to see the spice markets, we decided to take a cycle-rickshaw ride there together, which was great fun for us but hard work for the men had to frantically peddle to get us there. Although these three-wheel modes of transport are designed to seat two, we felt we should hire both the men were vying for our business rather than just one of them. On the way to the markets, we had to stop off at one of their cousin's shops to look at some expensive clothing and at another cousin's rug shop, as they were currently being sold for what they called a 'very best deal', and finally to a sitar shop, which not surprisingly was owned by yet another cousin. I wondered whether I could play anything recognizable on a sitar so gave it my best shot and attempted *Waltzing Matilda.* When Ruth gave me an encouraging nod, it gave me the confidence to then try Led Zeppelin's *Whole Lotta Love.*

After we'd finished this impromptu jam, the shop owner handed me a massive joint and not wishing to appear rude, I took the spliff from him. The effect was almost immediate. 'This is some heavy-duty hash man!' I said spluttering, which made him laugh. I handed the joint to Ruth who took a long drag, nodded at me, took a second drag and came up with the ridiculous idea we should swop places with our rickshaw-wallahs and allow them to sit in the back while we did the peddling back to our hotel instead.

After about three miles we were completely lost but our new friends were having a ball behind our backs and couldn't stop laughing, which is hardly surprising as we were paying them and doing their job. When we eventually reached our destination, my happy passenger pointed at my Rod Stewart concert tee shirt and nodded at me while pointing at his chest. I couldn't believe it. He literally wanted the shirt off my back.

When Steve saw us walk into the lobby, looking stoned and knackered in equal measures, he said, 'Strewth Ruth! What the F…have you been up to?' and how she got her nickname for the rest of the trip.

After seeing the fortified city of Fatehpur Sikri west of Agra, we drove on to Jaipur and stayed at the Khetri House Hotel in the oldest part of the city, where we were served saffron chai, which had a unique scent and tasted like grass but the kind you mow not smoke. Saffron is also known as the 'sunshine spice' as it can allegedly improve your mood. I wasn't as mad about saffron as some of the others initially but after a while its magic did seem to be working so when my companions started singing Donovan's song *Mellow Yellow,* I joined in. Well, it would have been rude not to.

In the morning, Strewth Ruth and I shared an elephant ride up to the Amber Fort. When we got off at the top of the steep hill, I wished we had walked up instead as it looked to me like the elephants were really suffering. I decided I would never ride one again.

The white marble and red sandstone of the Amber Fort was very impressive and when I looked down at Maota Lake, the main water source for the palace, I could easily imagine Raja Man Singh saying he was the King of the Castle. Well, the Kachwaha King of the Amber anyway. Being exposed to so many new and interesting experiences each day made me feel very creative and although I wouldn't know for sure whether my photographs were any good until I got back to the UK and had the transparencies processed, I instinctively felt my skills were improving, especially with my understanding of natural light but most importantly being able to tell a visual story.

When one of the coach tyres burst on the outskirts of Delhi, we had to stop so Ecka and Sid could change it but as it took ages to fix, we didn't arrive at the YMCA until well after dark.

The next morning, Ruth and I took ourselves into Old Delhi, the most historic part of the city and after wandering the streets for a while, we went to see the Red Fort's impressive red sandstone walls. The architecture was a mix of traditions and I loved the delicate flower and leaf designs had been carved into some of the walls. In contrast, New Delhi had a very different atmosphere to it, mainly due to Edwin Lutyens wonderful architecture especially the Viceroy's House or Rashtrapati Bhavan as it has been called since 1947 when India became independent. We then went to the infamous Kwality restaurant, which first opened its doors in 1940 and had since become a favourite with tourists, mainly for their delicious ice-cream.

When we returned to the hotel, one of the Americans in our group said, 'Did you hear the awful news? Ronnie Van Zant is dead!' Apparently, the plane which had been flying Lynyrd Skynyrd to their next gig in the USA had run out of fuel and crashed a couple of days earlier, killing their brilliant singer songwriter, guitarist Steve Gaines, his sister Cassie, the group's assistant road manager Dean Kilpatrick and both the pilots. I was totally devastated. As soon as we got back on the coach and started our long drive to Srinagar, I listened to *One More from the Road* from start to finish. When I finally got to *Free Bird,* I realised this song now had a whole new meaning for me and the tears I had been holding back now ran freely down my cheeks. It was sad to think there would be no more meaningful songs written by this magical musical storyteller.

'If I leave here tomorrow, would you still remember me? For I must be traveling on now 'cause there's too many places I've got to see.'

There were still many places I had to see too.

The next one was Kashmir.

*I travel because it makes me realize how much I haven't seen,*
*how much I'm not going to see, and how much I still need to see.*

Carew Paprit

## CHAPTER 12: KASHMIR

Srinagar is one of the most beautiful places in the world. As soon as I saw the wooden houseboats all moored in a row with the snow-capped mountains in the distance, I knew I would remember this majestic scene forever. It was easy to see why it was so popular in the days of the British Raj and why Mughal Emperor Jahangir called it 'Paradise on Earth'.

After taking our 'photo opportunity', Sid broke us up into small groups and put each one onto a different houseboat. Ruth and I were taken to ours on a small flat-bottomed shikara. As soon as we stepped onto the deck of The Bambri Palace we fell in love with it. It was built in the early 1900's, and featured a beautifully carved wooden interior full of ornate furniture, which was not what we expected to find at all.

In the evening, we put on our smartest clothes and met at 6pm for pre-dinner drinks on the top deck, which sounded very civilised and was somewhat of a contrast to the way we'd been living over the last few weeks. When we suddenly heard the distinct rhythmic opening riff to Led Zeppelin's *Kashmir* blaring over the houseboat speakers, we all started to laugh as we thought Sid must have put the record on as a joke simply because we were now actually in Kashmir, but to our delight, we discovered it wasn't our tour leader but the Indian cook currently making our dinner who was a fan of the heavy rock band. Apparently, he owned a copy of their double album *Physical Graffiti* as well as numerous other classic LPs recorded in the 60s and 70s, so our evening's entertainment was assured.

After drinking a wee dram of whisky, we went downstairs to the dining room, where we were served roast lamb, peas and potatoes with a choice of red or white wine. And when the plates were cleared away, we were offered brandy and cigars. As I said, very civilised!

Although I loved travelling on my own from Bali to Bangkok, I must admit I was rather enjoying being with this small group of like-minded, easy-going, positive thinking people. However, I also found it a bit tiring and wanted some time alone before I went to bed, so after everyone else retired to their rooms I went back on the top deck, collapsed on an ancient looking armchair and listened to some music on my headphones.

One of the cassettes I'd brought with me was *Diamantina Cocktail* by The Little River Band, an Aussie soft rock outfit who sounded even more laidback than The Eagles, so hearing a few of their songs was the perfect way to relax, unwind and re-charge my batteries.

It was quite chilly the next morning but the view from our houseboat was so spectacular the crisp air on my skin couldn't detract from the natural beauty. Ruth and I took a shikara across Dal Lake, which was both incredibly relaxing as well as being a photographer's paradise. Seeing the mirror-like reflection of the sky on the lake's surface made me feel as though I was floating on clouds.

I think this must have been the first time I ever appreciated what it felt like to be truly happy in the present moment, which was a momentous realisation. Being in the middle of this stunning lake surrounded by so much natural beauty made me feel I was in the 'here and now', so any concerns I might have been harbouring in my subconscious about my past and future were absolutely pointless. This awareness of being in the 'Now' made me feel totally at peace and it almost felt like some kind of a religious experience and the tranquil location certainly looked and felt like Heaven on Earth.

Up until this day music had been my only safe place but I now knew I could also feel secure when I was at one with nature. This knowledge made me feel very happy and as if to acknowledge my joy, a kingfisher flew past me dipping its wings like the Spitfire pilots did in WW2 to acknowledge someone on the ground. This fleeting vision made me think of my father and how happy he would have been to know I was too.

On the way to Amritsar, we were forced to make regular stops as nearly everyone in our group eventually succumbed to food poisoning with what can only be described politely as frequent watery bowel movements and vigorous vomiting, quite often at the same time. The only cure for it was a drug called Lomotil, which fortunately I'd had the foresight to bring with me.

Some of the group decided to stay in the hotel to recover from their previous day's odious ordeal but the rest of us walked into the middle of Amritsar to see the Harmandir Sahib, better known as the Golden Temple, which was exactly as advertised as apart from the golden domes on the top of the Sikh shrine, all the inner walls and door panels were gold as well.

In the evening, those of us in our group who were still standing, as opposed still squatting, decided to look for somewhere to have dinner together which served genuine Punjabi food. We wandered the narrow streets surrounding our hotel until we found a restaurant which looked promising as local dishes were on its menu. I ordered a chicken curry made with chilli, ginger, turmeric and coriander, which was very tasty but in hindsight maybe I should have ordered something less rich to eat. Just as our plates were been cleared away, I realised I needed to go to the loo, so made my way to the back of the restaurant where the toilets were situated.

When I got there, I was dismayed to discover it was just a hole in the ground, which would have been fine as I'd used a long drop before in Australia, but this one was extremely full and bared a striking resemblance to an Egyptian pyramid but made from excrement.

To make matters worse there were thousands of flies hovering over the pile of other people's poo. I didn't fancy the idea of having to 'do my business' here but there was little option and as they say, needs must. On the way back to our table, I bumped into the restaurant manager and suggested it might be an idea to get someone to empty the hole once in a while. As an after-thought I asked, 'By the way, is there a time you can go to the toilet when there are less flies?'

'Oh yes sir,' he replied with a knowing smile, 'Please be going at lunch time.'

'At lunch time? For pity's sake why then of all times?' I asked fearing the answer.

'Because at lunch time all the flies are in the kitchen!'

When we got out of the coach in Lahore it appeared the flies decided to follow us all the way to Pakistan, which didn't bode well for our new abode. As the Country Club only had three rooms left, it meant seven of us would have to squeeze into each room. I thought spending time on my own the next day might be a wise decision and would also make a welcome change. It was both. Having discovered I quite enjoyed my own company when I was in Far North Queensland and also when I was travelling solo from Sydney to Bangkok, I was excited to go exploring alone once more but this time I wanted to walk in Rudyard Kipling's footsteps.

Lahore was the setting for some of Kipling's stories, which he wrote while working here as an assistant editor for The Civil and Military Gazette. I always wondered what he meant in his great poem *If-*, when he wrote about triumph and disaster being two imposters, we should treat the same. Maybe he meant when something good happens to us, we shouldn't get too cocky because soon enough something bad could also occur and therefore we should try to see both as equal moments in time and not dwell on either but simply get on with our lives? I still hadn't come to a conclusion by the time I reached Lahore Fort.

After I'd taken a few photos, I continued walking until I arrived at the Mosque of Wazir Khan, which I found far more captivating. The intricate detail in the Islamic designs made the mosque very special in my eyes. Kipling said this site was 'full of beauty even when the noonday heat silences the voices of men and puts the pigeons of the mosque to sleep.' He wasn't wrong, apart from the pigeons.... and the constant honking of car horns, although in fairness to our feathered friends would have made sleep impossible.

Peshawar was the next stop on our itinerary. It is one of the oldest cities in Pakistan and an important trade route between India and Central Asia. It was also unexpectedly beautiful.

The first thing I saw as we entered the city was a 7th Century fort. In 1834, the Sikhs called it Sameer Garh, which they then re-named

Bala Hissar before the Mughals changed it to Bagram Fort. As I was feeling overloaded with too many historical facts and couldn't digest anymore, I decided to risk a new gastronomical experience instead. A small group of us found a restaurant which served our driver Ecka's favourite, Dum Pukht. It was a delicious beef dish made with potatoes, onions, cardamom, garam masala, garlic and yoghurt. It felt good to finally have a decent meal and not have any unpleasant effects afterwards.

On the 1st of November, we drove through the legendary Khyber Pass, the road which links Pakistan to Afghanistan. It was quite daunting as there were men with guns everywhere, AK47s I think, although I can't be certain as I didn't feel comfortable staring at them for too long. As we came to a halt, I saw a sign which read.

*CAUTION. All travellers are requested to cross the Khyber Pass & reach Torkham before the hours of darkness. Please note that stopping/camping is prohibited in the pass during the darkness. By order.*

Sid told us we could get off but to stay near the coach while he paid for our safe passage to get through. I managed to take one quick photo of three men walking into the rugged mountains but wanted to take more as it was like a scene from a movie. Once we were all safely back on board, Sid explained he was forced to pay a fine as there were so many of us travelling together. For 'fine' read 'bribe'.

As soon as we arrived in Kabul, Sid went to reception to check us in at the Metropolitan Hotel but before we got the opportunity to go inside, he came back and said, 'Sorry guys, it's going to be a tight squeeze again tonight, as they will only give us three rooms.'

After we checked out how many beds there were in each room and arranged for a few extra mattresses and blankets, a group of us went to Chicken Street, famous on the hippie trail and recommended to us by some travellers we met going in the opposite direction to us.

When we arrived at Sigi's Hotel restaurant, I saw a sign saying 'Good Food & Rice Pudding', which I took as a good omen. The Doors *Five to One* was blaring through the speakers, which was somewhat of a surprise but a welcome one, until I remembered the lyrics included 'No one here gets out alive.' I needn't have worried because it looked like Jim Morrison's immortal words only applied to poultry, or so I hoped when I noticed Vienna Schnitzel, made with chicken rather than veal, was on the menu. After eating chicken cooked with garlic and rice pudding flavoured with cinnamon, I was more than ready for a cup of mint tea, which I decided to have in the garden where there was a huge chess board painted on the ground. Each square was about the size of an LP cover and the chess pieces came right up to my waist. I was never very good at the game but it would have been rude not to have a go, so I challenged Strewth Ruth to a match but was easily beaten, as was everyone else who dared to take her on.

Wandering the streets on my own was a mistake. While I was lining up a good shot of three men crouching, talking and drinking chai together, one of them saw me, got up quickly and ran towards me brandishing a knife. I wasn't sure if he wanted to steal my camera or whether he'd simply got out of the wrong side of bed and wanted to kill the first person he saw. I didn't think it wise to hang around and find out so ran as fast as I could back to the hotel.

On the 3rd of November, I celebrated my 23rd birthday by going for an early walk. It felt odd to be listening to Peter Frampton sing *Baby, I Love Your Way* on my headphones while watching the local women walk past me in their traditional attire. Most of them wore a head covering called a hijab but some were wearing full burqas which covered them completely so I couldn't see their faces at all.

As I made my way to Sigi's for breakfast, I saw a street kid selling cigarettes from a tray around his neck, so stopped and bought some from him. I then got the surprise of my life when he asked me in perfect English if I liked AC/DC. Having met a fellow fan of Australia's greatest rock band, he was more than happy for me to take a photo of him and as I did so, his mates then turned up and all wanted their photos taken as well, so I dutifully obliged. Before heading back to our hotel, I asked him what his favourite AC/DC song was. The boy replied without any hesitation, *'Hell Ain't a Bad Place to Be.'* I decided to take his word for it.

In the afternoon, we were taken to the equivalent of the F.A Cup Final of the Afghan national sport, Buzkashi. The ancient game comprises of two teams of ten very skilled but highly aggressive horsemen and a headless goat, which has to be grabbed, picked up and either carried or wedged under one leg to keep the hands free, to a specific scoring circle while being hit repeatedly by the other men wielding whips and galloping at full pelt at the same time.

Although somewhat brutal and rather gory at times, it was an exciting spectacle to watch and so much easier to describe than cricket. The winners got a cup from President Mohammed Daoud Khan who was sitting just a few seats away from us and looked a lot like the actor who played Kojak and immortalised the catchphrase, 'Who loves ya, baby!'

Our next destination was a ten-hour drive from Kabul, so it was just as well I brought my cassette player with me and enough spare batteries for the duration of the trip. The album which kept me sane while we drove though the desert was *Even in the Quietest Moments* by Supertramp. Listening to Winston Churchill's inspiring speeches during the introduction to the lengthy track *Fool's Overture,* while looking at a caravan of camels carrying heavy loads through the coach window, is a magical music-travel experience I will remember forever. Apparently, camels can survive for 15 days without water. I would be lucky to last until we got to Kandahar.

The following day we passed through the Dasht-e Margo, a desert region near the province of Helmand. This desolate wasteland was the most inhospitable place I'd ever seen. As I gazed over this unwelcoming landscape I thought, no wonder westerners call it the Desert of Death. There was an oppressive atmosphere all around me so I was glad to hear, despite the ridiculous length of the journey, we were not going to stop until we got to Herat. But then we did. In fact, we were forced to stop several times over the next few hours as our coach was losing oil on a regular basis and we started to wonder whether we would make it to our intended destination. We eventually arrived in Herat at dusk and even though the Hotel Super didn't live up to its name, we were extremely happy and somewhat relieved to be there.

Ecka told us he would sort out the oil problem in the morning, so while he was busy being a part-time mechanic, a small group of us made our way to the Great Mosque. It is also known as the Blue Mosque and the reason became evident when we got there.

As soon as I saw this beautiful building, I felt eternally grateful to get such an unexpected opportunity, as it contained some of the best examples of Islamic architecture, I would ever get the chance to see, especially the repetitive elements which appealed to my sense of order.

It didn't take long for us to get to the Iranian border but it took ages to get into Iran. This was because the guards at both borders made us take our bags off and search them before allowing us to continue our journey. I suspect Sid also paid more 'fines' on our behalf.

We spent a night in Mashhad before continuing on to Gorgan with enough time for a walk on the shore of the Caspian Sea, the largest inland body of water in the world, before heading to Iran's capital, Tehran.

On the way there we saw some more snow-capped mountains and this was when Strewth Ruth told me she'd never touched snow before, so when we saw some by the side of the road a few miles further on, there was only one thing to do. Snow fight!

In Tehran we were taken to see the crown jewels and the famous peacock throne, which was once the seat of the emperors of the Mughal Empire in India. We only spent one day there before travelling on to Isfahan where a few of my fellow travellers and I got up early the next morning to see the Shah Mosque. It has been described as one of the best examples of Persian architecture. It was decorated with a variety of coloured tiles, mainly in blue and turquoise, which formed stunning mosaic patterns. Afterwards we went to the old bazaar and drank tea in a glass with a piece of toffee instead of sugar and ate some Gaz nougat.

In the evening I met two local men at a hotel bar who were part of the Iranian film crew working on the feature film version of James Mitchener's *Caravans*, which was being shot nearby. They introduced me to the art director, Peter Williams, and $2^{nd}$ unit director, Gordi Baker and after a few drinks they invited me on set the next day.

I got up at 5am as arranged and was driven to the location, where I was introduced to the director James Fargo and legendary cameraman Douglas Slocombe who shot some of my favourite films including *Kind Hearts and Coronets, The Lavender Hill Mob, The Blue Max, The Italian Job* and *The Great Gatsby*. I was told I could take as many photos as I wanted but to stick close to Gordi.

An hour later we were standing at the top of a rocky hill looking down at a group of black tents dotted around the base of some rather inhospitable looking mountains. As I focused my lens on the tents below, I heard someone shout an instruction through a megaphone. Suddenly all the tents rose as one, revealing a dozen pairs of men's bare feet under each one. After another instruction, the feet all moved in unison a few paces north before being set down again. This rather entertaining action happened another three times in succession before the cameraman said he was happy and they were all in the right place to catch the sun to look at their most dramatic against the dark mountainside.

The cast included Anthony Quinn, Michael Sarrazin and Jennifer O'Neill but the actors were too far away for me to see from our high vantage point. When we broke for lunch, I asked if I could stand a bit closer to the action during the afternoon shoot and while I was waiting for approval, one of the Iranian crew offered me a sip from his bottle of coke. This simple act of kindness would have some rather unpleasant ramifications a few weeks later.

I didn't see much on our drive to Hamadan, as I was exhausted and slept most of the way there. It took even longer to get to Tabriz by which time I was feeling unwell, my temperature was high and my joints and muscles were aching.

As soon as we crossed the border into Turkey, we noticed a

difference. There were people wearing colourful clothes everywhere and we could smell wonderful aromas of the food being cooked at the side of the road.

In Erzerum we found a restaurant where we were invited to go into the kitchen and choose what we wanted to eat from one of the bubbling pots of stew on the stove and when we got to Erzincan we were equally spoilt for choice and the meatloaf was out of this world.

The drive to Göreme via Ürgüp was very scenic. The town was once ruled by Alexander the Great and his successors until the Romans invaded in 27BC, which is when a number of underground cities in Cappadocia were built by Christians being persecuted for their faith. When we explored the network of caves and cave churches ourselves the following day, it was easy to imagine what it must have been like for anyone trying to protect themselves from Muslim Arabs during the Arab-Byzantine Wars.

In Zelve we saw a monastery which was carved into the rock in the Byzantine era. The scenery looked like we were on another planet because of its distinctive rock formations, including hundreds of what were described by our guide as 'fairy chimneys' eroded by wind and water, leaving the hard cap rock on top of pillars but to us they simply looked like 'rock willies.'

Our campsite was made up of small chalets, which made a pleasant change to being cramped in rundown hotels. In the evening we were treated to lamb on a spit for dinner and a Turkish band played some wonderful music, which made us all want to dance the night away.

With sore heads but happy hearts from the excesses of the night before, we got on our coach and went to Kaymaklõ, the largest underground city in the region with an impressive eight floors below ground; although not all of them were open to the public. Much to our relief, there was a ventilation shaft so despite feeling slightly queasy from our Raki-thon, there was enough air to enjoy this fascinating experience without passing out. We walked through the maze of tunnels for about an hour bent in half as the ceilings were so low.

Istanbul was everything I hoped it would be and so much more. Although the Hagia Sophia Grand Mosque and the Blue Mosque were both impressive examples of Byzantine architecture, it was the Grand Bazaar I enjoyed the most because it was full of colour and movement. The enormous covered market was full of fascinating people with interesting faces and colourful clothes buying even more colourful fabrics, exotic carpets, handmade plates and bowls and mosaic lamps. Steve decided to buy himself a pouf... as you do.

The Bazaar felt truly alive and I loved witnessing the hustle and bustle. It felt as though I'd just wandered onto the set of the 1963 Bond movie *From Russia with Love* where 007 is sent to Istanbul on a mission to obtain the Lektor decoder device from Russian defector Tatiana 'My friends call me Tania' Romanova, played by the delectable Daniela Bianchi.

The Bosphorus Strait was just as active with dozens of ferries and other boats of all shapes and sizes. As I walked across the Galata Bridge, I could smell the fresh sardines and mackerel recently been caught by the local fishermen all lined up next to each other flinging their rods into the water below. I could have watched them for ages but having agreed to meet a couple of my travel companions at a shop which boasted it was the oldest producer of Turkish delight in Turkey, I left the iconic scene behind and made my way there. I'd never eaten real Turkish delight before and couldn't believe how delicious it was. The chewy gel-like sweet or Lokum, as they call it locally, was made from cornflour and sugar and flavoured with rosewater and a hint of lemon. When Ruth let me have a bite of one of her pieces, I discovered it contained pistachio, which was heavenly.

At the Topkapi Palace I saw a young boy at the entrance giving an elderly gentleman a shoeshine, so stopped to take a photograph. As I did so, the lad pointed at my shoes and shouted, 'I promise three-year guarantee sir!'

Before going back to the hotel, Steve told me he wanted to go back to the bazaar, so I went with him. I didn't buy anything this time but

Steve wanted to buy another pouf. Well, you can never have too many can you? We thought the first vendor was a bit dodgy and his prices were definitely too high, so we walked a bit further into the market to look for another shop. When Steve told the next pouf salesman about the previous one, the man said, 'I do not trust that man. He has something strange in his behind!'

After we recovered from our giggling fit, and realised he meant the other vendor had a dubious past, Steve bought his pouf and we went back to the hotel to collect our bags and get back on the coach. Next stop Greece. After finding a seafood restaurant in the small fishing village of Kavala, we ate some delicious sea bream, which Steve announced was the best meal he'd eaten on the whole trip. When we got back to our hotel, he generously, although ill-advisedly, agreed to share the duty-free bottle of Glenfiddich he bought when we crossed the border earlier in the day. We polished most of it off while attempting to learn how to pronounce Slàinte Mhath properly. To save you a massive headache, its Slanj-a-va.

It was a really long drive the next day and about two hours into our journey, I started to feel unwell. This time I felt nauseous but put it down to the food we ate the night before. After we crossed the border into Yugoslavia, we stopped off at the hillside village of Predejane for a quick break before continuing onto Belgrade and finally Zagreb by which time I was feeling sleepy but slightly better health-wise. We arrived so late the hotel presumed we weren't coming and gave away our rooms to other tourists. Fortunately, the ever-resourceful Sid found us another hotel nearby. Twelve of us were forced to share a dormitory but we were all so tired it didn't matter as we were leaving at 5am the next day anyway.

In Austria, our accommodation couldn't have been more different from the previous night. Club Habitat in Kirchenberg was quite classy and I got to share a room with two pretty Australian girls, who after a few cold beers too many began to get quite amorous. But unfortunately, with each other and not with me.

There was so much snow in the morning, I could hear it crunch under my feet as I walked to the restaurant for breakfast. The food looked wonderful, but as soon as I looked at it, I started to feel nauseous, which lasted for the next few hours and made the drive through Germany to Heidelberg seem much longer than it really was. When we got to Ostend, there was just enough time for dinner before catching the midnight ferry to Dover, but I felt too unwell to eat anything.

During the overnight crossing I looked at my travel diary and went over my journey from start to finish to see if I had written anything, which might indicate how, or even if, the overland adventure had changed me in any way. I had enjoyed meeting new people, being exposed to different cultures and embracing their differences and similarities but the main conclusion I made was how I now had more respect for other people's points of view and felt it was more important to be kind than right.

I got back to Blighty at 4am on the 28th of November, took the first train to London, caught the tube to South Kensington and then walked to my old friend Vicki's house where I planned to stay the night. The minute she saw me she shrieked, 'You're yellow!'

When I saw my reflection in the mirror, I realised immediately something was very wrong and it wasn't just exhaustion. My skin was completely yellow. When I took a closer look, I noticed my eyes were also yellow. Thinking I must have jaundice, Vicki decided she would drive me straight to my parent's house in Hampshire, which was not only very kind of her but also quite brave of her as I might have been contagious.

Although my mother was pleased to see me, she realised immediately I was in a bad way, so she rang the local doctor and relayed my symptoms to him. My temperature was now a hundred and five degrees, my pee was as dark Guinness and my poo was a whiter shade of pale. Too much information? It gets worse.

*Analysis of death is not for the sake of becoming fearful but to appreciate this precious lifetime.*

Dalai Lama

## CHAPTER 13: THE KIDS ARE ALRIGHT

When my tests came back from the lab, the results showed I had Hepatitis A (HAV). As it normally takes four to five weeks for the symptoms to appear, I looked in my diary to check the dates and worked out I must have caught the liver infection when I was visiting the set of the movie *Caravans*. The doctor said it could either have been transmitted though ingestion of contaminated food or through direct contact with an infectious person, so I think it might have been passed it on to me when I drank out of the same Coke bottle as one of the Iranian film crew members. Perhaps, he was already infected with the disease and unknowingly passed it on to me. I would never know for certain but it didn't stop me feeling angry and frustrated at having caught the disease. I tried my best to keep my emotions in check but the psychological consequences were harder to keep to myself, as I felt so embarrassed and humiliated at having to explain to my friends, I hadn't caught it because of taking drugs or having anal intercourse. That was Hepatitis B and C. I knew my mates were most probably just trying to make light of my situation but their snide comments just made me want to stop talking to them on the phone. I was still contagious so nobody was allowed to visit me anyway and it was left to my poor mother to care for me by mopping my fevered brow and emptying my sick bowl when required. The constant nausea, stomach aches and high temperatures made me delirious, which is when I started to experience some seriously weird dreams.

*I see a gap at the bottom of my bedroom window and as I am now so emaciated from the disease festering inside me, I am able to squeeze through it with ease. I then leap into the air and fly over the fields between our house and the sea. It feels as if I have always been able to do this. I am a free bird. I am flying at such a low level I can almost touch the tall grasses with my outstretched hands as I glide over them. When I reach the sea, I look down at the waves sparkling magically below me. The bright lights make me squint and have to close my eyes for a moment. When I re-open them, I discover to my surprise I am now inside a brightly lit liquid tunnel. For a moment everything goes pitch black but when I am able to see again, I realise I am no longer flying but back inside my bedroom, walking upside-down across the ceiling like a gecko. When I look down, I can see my mother shaking an unfamiliar version of me lying in a bed and trying desperately to wake me up. It feels completely normal to see myself from this high vantage point. Perhaps I have been here before. I then hear my mother's voice telling me to wake up. And eventually... I do.*

Quite how close to complete liver failure I was, I will never be quite sure but it was a scary time for me. The emotional consequence was having a sense of loneliness and isolation and I missed my mates terribly but at the same time I felt ashamed, as if it was all my fault for catching the virus.

A week before Christmas, I stood on the bathroom scales and was shocked to discover I now only weighed seven stone. (98lbs). My usual weight was just under eleven. I was also now almost completely bald. To add salt to the wound, my doctor told me I had to stop drinking for at least a year to allow time for my liver to recover. I spent the whole of Christmas and New Year feeling very sorry for myself. If it wasn't for my love of music, I would have gone bonkers.

In the first week of 1978, my friend Nicol lent me his copy of the Electric Light Orchestra's double album *Out of the Blue*, which cheered me up enormously as their music was so uplifting. I especially liked the songs *Turn to Stone, Sweet Talkin' Woman* and *Mr. Blue Sky*, which ends with the words 'Please turn me over' sung through a vocoder by keyboard maestro Richard Tandy. After dutifully flipping the LP over, I listened to side four, which ends with the emotive song *Wild West Hero*. Jeff Lynne's wonderful music made me feel much better, which was just what the doctor ordered.

As soon as I was no longer contagious and well enough to get up and go shopping, I bought Santana's double album *Moonflower*, which was a combination of some impressive live recordings including *Let the Children Play, Black Magic Woman/Gypsy Queen* and *Soul Sacrifice/Heads, Hands and Feet* plus some beautiful studio tracks like Flor d'Luna and an energetic cover of Rod Argent's *She's Not There*. However, it was another double live album which really helped me get back on my feet. *Waiting for Columbus* by Little Feat, which captured the spirit of the band performing live perfectly, particularly on *Dixie Chicken* and *Triple Face Boogie*.

Although I still wasn't back to full strength and felt fatigued a lot of the time, I didn't want to stay at home and bludge off my parents and decided it was time to get my career back on track as soon as possible. But before I was allowed to work in the British Film industry again, I would have to obtain a Union card. This involved taking the train up to London and going to The Association of Cinematograph, Television and Allied Technicians (ACTT) office in Soho to sort it out. To my amazement, it was relatively easy because my decision to spend a year in Australia had been the right one and as a result of taking the risk and gaining more experience my restriction was lifted and I was now free to work for anyone who was willing to hire me.

As the ACTT office posted upcoming jobs on their board every week, I applied for everything I thought I might be suitable for and a week later got an interview to work as an assistant editor on a movie called *The Kids Are Alright*, about The Who, which was named after one of the songs on their first album *My Generation*. I couldn't believe my luck. Having no income for the last few months I was now on the verge of being paid to work on a feature-length rockumentary about my favourite band.

When I met the director, a young American called Jeff Stein, he told me he had no previous experience of making a feature length movie and was happy to hear I was a fellow fan of The Who and knew their songs, as it could prove useful during the editing process. I liked him straightaway for his evident passion for The Who. I then met Sydney Rose, the Executive Producer, who had worked with some of the biggest names in the entertainment industry, including Sammy Davies Jnr, Frank Sinatra and Dean Martin. I was a bit nervous being interviewed by such a successful man but I must have said the right things, as to my immense relief I got the job.

Now all I needed was somewhere to live. My accommodation problem was solved overnight after catching up with my friend Vicki for a drink at a pub called The Scarsdale in West Kensington. When we were on our second G&T, she told me she lived in the attic flat at her parents three-storey house in Addison Road, which was a short walk from the pub, but more importantly there was also a granny flat at the bottom of the house, which was currently empty. After a quick conversation with her mother about how much the rent was, I was able to move in straightaway, and as the job was in Soho the location of my new abode was absolutely perfect.

I started working on *The Kids Are Alright* on the 1st of February 1978. The first thing Jeff Stein did was to introduce me to his American editor, Ed Rothkowitz who quietly explained the film was going to include various interviews, TV clips and concert footage and then for some unexplained reason suddenly raised his voice and yelled. 'And I want you to fucking library everything man!'

The first assistant editor, Bob Gavin, showed me how I should organise the cutting room by putting labels on each of the shelves and by marking up all the film cans which would be arriving later, so when Ed asked for a specific film can or film clip, I knew exactly where 'fucking everything' was and could find it quickly for him. It was the perfect job as putting everything in alphabetical order was second nature to me.

One of my first tasks was to look at footage of a special one-off show by The Who shot on a stage in Kilburn at the end of the previous year. I loved every minute of it but for some reason Ed thought it wasn't good enough to be included in the movie but just in case they changed their minds, I broke down each song and put them in separate cans all marked up clearly so they could be found in an instant.

The first time I met Keith Moon, he was wearing a rather natty pin-stripe suit and I was a bit surprised at how well-dressed, polite and charming he was. As he shook my hand he smiled and said, 'Hello,

I'm Keith. Who are you, dear boy?'

I introduced myself and after mentioning I'd recently returned from Australia, he told me The Who performed there ten years earlier when they did a tour with the Small Faces and Paul Jones, and then added with a wry smile. 'It didn't go well!'

The second time I met Keith, it was obvious he was pissed. It was only 10am when he waltzed into the cutting room with a half-bottle of Remy Martin in one hand, the other half having already been consumed, presumably as a breakfast substitute. He then asked me in the distinctive voice of Peter Sellars' immortal character Bluebottle, 'Where did it went? Do you remember Eccles?'

Luckily, I was a fan of The Goon Show so knew the next line off by heart and replied doing a rather poor impersonation of Spike Milligan's character Eccles, 'Oh yeah, I remember Eccles!'

'Fucking brilliant! I thought you might be a Goons fan,' He said shaking my hand warmly, 'Have a drink with me, dear boy.'

Having been advised by my doctor not to drink for a year to allow my liver a chance to recover, I turned the offer down, but in hindsight I wish I hadn't, as then I would have been able to claim I had once got drunk with the infamous 'Moon the Loon'.

The third time I met Keith, he appeared to be sober and was wearing a light grey three-piece suit, which made him look very smart, so I asked if I could take a photo of him and he kindly agreed. I then asked him to hold some 16mm film trims in one hand, which looked a bit like spaghetti and combined with his elegant attire gave him the look like an Italian gangster. He thought this was a real laugh and when Jeff and Ed came to see what all the laughter was about, they all agreed to pose for a group photo with me and Keith. Bob was roped in to take the photo and it is one of my prized possessions.

Our editing suites were in the same building as another movie being edited at the same time called *Wings over the World,* which also featured archive footage but theirs was shot during Paul McCartney's band Wings tour of England, Australia and America in 1975-76. It was being edited by Thelma Schoonmaker who was one of the editors on the film *Woodstock*. Martin Scorsese was one of the other editors. I couldn't wait to meet her and it didn't take long before I got the opportunity.

One day Paul popped his head around the door and asked if he could watch what we were doing with the archive footage of The Who. Jeff of course said yes and I was then sent off to make everyone a cup of tea. This gave me the perfect excuse to go to Thelma's edit suite to see if she would like a cup of tea, and after I made one for her, I then felt brave enough to ask if I could watch her work for a while. She was more than happy for me to do so and encouraged me to ask questions, which was very generous of her, so I did. I was keen to know how they did the split screen for *Woodstock*. After she explained to me how they were done, she then told me they nearly didn't happen at all, as the director was forced to fight the studio to use split screen, as they thought the technique was over-used at the time. But they changed their mind after the director projected two images of The Who's performance at the festival on the same screen, shot on separate cameras, and this split screen test was enough to convince them to change their mind.

After Linda McCartney walked into the room and asked where Paul was, I offered to get him for her but she just wanted to know his whereabouts and seemed quite content to wait for him with Thelma. I didn't want to overstay my welcome so left them to have a chat and went back to what I should have been doing and was being paid £75 a week to do.

One day Thelma invited me for a lunchtime drink at a nearby pub called The Ship in Wardour Street and introduced me to a man called Cliff Culley, who supervised the matte paintings for some of the James Bond movies I loved so much, including *From Russia with Love*. He explained how a matte painting composited with live-action allowed the director to create the illusion of an environment which isn't really there and was either filmed on location so they looked like part of the set or simply combined with the live footage at the film laboratory.

Cliff then gave me a 'for instance'. The ornate ceiling in the wide shot of the room where Kronsteen's chess match took place in this particular Bond film, was actually something= he painted on a piece of glass. He said it was done in such a way the bottom of his painting lined up perfectly with the top of the set when viewed through the lens of the matte camera. They then did a front-lit pass of his painted ceiling, leaving the area where the live-action would take place clear and black, which they did by hanging a black drape behind the glass. They then re-wound the film in the camera, put a white cyclorama behind the glass and light it in a way the painting became a silhouette.

'With me so far?' he asked. I was completely out of my depth of course, but didn't want to admit it, especially as he was on a roll. But being the kind man he was, he persevered and tried to explain in layman's terms after the live-action was shot, they would then combine the two elements together and they would, or at least should look seamless. My interest in visual effects was now piqued and I was determined I would try to put this knowledge to good use one day.

On the way to our cutting rooms, I saw Paul and Linda McCartney on the other side of Dean Street being followed by some fans screaming, 'Look it's Paul...it's Paul!' Linda must have recognised me and gave me a quick wave. Paul then pointed at me and yelled, 'Look it's Jamie!' and as their fans turned to see who he was talking about, they ducked into our building, leaving me to face the mob of confused faces who after realising I was a nobody quickly dispersed and left me on my own.

On the 26th of February, I took Vicki to see Be Bop Deluxe at the Hammersmith Odeon. Bill Nelson's guitar style was totally unique, which made some of the songs on the albums a bit hard to replicate live but there were others which seemed to work even better on stage such as *Sister Seagull* and *Blazing Apostle*. It was an amazing feeling to be able to go to a live gig again, as when I was at my lowest point suffering from the effects of hepatitis, I did wonder whether I might not live long enough to attend another.

Now my film career was back on track, I was in a much better place emotionally but my health issues were still holding me back physically. I managed to get through each day without too many problems but by the time I got home in the evening I felt totally exhausted, and often experienced headaches and muscle pains and occasional bouts of nausea. My body was obviously trying to tell me something wasn't quite right, so I agreed to have more tests done.

A few days later, my doctor rang to tell me the results indicated my colon was 'playing up' most likely due to some small ulcers on the lining of my large intestine, or something along those lines anyway. However, the bigger problem was whatever my ailments were, they were causing my body's immune system to attack healthy tissue as well as fight any infections I might have.

'So basically, you're fucked!' by friend and self-appointed medical expert, Nicol, told me as he sipped his pint of bitter while I nursed a glass of overly sweet tasting orange juice. It may not have been the correct technical term but a fairly accurate description none the less. Apparently, there was no cure for autoimmune disorders but it could be controlled by having a healthy diet, getting regular exercise and plenty of rest. All more than possible to achieve but not easy to do while working so many hours a week on the film, so I would just have to take it day by day and try not to worry about it too much.

Over the next few weeks, I would sometimes wake up in a sweat in the middle of the night and not know where I was, and I would lose concentration at work, which wasn't good but thankfully I didn't make any major mistakes.

On the 9th of March Vicki and I went to see the musical *Elvis* at the Astoria Theatre. Bogdan Kominowski, PJ Proby and Shakin' Stevens played Presley at three different times of his life. I thought Stevens, as the young Elvis, was sensational and the charismatic singer-dancer who also played the dance captain was definitely going to become a big star one day, so I made a note of her name in my diary. Tracey Ullman.

After a rather boozy lunch with Moonie, Ed came back to the edit suite absolutely plastered and then slumped on the floor, fell asleep and started snoring his big American heart out. There were half empty glasses of red wine on his editing bench and all the ashtrays were full, so I took it upon myself to clean the room as quickly as possible and then make our esteemed editor a cup of extra strong coffee. When he sobered up enough to be coherent, he stood up and politely announced, 'Excuse me but I need to use the vomit room!' and then rushed out of the room.

In the morning, Ed was full of remorse and thanked me for not only clearing up after him, but for looking after him as well. When I asked him how the edit was going, he admitted it wasn't quite working for them yet. Jeff thought the Kilburn footage didn't show the band at their best and wanted The Who to do another live performance so they would have some better material to work with, but Pete Townshend was reluctant to do anymore filming.

When Bob Gavin told me we had been asked to take an unpaid break for a week, so the producers could work out what to do next, I wasn't too fussed as by pure chance I had just been approached by a company called Meard Street Movies to sync some rushes for a documentary directed by Diane Cilento. The Australian actress was great fun and when I told her I'd been working in Australia the previous year she wanted me to tell her all about my antipodean adventures. I was surprised when she mentioned she was Sean Connery's ex-wife, and even more so when she confided to me one day he abused her both mentally and physically, which was very sad to hear and made me view my favourite Bond in a much less favourable way from then on.

On the day the edit for *The Kids Are Alright* was supposed to resume, Ed told me they might not require my services for much longer, as Jeff decided to wait until they were given a green light to shoot another performance before doing anymore major editing, so I wasn't sure what I would do if I was suddenly 'let go.'

The answer came from my doctor, after he looked at my latest lab tests.

'You have autoimmune hepatitis, which is causing chronic inflammation with your liver and although the symptoms shouldn't be as acute as you had before, you may still feel unwell for quite a while. In hindsight, I think you have gone back to work a bit too soon and I suggest you consider taking a long holiday, preferably somewhere warm where you can get some Vitamin D on your body, which will aid your recovery.'

It was a bit of a shock but the test results did explain why I was still experiencing nausea and stomach pains. The doctor asked me if I had been social distancing myself from my friends, which I was surprised he knew about but apparently this was quite a common thing to do after an illness like mine, as my avoiding interaction I didn't have to explain what my condition was every time someone asked.

At the end of March, I went to see Tangerine Dream at Hammersmith Odeon with Vicki and we smoked a huge joint before the gig started. The *Cyclone* tour, as it was billed, included a Laserium light show, which might be considered rather unsophisticated by today's standards but at the time it was mesmerising. Although, our state of wonder may have simply been the effect of the dope. During the concert, which comprised of very long improvised soundscapes, my mind wandered off and I started to visualise about travelling overland across both North and Central America. By the time I got home, I decided to make this dream become a reality.

When I told Bob I was going travelling if the film was put on hold indefinitely, he advised me not to wait and to go whenever I was ready, as there wasn't much more I could do on the film until they shot more footage anyway, so I handed in my notice the next day. Jeff was very understanding and thanked me for all my hard work. He had tried to persuade the band to do another live performance but they just weren't interested, so he would just have to make the most of what he had got already and hope it was enough.

When I told Vicki I was about to leave the job, give up her parent's flat and travel to North America for the next couple of months and then go on to Mexico and Guatemala, she asked if she could come with me. I was reluctant at first, as I really wanted to travel by myself and as Vicki was only nineteen, I didn't want to end up being a chaperone to someone who I thought of as a little sister. My mother on the other hand thought it was a great idea, as she thought Vicki would look after me if I had another relapse. In the end, we agreed to travel together across America and Canada and then when I crossed the border into Mexico, she would fly back to the UK on her own.

At the end of April, Jeff Stein kindly hosted a farewell party for me at his house, which was very generous of him considering I was just a lowly assistant editor. As he handed me a bottle of Coke, he told me he would not only make sure I got paid for the week I was laid off, as it wasn't my fault, but I would also get an extra week's pay as a bonus and as a thank you for my hard work. He then gave me an address of a friend of his who was willing to put Vicki and I up for a night when we were in Boston, which was very decent of him. It was a great party, but I felt mixed emotions all evening, as although I was excited at the idea of travelling again, I was also going to miss being part of Jeff's team, even if I was just a tiny cog in the machine.

There was still time for one more live gig before heading overseas, so Vicki and I went to see Jethro Tull at Hammersmith Odeon. On this tour they were promoting their *Heavy Horses* album. Apart from performing a great rendition of the title track, they also played *No Lullaby* and *One Brown Mouse* before treating us to a best of the rest which included *Songs from the Wood, Minstrel in the Gallery, Thick as a Brick* and *Aqualung.*

A few days later I was invited to the premiere of *The Irishman* in Leicester Square. Producer Tony Buckley and director Donald Crombie were both there as well the film's star Michael Craig. I enjoyed watching the film and I thought the score by Charles Marawood was perfect. And I must admit it was a bit of a thrill to see my name in the credits for the first time.

A week before Vicki and I flew to New York, I went into *The Kids Are Alright* cutting rooms to say goodbye to everyone. Jeff told me The Who had finally agreed to do one more live show, which they would film at Shepperton. I was really pleased for him, but I felt really disappointed not to be invited, as I would have loved to have seen the band perform one last time.

Just as I was about to go, Keith Moon walked into the edit suite and presented me with a box of Romeo y Julieta wide cigars. I was amazed, as I was only a lowly assistant editor on the film, so hardly deserved such an expensive going away gift. Before I'd the chance to say thank you, he said, 'Go on then, dear boy. Open the bloody box!' So, I did, and to my astonishment there were no cigars in it at all. Instead, there were ten hand-rolled joints all beautifully lined up in a row. And this was the last time I ever saw the greatest drummer in the history of rock 'n' roll.

I was now going to put my film career on hold for a few months and concentrate on improving my health. My doctor said travelling would reduce my stress levels by removing me from my daily routine and allow me to experience new things every day, which would hopefully also boost my mental health at the same time. What better way to get well than to go on another adventure.

It was time to visit 'The Americas'.

*The world is a book, and those who do not travel read only one page.*

Saint Augustine

## CHAPTER 14: PROVE IT ALL NIGHT

On the 30th of May 1978, Vicki and I flew to New York on a Jumbo Jet. On the five-hour flight, I listened to the new Tom Petty & The Heartbreakers album *You're Gonna Get it!* on my headphones. There was one track called *No Second Thoughts* but apparently there were, as I found out later the record was originally going to be called *Terminal Romance*. I was also having second thoughts about travelling with my honorary little sister, which as any elder brother who has ever been made to chaperone a younger sibling will understand is not something you take on willingly, but I was determined to make our American adventure as much fun as possible... for both of us.

After landing at John F. Kennedy airport, we took a coach to Asbury Park, a small seaside city in New Jersey, where we met up with Vicki's cousin June. The Atlantic Ocean looked inviting so we went for a quick dip and then ate fish & chips and told her about our travel plans. The beachfront was almost identical to the seafront in Brighton... apart from having clean sand rather than pebbles and warm sunshine rather than constant drizzle. But apart from that... almost identical.

The following day, we took the coach into New York and it was everything I imagined it would be like...but bigger, taller and noisier. We took the subway and were surprised to discover the trains were completely covered in graffiti inside and out.

Although I was excited to be travelling again, I was also aware my damaged liver was still in recovery mode so I was going to have to be careful what I ate and drank. Easier said than done in a place like Manhattan, which was full of good, cheap food from every part of the globe. The smell of caramelised onions wafting from a hot dog stand was too hard to resist so Vicki and I bought a couple of frankfurters covered in a criss-cross pattern of tomato sauce and American mustard before heading to our first tourist attraction.

While we were waiting for the elevator at the Empire State

Building, everyone in the queue was chatting away contentedly but as soon as the next lift arrived and a handful of us got in, it went completely silent. Until, some joker said in a loud voice. 'Did you know Jackie Onassis lost her virginity in an elevator?' We were still giggling when we finally arrived at the 102nd floor. The view from the Top Deck was breathtaking. Seeing Manhattan spread out beneath us was like something out of a movie. Looking over the edge and seeing the people so far below was quite bizarre. Everyone was rushing around and from our great height, they looked like ants.

Although my film career was on hold, this holiday was the perfect excuse to indulge in my passion for photography and there were endless photo opportunities in New York. Over the next two days, we did all the things you do as tourist when you are in the Big Apple. We went to 5th Avenue, the Metropolitan and Guggenheim Museums, walked around Greenwich Village and Chinatown and afterwards we took the Staten Island Ferry.

As Vicki wanted to sleep in and I was keen to make the most of the short time allocated for each destination, I went back into Manhattan on my own the next morning to see more sights and take more photos, but before I left. we arranged to meet for lunch at the same hot dog stand as the day before. We went to the matinee session of *The Wiz* on Broadway together, which featured the amazing singer-dancer Kenneth Kamal Scott.

Karen, a friend of Vicki's family who also lived New Jersey, let us stay for the next couple of days in her flat Springfield. One of her flatmates, an attractive girl called Betty Jo produced a copy of Bruce Springsteen's latest album *Darkness on the Edge of Town*, so we listened to the LP all the way through. I particularly liked *Prove It All Night* a song which conveys 'success means sacrifice', which is something I suspect we all discover eventually. Afterwards, I decided to take a shower before going to bed and was given a rather pleasant surprise when BJ, as she preferred to be called, walked into the bathroom, took off her clothes and stepped into the cubicle with me. Things then got... a bit steamy. Although my liver hadn't fully recovered yet, it was good to know everything else appeared to be in working order. When BJ put Aerosmith's album *Rocks* on the turntable while we ate our breakfast, I couldn't help but smile. The opening track was called *Back in the Saddle*.

It took about five hours to get to Boston, which gave me plenty of time to listen to music on the way. One of the cassettes I brought with me was *Drastic Plastic,* the fifth album by Be-Bop Deluxe. I didn't like their new electronic sound nearly as much as their previous guitar-heavy one but admired Bill Nelson's decision to not be complacent and try something new. *Panic in the World* was my favourite track and the lyrics, 'Above our heads, in fiery red, the clouds, they bleed like open wounds across the sky,' will always resonate with me as we arrived in Boston just as the sun was setting.

In the morning, we looked at the impressive John Hancock Tower and the imposing Christian Science church before making our way to the apartment of a couple of Vicki's friends, who were willing to put us up for the night. Charlie and Trixie were what American's call 'stoners.' They were already fairly 'stoned' when we arrived but compos mentis enough to greet us warmly and to my delight, they invited us to go with them to see Cheap Trick at the Paradise. Charlie told us the band's original name was *Sick Man of Europe*, which for some unknown reason didn't take off, so they changed it after attending a concert by Slade where their bassist Tom Petersson commented the British band used 'every cheap trick in the book' as part of their act. Cheap Trick gave a terrific performance and Rick Nielson was the ultimate showman playing some blazing guitar solos. Although I liked their original songs, it was the cover of The Move's *California Man*, I enjoyed the most because it included an instrumental break based on the riff from *Brontosaurus,* another classic penned by Roy Wood who they obviously admired and respected as much as I did, which made the band a class act in my book.

We got back to the apartment at around midnight and went straight to sleep but an hour later, we were abruptly woken up by Trixie who was shrieking at us to get dressed and leave the apartment as quickly as possible.

The rest of what she said was completely incomprehensible but the gist of it was someone's mother was coming to get money for Charlie, or from Charlie, I wasn't quite sure which, and therefore we needed to leave. Vicki and I looked at each other in total confusion. Charlie then explained in a much calmer voice, 'We owe a really bad motherfucker a couple of grand for cocaine... and as we haven't been able to pay off the debt yet he is sending someone over here to collect it right now, so things could turn a bit ugly. It was awesome to meet you guys but if you don't mind, I really want you to fuck off now!'

Not needing to be told anything thrice, we quickly packed our backpacks and made our way down the external fire escape to the main road six floors below, while our new but rather short-term friends stayed to face the music.

Luckily for us, the Greyhound coach station was close by, so we waited there until the morning before continuing our journey. The drive to Vermont took over eight hours so we were able to catch up on our sleep before arriving in Stowe where some friends of Vicki's parents kindly put us up for a night.

We did try calling Trixie the next day to make sure she and Charlie were okay, but the phone line was dead. We prayed they weren't too.

The following evening, we took the night coach across the border into Canada.

My mother's younger brother Anthony was there to greet us in Montreal and as we were staying with him for the next three days, I got the chance to go sightseeing with his children, Michael and Jennifer. On the last day, Vicki and I decided to do a day trip to Quebec, where we discovered they spoke Québécois, a more informal version of French, so I got away with speaking my schoolboy French, which I wouldn't have got away with in Paris. I took photos of Chateau Frontenac and Rue du Petit Champlain and then as we couldn't afford to go to an expensive restaurant for lunch, we each bought a Tourtière from a street stall in Old Quebec. The pies were delicious and made from minced pork, veal and potatoes.

After saying our goodbyes to my uncle and his family, we decided to try our hand, or thumbs at least, at hitchhiking our way from Montreal to Ottawa.

The first time it went so smoothly we got to our destination in just two rides, so when we stood at the side of the road the following day hoping to hitch a ride all the way to Toronto, we were hopeful of a similar experience but it wasn't to be. After about twenty minutes a car finally stopped and the driver, who told us he was a travelling salesman, offered to take us as far as Kingston, which wasn't the most direct route but at least we would be heading in the right direction, so we got in. After he dropped us off, we then got a ride with a rather strange middle-aged man who played us a home-recorded cassette of his wife singing over the top of some well-known pop songs. I think the word 'excruciating' must have been specifically created to describe moments like this. However, it was our next lift which was the most memorable but for all the wrong reasons.

I should have realised we made a big mistake much earlier. The bullet holes in the side panels and windscreen of the old Chevrolet pickup truck should have been an obvious sign, if not an ominous warning. The deformed cowboy hat, sweaty appearance, beady eyes and toothless grin of the driver another. It wasn't until Vicki and our two backpacks were in the back of the truck and I was sitting in the front, when I noticed a large pile of empty beer cans at my feet and by then it was too late. Before I even closed the passenger door, our drunk driver took off at speed cutting across three lanes of busy traffic without indicating or glancing in any of his mirrors even once. When we told him we were from England, he started to ask me questions, which would have been fine if he kept his eyes on the road and not looked directly at me while he asked them. He then began driving even faster, swerving in and out of lanes and getting so close to the rear bumper of other cars I began to fear for our lives.

So… what do you do with a drunken cowboy? The only answer I could think of was to use some previously untried and certainly untrained child psychology, so when he got too close to the car in front of us again, I blamed the driver of the other car for their stupidity and suggested we should back off and slow down as 'they' might cause an accident. Thankfully this tactic seemed to work and he slowed down. Eventually we managed to persuade him to pull over and drop us off at the next gas station, where Vicki clambered out of the back of the car and immediately threw up.

My travel companion's reluctance to do anymore hitching was understandable, but as we were nowhere near a coach or train station, we didn't have much option. Fortunately for us, our next lift was with a sober, slower and much safer driver who took us all the way to Kitchener, where one of the couples I met on the previous year's overland trip lived and worked. After hearing all about our jeopardous journey, Dave and Lynda suggested Vicki have a long soak in their bath to recover from the ordeal, while they showed me photos from our shared adventure through Asia and we swopped travel experiences.

It was fascinating to hear how their perspective of our coach trip differed from my own. It was almost as though we were on different tours. We all discovered new and exciting things along the route but they only remembered the historical facts about each place we visited, whereas my memories were more about the personal experience, how it made me feel at the time and how I'd grown as a person. Travelling overland from Kathmandu to London made me more compassionate, empathetic and open to new ideas but was I getting the same kind of benefits from this trip? The answer was no, so I would have to start thinking about why this was and what I could or should do about it. But the answer could wait until the morning.

After thinking about the question all night, I came up with three reasons the trip wasn't giving me the same joy as my trip had the previous year. The first was obvious. I was having to act as a chaperone to Vicki, so my personal freedom was more restricted than if I had been travelling alone. The second was because American culture wasn't that different to ours and certainly not as exciting as the cultures had been on my adventure through Asia, so I wasn't experiencing anything dramatically different. The final reason was because we were trying to fit in far too much in too short a time, so I decided to forget the tight schedule we had originally planned from now on and try to go with the flow.

Talking of which, the Niagara Falls were truly spectacular, but despite taking numerous photos of the impressive sight, they didn't inspire me enough to want to walk across them on a tightrope or go over them in a barrel, so I just took some photos. Dave was full of facts about the falls, the most interesting being how the continuous flow on both sides of the fall were stopped for a few months in 1969, so 'the powers that be' could decide whether removing huge amounts of loose rock at the base would make the falls more attractive. In the end the excessive cost put an end to the nonsensical idea.

The following morning, Dave suggested we should backtrack east and spend a day in Toronto before catching the night coach to cross the border back into America, so we took his advice before continuing our trek west.

Spending so many hours travelling on coaches can be pretty boring but I find listening to relaxing music always helps to reduce my stress levels, so I was glad I brought an album by Ralph Vaughan Williams with me, which included *Fantasia On A Theme By Thomas Tallis* and *The Lark Ascending,* which according to the liner notes of the cassette was composed in 1914 but because of the outbreak of WW1, the divine piece of music wasn't heard until 1920 and even then it was only performed on violin and piano. The orchestral version wasn't played until 1921. The delay must have been frustrating for the visionary composer and made me appreciate how grateful I should be, as my career was only on hold for the next few months not years. Well, this was the plan anyway.

We arrived in Chicago at the crack of dawn and found somewhere open to have breakfast despite the early hour. One of the many things I love about America is there is always somewhere open for food. Vicki ordered pancakes with maple syrup and a chocolate milkshake, so she was in seventh heaven. Afterwards, we wandered the streets of the aptly named Windy City until I found an old record store, which was not only open but also full of LPs by famous Chicago Bluesmen, all stacked in alphabetical order, so it was now my turn for a heavenly experience. While I read the sleeve notes of records by Luther Allison, Willie Dixon, Buddy Guy, Elmore James, Muddy Waters and Howlin' Wolf, Vicki went to look for a 'clean loo' and then we walked back to the Greyhound station to get on another coach to Manitowoc in Wisconsin, where we arranged to stay with Christine, one of my other fellow travellers from the previous year's overland adventure. When we arrived the family were watching *Saturday Night Live*, a comedy show, which featured Dan Ackroyd and John Belushi. Vicki and I became instant fans.

On the 4$^{th}$ of July, Christine's family lent us a couple of bikes and the whole family went for a long ride followed by a game of baseball before attending a special Independence Day BBQ and watching the fireworks by Lake Michigan. From there we made good use of our Greyhound pass stopping off in Minneapolis-St Paul before crossing the border back into Canada where we stayed with a distant cousin of Vicki's, who was a senior policeman called Roland Stoneham based in Regina, Saskatchewan.

After dinner, Roland, who was quite a character, told us a few anecdotes about when he 'walked the beat' in the 1950s, and then proudly showed us the huge arsenal of weapons he kept in his basement. I hate guns but our host clearly loved them and as I didn't want to appear rude, I just nodded my appreciation as each weapon was presented for me to inspect. When he produced a particularly nasty looking telescopic rifle and said without a hint of a smile, 'And this is the one I've done the most kills with!' I was more than a little freaked out, as I'm pretty sure he wasn't talking about the animals he hunted on his days off but meant the 'bad guys he'd wasted' in the line of duty. Both Vicki and I were far too scared to ask and as we didn't want to overstay our welcome, we left straight after breakfast the following morning.

The main reason to go to Calgary was to attend the Stampede. The annual rodeo featured bull riding and bareback riding at its very best. Seeing so many cowboys and cowgirls in one place was quite a sight and I got through a whole roll of film in the first hour. We then went from the Rodeo to the Rockies, which were absolutely stunning especially Lake Louise, which like Dal Lake in Kathmandu is one of the most beautiful places on Earth, I wanted to spend much longer there but the idea of our whirlwind trip through North America was to 'see a bit of everything' rather than to 'see everything', and I could always come back another day with more time and a bigger budget, so we continued west.

In Vancouver, we stayed with my father's best friend George Paterson who was at Edinburgh University with him before and after WW2 when they were both studying forestry. George was a Canadian S.O.E agent in the war who was captured five times and escaped five times in occupied territory, receiving the Military Cross and two bars for his heroic actions in Italy. When we first met him, he was self-depreciating and gave no hint of the terrible things he must have endured during those awful years. His wife Oogie, was equally delightful and took Vicki into the kitchen to help her prepare dinner, allowing me the opportunity to talk to someone who knew my father when he was alive and I found the experience very emotional.

'Everyone finds it hard to talk about someone who is dead,' George said while pouring us both a dram of Canadian whisky, 'yet we all have to experience it at some stage in our lives, some more than others. Talking about them keeps their memory alive, which is a good thing in my book.'

'Did you get on well with my father?' I asked.

'Oh yes...well everyone did, as he could be very charming. Your father was also a very compassionate man and after the war both he and your mother looked after me like family. I'll never forget their kindness... ever.'

After telling George about my adventures in Australia and my dream to work in Hollywood one day, he told me how he thought my

Dad would be proud of me, which was very touching to say the least. Although, he wasn't a physical presence in my life, I often felt my father was looking down on me to check I was doing alright, so to hear his best friend say those kind words meant a great deal to me.

In the morning, Vicki wanted to spend the day writing postcards and catching up with her washing, so George suggested I meet his neighbour Osmond Borrowdale, who was the cameraman on *Elephant Boy, The Drum* and *The Four Feathers*, which he won an Oscar for in 1939 and now used as a doorstop in the downstairs loo.

'Call me Bordi' he insisted when I arrived at his front door. Over a cup of coffee, he told me stories about the various films he had worked on, including the aerial sequences for the movie *Hell's Angels* and how the director, Howard Hughes, was also his pilot. When I asked him if he could give me some advice, he smiled and said, 'You only need two things to be successful in this business.'

Only two? I was intrigued, 'What are they?' I asked.

'Restrained arrogance and eternal optimism!' Bordi replied with a twinkle in his eye.

I would have to work at both.

As I was now on my own for the first time in weeks, I decided call a woman whose number I was given by one of the production team on *The Kids Are Alright* and ask her if she was free for lunch. Luckily for me, Nuala was free and agreed to meet me. There was an immediate mutual attraction and we flirted outrageously with each other all though lunch. Afterwards, we went back to her apartment for coffee and then one thing led to another, well 'the other' anyway.

Playing 'doctors and nurses' in the afternoon was definitely an indication my health was improving, I thought to myself as I made my way back to the Paterson's house in West Vancouver.

While I was out, George's son Alan arrived home to see his parents. He was only a year younger than me and we liked each other straight away as we liked the same bands. It was fun to think our fathers were such good pals before and after the war. I was sure we would become good mates too.

When Alan said he wanted to take us to Gambia Island in Howe Sound on his motorboat to stay at a friend's holiday home for the weekend, I asked if he would mind me bringing Nuala along. He didn't mind at all and once we were all on the island we went exploring. It was very peaceful walking in the forest and swimming in the clear, cool water during the day and in the evenings, we ate our dinner outside and then cuddled up in front of a huge log fire. It was absolute bliss.

When we got back to the mainland we stayed with George and Oogie for one more night and then as Alan wanted to see his sister Theresa and her family in Seattle we decided to travel together. Alan drove us to the border in his old Datsun B210 and then to my surprise let me drive it from there for the rest of the way. This was the second time I got to drive an automatic but the first having to drive on the right side of the road, the opposite to the UK and Australia where we drive on the left, so it took me a while to get used to but we arrived safely and then went straight to the Space Needle so we could take photos of the spectacular view of the city from the 360-degree tower with Mount Rainier in the distance. From there we walked from Pike Street Market to buy some flowers for Theresa and her husband Tom's who kindly agreed for us all to stay the night. We arrived just in time to watch *Saturday Night Live* with them. Steve Martin was the special guest. Afterwards, I understood what every American already knew, this comedy genius really was 'a wild and crazy guy!'

On the way south, we stopped off in Portland and Eureka and walked amongst the Giant Redwoods, which were truly spectacular and driving over the magnificent Golden Gate Bridge into San Francisco for the first time, was a huge thrill. Our coach driver told us over his loudspeaker, how the U.S Navy suggested the bridge be painted in blue and yellow stripes when it was first built to help increase its visibility but thankfully the decision was made to leave it the burnt red hue the steel was primed in when it first arrived.

Having been lucky to have stayed with friends for free for so much of our journey, we decided to splash our cash and have two nights in a fancy hotel downtown so we could walk to all the tourist spots with ease like Lombard Street and Fisherman's Wharf.

I loved walking up and down the streets of San Francisco, and taking the cable car made us feel we were in a movie. 'San Fran' was the backdrop for two of my favourite films. *Vertigo*, the 1958 Alfred Hitchcock movie starring James Stewart and *Bullitt*, the 1968 thriller starring Steve McQueen, which features one of the best car chase sequences of all-time. Frank P. Keller won an Oscar in 1968 for best editing, mainly due to the way he made the 10-minute chase, which was shot over three weeks, look as though it was all shot in real time. Although, I was still prioritising my health while I was on the road, my dream of working on feature films was never too far away. At least I would be able to visit Hollywood when we reached L.A.

When we did finally get to Los Angeles, we then took a local bus to Long Beach where we were met by father's cousin Elmar Baxter, who was a successful travel writer and an exceptional photographer but now worked in PR for the Port of Long Beach.

In the evening we met his wife Jeanne, son Ken and daughter Jamie, who apart from sharing the same name as me was also a budding photographer, so we all got on like a house on fire. Uncle Elmar was the perfect host and in the morning drove us to Long Beach where we went on board the legendary ocean liner The Queen Mary, which he was responsible for getting to its final resting place as a floating hotel and tourist attraction.

His son Ken and wife Jodi took us to see Disneyland the next day. Vicki insisted going on the infamous indoor roller-coaster Space Mountain but felt sick for the rest of the day, which wasn't much for her. Pirates of the Caribbean was the best ride but seeing the fireworks over the Sleeping Beauty Castle was the highlight of the day.

After telling Elmar about my dream of working in Hollywood, he left the room, made a quick call and five minutes later told me I had just been invited by Dinty, one of his friends who worked as accountant at Warner Brothers and Burbank Studios, to have a look around the backlot the following day and then stay with he and his wife the night at their house. Meanwhile, he and Jeanne would entertain Vicki while I was away.

I was so excited I could hardly sleep. I was finally going to get a taste of Hollywood.

By the way all the staff at Warner Brothers treated Bryan 'Dinty' Moore, he was clearly a bit more important than 'just' an accountant and after giving me a guided tour around the studio lots he introduced me to David L. Wolper, who was the producer responsible for *Roots,* which was a huge success on television the previous year. He was a charming man and despite being busy took the time to talk to me about my aspirations in the film industry and gave me some interesting advice, 'If you do end up making films, make sure you try to educate and entertain people at the same time.' I would never forget those words.

While I was at the studio, I was allowed to watch an episode of *The Waltons* being filmed and then saw the stunning actress Natalie Wood being driven to the set of whatever film she was currently working on in a buggy.

On the way to his house in La Canada, Dinty took me to Griffith Park, so I could see the huge 50 feet high Hollywood sign. As I took a photo of it, I made a wish to be able to come back and work in the film industry... one day.

I wasn't sure when I would next get the chance to further my film career but at least my health was improving daily, so I wouldn't have too long to wait I was certain. Meanwhile, I would focus on my photography.

When I got back to Long Beach, Elmar let me drive his Pontiac Firebird to Huntington Beach, which was an ideal spot for an impromptu photography lesson. His camera was much more expensive than mine but he put my mind at rest when he said, 'It's not the cost of the camera Jamie, it's the person behind the lens which makes the difference.'

After lunch, Vicki and I our goodbyes and we boarded a coach to San Diego where we went sightseeing for a couple of days. At

SeaWorld, we saw Shamu the Killer whale doing various clever tricks but although it was entertaining to watch, I couldn't help thinking keeping sea creatures in captivity wasn't the right thing to do. My empathy for any wild animals taken out of their natural environment and placed in captivity was becoming stronger every day. However, I could also appreciate how most of us would only ever become aware of the existence of some of our rarest creatures by being able to see them in zoos, wildlife parks and aquariums, so perhaps there was some justification for these places, as long as the animals were treated well and not exploited. It was food for thought.

Our next stop was Las Vegas, where we were advised to stay at the Victory Motel because it was walking distance from the Greyhound bus station, somewhere safe to sleep during the day while we went gambling at night, and cheaper than everywhere else. A courtesy bus took us to the sunset strip and the first thing we saw was a huge neon cowboy next to a sign for Caesar's Palace. It was quite surreal to see so many slot machines with people staring hopefully at the spinning cards and fruits in front of them. We were offered a free drink and some bar snacks if we used one of the slot machines, so we did and instantly won but as neither of us were interested in gambling, we used our winnings to buy some coffee and then went back to the hotel for a quick nap before getting our next coach from Nevada to Arizona.

When we got to the Grand Canyon, we bought some water at the visitor centre and looked at the maps showing the various trails we could take. I was keen to walk to the bottom and back in a day but was advised by a group of young and fit looking tourists from Israel, who were topping up their water bottles, to only hike as far as a rest house about three miles down, as to go all the way to the river would take me four hours to get there and then at least six or seven to get back up to the top due to the steepness. I decided to take their advice and as Vicki wasn't interested to come with me, I was pleased when she accepted their invitation to spend the day with them while I walked the trail. As I hadn't drunk any alcohol since I'd been ill, my fitness level was at an all-time high, so I found the descent fairly easy but coming back up was much harder. It was also thirsty work so when I eventually got back to the top and was offered an ice-cold beer while we watched the spectacular sunset together, I was sorely tempted.

While I had been voluntarily sweating my guts out, not something I would consider repeating anytime soon, Vicki seemed to have become great mates with the young Israelis, who she told me were planning to drive to the East coast in their matching Merino yellow rental VW camper vans and had asked her if she would like to go with them. It was fairly obvious Vicki had taken a shine to one of the lads, who looked equally smitten with her, so I told her it was fine by me if she wanted like to travel to New York with them, as it would then allow me to travel through Mexico and Guatemala on my own.

Understandably, Vicki wasn't a hundred percent sure about travelling into the unknown with these virtual strangers and neither was I initially, but after spending a really enjoyable evening with them chatting about everything under the sun, I changed my mind as I felt they were all trustworthy, kind and compassionate people, so it might actually be good for her to travel with them for a while. She might even have a bit of romance along the way, which she thoroughly deserved, so I suggested she sleep on it and make a decision in the morning. The choice was completely up to her. If she decided not to go with them, I could always go to Central America another day.

To my surprise… and suppressed delight, she decided she did want to travel with the group…or at least with the handsome young man she had taken such a fancy to, so after having a serious 'big brother' chat to her new travel companions to ask them to look after Vicki and make sure she got safely onto a plane when they arrived in New York, which they swore solemnly to do, we went our separate ways.

As I stood on the edge of the Grand Canyon, a lone tumbleweed blew right past me and over the edge. I hoped it wasn't an omen of things to come.

'Did you know Tumbleweeds aren't native to America?' said an elderly man with a wizened face who suddenly appeared by my side as if by magic, 'A shipment of flax seeds arrived by accident from

Russia in South Dakota in 1870 and since then have spread from coast to coast.'

'Well, I'll be darned!'... is what I wanted to say, using the same Texan drawl as the old man had, but what I actually said was, 'Gosh! How fascinating.'

Another tumbleweed then rolled over the edge, as if it was so disappointed with my feeble response it could take no more and decided to end it all right now.

Before making my way back to Tijuana where I would cross into Mexico, I stopped off in Tucson, Arizona for a couple of days to see my second cousin Robin who worked there as a park ranger. I noticed he only had one leg like my father, but was able to get around quite easily with his prosthetic. In fact, when we went for a walk in the Saguaro National Park to look at the huge cacti, I was having difficulty keeping up with him. These amazing plants looked really impressive when silhouetted against the bright orange sunset, so I took a couple of photographs to add to my ever-growing collection. When his brother Tony joined us later in the day we decided to drive to California in the morning to look for a camping spot in the Anza Borrega National Park, not far from the Mexican border.

As soon as we arrived, we collected some dry wood and prepared a fire so we could cook our dinner on it. The desert was beautiful but not somewhere you would want to break down or get lost in, so I was glad to be with my cousins who were both experienced campers and knew what to do and not do in the wild.

After cooking our steaks and sinking a few beers we then swopped travel stories around the campfire. When it was my turn, I told a few anecdotes about my adventures in Australia and afterwards Robin complemented me on being a natural storyteller, which was high praise indeed after hearing about some of his entertaining exploits.

As I looked up at the stars, my cousin's comment made me recall the time my old art teacher asked me if I wanted to tell stories with my art. This was a similar light-bulb moment, as I suddenly knew exactly what I wanted to do when I resumed my career. I would no longer be content with just being an assistant editor; I now wanted to be a storyteller…a visual storyteller. My new goal was to work my way up the ladder and eventually become a film director. As to how I would achieve this lofty ambition wasn't exactly clear, so I had some serious thinking to do over the next few weeks, but first there was a new adventure to experience South of the Border (Down Mexico Way).

*Traveling – it leaves you speechless, then turns you into a storyteller.*

Ibn Battutah

## CHAPTER 15: EVEN IN THE QUIETEST MOMENTS

On the 1st of September 1978, my cousins dropped me off on the U.S side of the border; I carried my trusty backpack across the ridiculously busy crossing, also known as El Chaparral, got my passport stamped by a border official with a Pancho Villa moustache, and walked into Mexico.

Tijuana was not what I was expecting at all. Rather than Mariachi bands and flower sellers on every corner, as I was led to believe, there were homeless people everywhere. Apparently, there were extensive rains here in March which killed seven people and left more than 10,000 homeless. The only reason I discovered this information was because I decided to get my haircut and there was an old American newspaper at the barbers, which I browed through while waiting my turn. The article mentioned the Chinese community donated 500 hot meals to feed the refugees at the Army barracks and a local bakery donated a truckload of bread. There was also concern there might be an outbreak of cholera and typhoid in the area due to the water being contaminated. I felt desperately sad for all those people, so when I got to the bus station and was able to change some of my traveller's cheques into Mexican pesos, I made a small donation to a woman who was collecting funds to help the victims.

I always feel a bit guilty for being happy when I know others are suffering, as I am sure many other people do too. My mother told me this is a normal reaction and had often felt this way herself, especially during WW2 when so many people were killed, wounded and made homeless. Her advice was to just be grateful for your happiness and to try to share your joy with others whenever possible. Thinking about my Mum reminded me to buy some postcards as soon as I got to Mazatlán, as I hadn't written to her for ages.

Hotel Belmar was right by the sea, the beaches were sandy and the weather was warm, so I really couldn't ask for more. As I walked along the seafront, I saw some fishermen casting their nets into the ocean, so took some photos. After they caught enough, they degutted their catch and fed the entrails to the pelicans who were all standing nearby waiting their turn for any scraps. It was a sight to see. I then went in search of a suitable bar to watch the sunset, and couldn't resist a smile when I heard The Who's new single *Who Are You* blaring from a set of speakers. I took it as a positive sign and went inside to investigate.

At the bar there was a group of young students singing along to the song, so I joined in. After a quick round of 'who are you' I discovered they were all marine biology students researching algal blooms in Mazatlán Bay. We got on like a house on fire and listened to music while we watched the sunset, which was a reddish hue this particular evening, so I said the old adage, 'Red sky at night, sailor's delight!'

'It's actually red because the atmosphere is loaded with dust and moisture particles,' one of the men informed me in a deadly serious tone, 'so it looks red to us because the red wavelengths are breaking through the atmosphere.' I forgot they were scientists.

In the morning they gave me a guided tour around their laboratory, which I found fascinating and afterwards they showed me numerous photos of fish of all shapes and sizes with strange names like Amberjack, Corvina, Snook and Rooster. I thought their research would make an interesting documentary, which made me start to think how I would go about producing one. Before I left the UK, I presumed I would continue working as an assistant editor when I got back. The idea of becoming an assistant director hadn't really crossed my mind. It did now.

The four-hour bus journey to Tepic was breathtaking. On the way I saw lush green scenery, bananas and coconuts, birds and butterflies. I should have stayed the night there but as I was already booked at Posada Roger in Puerta Vallarta I kept going.

There were a number of sensational beaches to choose from, so on the first day I decided to just relax and listen to the soothing sound of the ocean waves but on the second I felt like getting some exercise and soon got roped into playing frisbee with some young Americans. Before leaving, they invited me to go dancing with them at the local disco in the evening, which was known as the City Dump but fortunately for us, it wasn't. I was never a big fan of disco music but had to admit the songs they played at this venue were really funky and I was more than happy to bop along to them all night. When I asked which record, we were listening to, I was told it was an album called *C'est Chic*, by Bernard Edwards and Nile Rodgers, better known as Chic. It was impressive and I realised I would have to broaden my tastes from now on and not be such a rock snob.

I flew to Guadalajara a couple of days later and stayed at a hotel near the main square. After so much sun and sand I felt it was time for some culture, so I went for a walk and took photos of the Cathedral, looked at a mural by Jose Clemente Orozco and wandered through the Mercado San Juan de Dios. On the way back to my hotel I saw a man selling newspapers with the headline, 'Moon esta Muerto!

I couldn't take it in to start with but when I saw a photo of Keith Moon next to the article dated the 7th of September 1978, I understood what had happened. My initial shock was followed by disbelief and then what I can only describe as a kind of numbness as I came to terms with the reality. The greatest rock'n'roll drummer of all time had passed away and we would never see his like again. Although I only met him a few times, I still felt incredibly sad and wept openly without shame.

It took over six hours to get to Pátzcuaro by coach and as soon as I arrived, I booked myself into a small hotel and went exploring the old paved streets. The buildings were colourful but also shabby, which were ideal subjects for my photographs but couldn't have been much fun to live in. After walking for about an hour, I eventually found a restaurant called El Patio which served fresh fish from the nearby lake.

In the middle of Lake Pátzcuaro is a tiny island called Janitzio, so in the morning I took a ferry and on the way there I took photos of fishermen doing their craft in the traditional way using huge butterfly shaped nets, which was a beautiful sight to behold and made me appreciate the beauty around me in the same way as when I was on Dal Lake in Kashmir.

I was experiencing the joy of being in the present moment again, which made me grin from ear to ear just like the Cheshire Cat and a certain drummer who I had been fortunate enough to know albeit for such a short time. When I got onto the island, I wandered the old streets and came upon an old blind man with a violin but had no idea whether he was playing traditional music or something he composed himself. Either way, it was rather haunting and made me appreciate the gifts of both sight and being able to hear music. I would never take either for granted ever again.

I decided to take the night train to Mexico and because I was so tired, I slept the whole way. When I arrived, it was like waking up in the year 1810 during the Mexican Revolution, as I was now surrounded by dozens of Banditos all wearing white clothing, red scarves and large sombreros and carrying guns with ammunition belts over their shoulders. It was a wee bit discombobulating to say the least. The reason for their stylish outfits was because the Mexican Independence Day was only two days away so thousands of people were on their way from the country to the city to celebrate the festival.

I had pre-booked the budget friendly Monte Carlo Hotel, knowing it would be too hard to find accommodation just by turning up on the day. It was a wise decision. In the morning, I took the metro to Bosque de Chapultepec where I saw the Monumento a los Ninos Heroes, which was built to commemorate six military cadets who were killed in the Mexican-American War in 1847. I visited the National Museum of Anthropology, which was one of the most fascinating buildings I had ever been to. It contained all sort of artifacts from Mexico's heritage including the Aztec sun stone, which is also called the Calendar Stone and was carved from solidified larva in the late 15$^{th}$ century. Visiting the museum made me interested to know more about Mexico's history, so I took a bus to Teotihuacan the next morning. The Aztecs constructed the ancient city on an island in Lake Texcoco and then built a system of canals and causeways to connect it to the mainland. Walking down the Avenue of the Dead and climbing up the three huge Pyramids, I could easily imagine this had once been the largest city in the pre-Columbian Americas. My guide told me at least 120,000 people lived there 'back in the day.'

Going to Xochimilco wasn't originally on my list of things to see in Mexico City, as I thought it might be a bit touristy. It was, but as I was a tourist it hardly mattered. The Aztecs had created a sophisticated agricultural system which included floating gardens made of mud and vegetation and it was fascinating to see a modern-day version. As I was taking some photos two young Mexican sisters asked me if I would take a portrait of them with their camera, so I duly obliged. Their names were Rocio and Sandy and they both spoke a little English. After asking them about where the best street food was in the area, they took it upon themselves to become my unofficial guides for the rest of the day. The girls suggested we eat some traditional Mexican food together, so I followed them to a local café where they served chicken enchiladas covered in cheese, lettuce, olives, onions, chilli and salsa.

'No Queso por favor!' was one of the two phrases I had learned since arriving in Mexico, and I needed to use it now as if I eat any cheese my throat constricts and I have to drink at least a pint of water before I can breathe properly again. The sisters explained my situation to the chef and he found an easy solution. Instead of cheese he simply added diced avocado and extra cilantro dressing. I then tried some pork tamales with a nutty flavoured sauce called mole all over them, which was disgusting but I managed to force it down. The other phrase I memorised was 'Dónde está el baño?', which means where is the bathroom? It was a wise choice, as I needed to find one *rápidamente*!

The girls took me to Plaza Garibaldi next to watch a Mariachi band play traditional folk songs. There were two men playing violins, two others with trumpets and three on guitars of varying sizes. The main singer also played a guitar. All the men wore matching black three-piece suits which were embroidered with red roses on them and they also wore bright red neck scarves and unusually wide-rimmed black sombreros with red roses printed on them. It was quite a spectacle.

We then went to a quirky cocktail bar, which had about fifty old vinyl records hanging from nylon wires from the ceiling. The girls ordered us all cocktails, which consisted of tequila, orange liqueur and lime juice and the glasses were served with salt on the rim. They were called Margaritas, which I had never heard of before and they tasted wonderful. However, in the morning I felt really nauseous and had pains in my abdomen so regretted my rash decision to drink the cocktail. My liver obviously wasn't ready to indulge my craving for alcohol yet and needed a bit more time to recover.

The 16th of September is Independence Day in Mexico and by the time I met the girls for lunch, thousands of people had already congregated in the main square to watch the upcoming procession of soldiers, cavalry, tanks, planes and helicopters. After about two hours of witnessing this event, I was roughly pushed to the front of the crowd but the timing could not have been better, as just as I raised my camera, the vehicle the Mexican President José López Portillo y Pacheco was standing in, drove right past me and he waved directly into my lens. After we had seen enough, the girls invited me back to their parent's house that was having a big party to celebrate the day. The food was fabulous, as it was all home-made. After dinner, everyone danced and watched the fireworks together. It was a wonderful night and I didn't get back to my hotel until early the next morning.

Having spent such a lovely time with these two lovely young senoritas, I wondered how Vicki was doing with her new friends and hoped she was having as much fun as I was.

My next stop was Cuernavaca and as soon as I got off the bus the heavens opened. I wasn't planning to stay there, as I was actually on my way to the former silver-mining city Taxco but apparently the roads were too dangerous to continue the journey because of the amount of rain, so I wandered the streets in search of a cheap hotel. Eventually I found somewhere affordable. It was dark and dingy but for one night it was more than adequate.

Before going to bed, I listened to *The Who by Numbers* on my portable cassette and when I got to the track *However Much I Booze,* I raised an imaginary glass of brandy as a toast to Keith Moon and then remembering his love of The Goons mimicked one of the show's character's catchphrases, 'And there's more where that came from.'

Two days later, I was at the ancient Mayan ruins in Palenque. When I arrived the early morning mist was still clinging to the overgrown jungle surrounding the site and I could hear the calls of howler monkeys and toucans. The ruins were abandoned in the 9th Century and only re-discovered in the 1950s. Climbing the stone steps up the pyramid and over the ruins of the palace made me feel like the fictional character Allan Quartermain in the 1950 Technicolor adventure film *King Solomon's Mines*. I tried to visualise what the city must have looked like at in its heyday when all the buildings would have been painted red and it was full of Mayans going about their daily business. My imagination went into overdrive and as I wandered through the courtyards, I could hear the voices of the original inhabitants in my head. It was a poignant reminder of how fragile and fleeting life really is.

The bus to San Cristóbal de las Casas broke down on the way there, so everyone on board chipped in whatever they could afford and we rented a van together which took us the rest of the way, including a quick stop off to look at the Agua Azul waterfalls and have a swim in the clear cool water. The Posada Colonial in San Cristóbal only charged one US dollar a night, so the unexpected cost of the van was soon forgotten. While wandering the streets, I bumped into another Englishman called Mike, who was working there as a teacher. As it was his birthday, he was inviting anyone who spoke English to come to his favourite bar after five o'clock to celebrate with him.

When I got to El Cerillo Bar, the party was already in full swing. A local musician was singing songs by Bob Dylan while accompanying himself on guitar. Noticing an extra acoustic guitar sitting on a stand next to him, I asked if I could have a jam. My musical skills were still a bit amateurish but I managed *Mr. Tambourine Man* and *Blowin' in the Wind* without embarrassing myself too much and then attempted a rather ambitious solo on *All Along the Watchtower*, which to my relief went down well with the small crowd. After my brief guest spot was over, a girl came up to me and told me she had seen me play guitar before, which I thought was highly unlikely. The girl told me her name was Gita and she had studied fashion at Bournemouth at the same time I was at film school, and her ex-boyfriend was in the year above me. Apparently, I played guitar at a party with one of their friends and she recognised me. Now, by pure coincidence, here we were all these years later in San Cristóbal de las Casas, an eleven-hour drive from Mexico City and about 4 hours from the Guatemalan border. It's a small world.

In the morning, I got on the bus to Guatemala but didn't get very far, as the driver crashed it after only ten minutes into the journey, which wasn't a good omen but fortunately it was a minor hiccup and we eventually crossed the border without any trouble, although the guards who were all carrying AK47s did look keen to use them, which was a bit concerning.

I stayed one night in Huehuetenango, and in the morning took a bus to Panajachel where I found myself a room at a small hotel called Santa Elena for one US dollar a night. It poured with rain non-stop for the rest of the day, so I bought myself a slice on fresh banana bread to eat and had an early night.

In the morning, I opened my door and saw the fog was sitting on the surface of Lake Atitlán, so took a photo. In the distance a cloud was just drifting over the top of the volcano so it looked like volcanic ash was erupting from it.

The half hour ferry trip across the lake to San Pedro was well worth taking. It was a pretty little village and as I walked past one of the larger houses, I saw a group of kids watching a young blindfolded boy, whose birthday it must have been, bashing a piñata until the sweets which were inside it fell to the ground for them to scavenge.

On Thursdays and Sundays, the village of Chichicastenango transforms into the largest and certainly the most colourful market in Central America, full of everything from pottery and textiles to flowers and live chickens. I took photos of all the locals in their bright coloured clothing and couldn't help but notice everyone was smiling and looked genuinely happy despite the evident poverty there. Their dignity was as inspiring as it was a humbling experience. Out of the corner of my eye, I saw an old lady kneel down and start swinging her incense so I tried to capture the moment on camera. This iconic image has hung in every house I have lived in ever since I took it, as a reminder to always be grateful for everything I have.

When I finally got on the bus, which would take me to Santiago Atitlán, it was not only full of local people but also three chickens and a pig, presumably on their way to the market. The locals found me as fascinating as I did them and stared at me quite openly. When I smiled at them, they smiled back, so I felt most welcome.

After we arrived at our destination, I went in search of somewhere open for breakfast and almost immediately got completely lost and somehow ended up in old cemetery with many colourful and ornately decorated structures, which I found out later housed the dead.

As I walked amongst the tombs I could hear *Even in the Quietest Moments,* the title song off Supertramp's 1977 album, being played somewhere in the distance. It was a bit weird listening to the song while I was in a graveyard as the last time I heard it was in the Desert of Death in Afghanistan. I followed the music until I came to what might have once been a half decent bar, so went inside to investigate. The owner, surprised to have a customer at this early hour waved at me to come in.

'Supertramp!' I said, giving him a thumbs up. The man gave me a huge smile in return before proudly showing me the rest of his small collection of LPs, which included Pink Floyd's *Dark Side of the Moon* and *Fly by Night* by the Canadian band Rush. One of the things I love about music is so much fun to share with other like-minded people, wherever they are from and whatever their background. Music crosses all boundaries and for the length of a few songs you become kindred spirits. Sitting next to the bar owner and appreciating the quality music Supertramp are famous for, is a special memory for me.

Every time I listen to the album now, I am no longer reminded of the inhospitable and desolate Afghan desert but of a peaceful little town nestled in a beautiful bay on Lake Atitlán in Guatemala.

I would have liked to have seen more of the country, especially the ruins of the ancient Mayan citadel of Tikal, but my funds were dwindling so I decided to get my archaeology fix in the Yucatan instead. I flew from Guatemala City to Merida on the 1st of October with the plan of seeing the ancient Mayan ruins at Uxmal and Chichen Itza and having a few days lying on a beach before heading back to England.

Uxmal is one of the best examples of pre-Columbian ruins in the whole of Mexico, and the tallest structure is called the Pyramid of the Magician. The steps were incredibly steep but the view at the top made it worthwhile. Nobody knows exactly when the Maya first settled here but it is thought about 15-20,000 people would have called Uxmal home in its heyday. It was abandoned after the Spanish conquest. I was impressed with the two-headed jaguar throne in front of the Governor's Palace and took a photo but the ball court was the most fascinating part of the site for me, as I could easily visualise the exciting ritual ball game played there in the time of the Mayans. My guide explained how the players had to keep a small heavy rubber ball in the air without using their heads, hands or feet but could use their upper arms, thighs and hips until one of them managed to get the ball through one of the round stone hoops on each side of the court. There are conflicting myths about whether it was the winning or losing captain who was sacrificed afterwards. Personally, I would have handed over the captain's armband before the game went into extra time, as I wouldn't have been happy to hear the Mayan equivalent of, 'They think it's all over...it is now!'

The Maya deserted Chichen Itza by 900 A.D and the Toltecs rebuilt it almost a hundred years later. The biggest structure is a four-sided pyramid called the Temple of Kukulcan, which is the Toltec name for Quetzalcoatl the plumed serpent God. It is 78 feet high and has 91 steps on each side, making 364. The upper platform makes it 365 as in the days of the year. One hour before sunset at the two equinoxes, the sun casts a shadow resembling a large undulating snake across the steps, which then connects with sculptures of serpent heads at the base, which I thought was brilliant. The Great ball court was even more impressive than the one at Uxmal, as it was at least three times the size and the hoops were much higher off the ground. This was the Mayan equivalent of Wembley, where all the big ball games took place and where the winner's captain was sacrificed by being de-capitated, or de-captained at the very least.

As my adventure would soon be coming to its end, I needed to start thinking about how to resurrect my film career when I got back to the UK. Looking at my union's job board was going to be my first port of call but whether there would be much available was anyone's guess, so I would just have to wait and see. However, after giving it some considerable thought over the last few weeks I now had a plan. I had already decided I wanted to become an assistant director but appreciated it wouldn't happen overnight, so my short-term plan was to take the first assistant editor job I was offered, so I had some regular income coming in, and then try to meet as many people in the industry as I could who might be in a position to help me make the next step up into directing. It may not sound like much of a plan but since travelling on my own through Central America I had grown in confidence and now felt anything and everything was possible. I just needed this sense of optimism to last.

Before heading back to London, I decided to have a couple of days R&R, so I caught a ferry to Islas de Mujeres, a tiny island in the middle of the Gulf of Mexico and the Caribbean Sea. There were very few hotels there, as the location was still a well-kept secret at the time, so apart from a handful of other adventurous tourists like me, I had the place to myself. The island was surrounded with corals and the ocean was crystal clear so it was the perfect place for swimming, snorkelling and scuba diving.

When I went snorkelling at Garrafon the next morning, the sea looked turquoise and felt lovely and warm. I could make out the shapes of lobsters, urchins and tiny colourful fish darting all around me but being so short-sighted everything was slightly out of focus, which was a pity but prescription goggles hadn't been invented yet. Hitching a ride on the back of a passing giant turtle as it glided effortlessly through the glass-like water was an incredible experience but while in my blissful state of being dragged along by this innocent sea creature, I lost my bearings and could no longer see the shore.

Something sharp suddenly touched my back and it felt like I had just been bitten, so I turned around to see what it was and was horrified to be confronted by a set of ferocious looking teeth, which were half in and half out of the water... and coming in my direction. I desperately looked around me trying to find the shoreline but could not see it anywhere. When I saw there were now a dozen creatures with similar looking bite-to-the bone gnashers right behind me, I started to swim for my life but the faster I swam, so did the monsters from the deep.

When I finally got back to the beach and was able to retrieve my glasses, I went back to the shoreline to look at whatever had been chasing me, which was now lying motionless on the sand. The scary sea creatures couldn't have harmed me, as my pursuers were just a half a dozen fish heads with their entrails hanging down below the surface, which had made them buoyant enough to float with their heads just breaking the surface. The local fishermen must have gutted the fish and thrown the heads and guts back into sea afterwards. The tide then carried the bits towards shore in the same direction I was heading. I felt such an idiot but had to laugh at myself.

I restored my self-confidence by eating the same kind of fish for dinner. Barracuda!

As soon as I got back to Merida, I went to the airport to buy a ticket to New York, which would allow me two more days to unwind before departing Mexico. The girl who sorted my ticket for me at the Aviateca counter told me her name was Monica and I thought she was really beautiful. I am not sure where I found the courage to ask her if she would like to come out for dinner with me, but I did and to my surprise she agreed to meet me at my hotel after she finished work.

My Spanish was still pretty awful and her English wasn't great either, but we managed to communicate with each other using the odd word in both languages as we walked into the old part of town. She told me she wanted to take me to a proper Mexican restaurant and not one used by tourists. The place was small but cosy and full of locals, which I thought was a good sign. It was intricately decorated and each table had a small vase of colourful flowers on it. I stared longingly into the greenest eyes I had ever seen and she stared longingly... at the menu.

The food was delicious and surprisingly not too spicy but there was a bowl of chillies in front of us which customers could add as they desired. Monica dared me to try one, which of course stupidly, I did. Mercifully, the chilli was not as spicy as I expected it to taste, which was a relief, but after a couple of minutes I suddenly began to perspire profusely. To stop the sweat pouring into my eyes I made the chilli rookie mistake of using the back of my hand to wipe it away. And this is where it all went terribly wrong. The chilli juice must have splashed onto the back of my hand and now the same hand connected to my eyelids. I should mention here I was wearing my contact lenses.

The following scene was something straight out of a bad TV comedy. I was in absolute agony so putting vanity aside; I grabbed the vase on the table, threw the flowers to the floor and poured the water directly over my eyes, losing one of my contact lenses in the process. But the excruciating stinging in my eyes was still too much, so I rushed to the *hombres* and put my head right under the cold tap until the effects of the chilli and my remaining contact lens were gone. When I eventually emerged, red eyed and now soaking wet, my beautiful dinner companion was explaining to the rest of the restaurant what just happened and I wasn't completely *loco* or any danger to them. I was just not used to Mexican chillies. I presumed was what she was saying anyway as everyone laughed *at* me, not *with* me, which made me feel so much better, or humiliated as we say in England.

I tried to explain to Monica in my feeble Spanish I had now lost both my contact lenses I was now legally blind. I then asked her if she would mind taking me back to my hotel, as I was incapable of doing so alone. She must have misunderstood me because not only did she take me back to my hotel but then kindly stayed with me until the morning. Perhaps she just wanted to make sure while my eyesight recovered, my other senses were still in working order.

I am glad to report they were.

*Anyone who lives within their means suffers from a lack of imagination.*

Lionel Stander

## CHAPTER 16: LONDON CALLING

I got back to London on the 12th of October 1978, which was the same day Sid Vicious, bassist for the Sex Pistols, was arrested for the murder of his girlfriend Nancy Spungen in New York, and then stuck to my plan by going straight to the ACTT office to look at the jobs board. I wrote to three companies looking for an assistant editor but didn't get a reply from any of them, which was a little disheartening, so I decided to take a risk and move into a shared flat in central London thinking if I was 'Johnny-on-the-spot' it might increase my chances of success.

Within a week of making this decision, I got an interview with a well-respected Producer called Jeremy Thomas who asked me if I would like to work as an assistant editor on a mockumentary about The Sex Pistols called *The Great Rock'n'Roll Swindle,* which Julien Temple was going to direct, so this was a very exciting opportunity. Unfortunately, the start date got put back, so I had to look for something else. When Jeremy rang to tell me the bad news I said, 'Never mind,' but after I'd put the phone down, I yelled, 'Bollocks!'

As I was back in London, I decided I should catch up with Vicki who I was relieved to hear had not only got home safely but had also experienced the time of her life travelling with the Israelis. Over dinner we swopped travel stories and it was interesting to see how much she had grown up since we had last seen each other. When I apologised to her mother for leaving her little girl in the middle of America with a group of strangers she laughed and said, 'we were amazed you lasted that long!'

A few days later Vicki and I went to see Santana at Wembley together. It was the *Definitive Inner Secrets* tour and they played a few songs off their latest album, including *Well All Right* and *One Chain (Don't Make No Prison)* as well as old favourites like *Black Magic Woman* and *Soul Sacrifice.*

I finally got a job a week later but as an editor rather than just as an assistant, which was a step up for me and also meant more money. I was back in business.

My client was Major John Blashford-Snell who founded the Scientific Exploration Society. The former British Army officer and explorer was easy to work with as he was a good communicator and his instructions were precise, so all I had to do was listen carefully and do what was asked of me. The film was about Prince Charles commissioning the Brigantine *Eye of the Wind*, part of Operation Drake which would later develop into Operation Raleigh, a round the world voyage which young people from many countries participated in. During our frequent tea breaks, the Major told me about his past adventures, which were inspiring and made me want to go on more of my own.

The next job I applied for was as the assistant editor on *The Muppet Movie*, which I was very excited about as I was such a fan of Kermit the Frog and Miss Piggy. I thought my interview was going really well until I was asked, 'What star sign are you?'

'Why on Earth would you need to know my star sign?' I asked politely, 'Surely that isn't important? Aren't you interested to know what feature film experience I have?'

'Well, we have to make sure you will be compatible with the rest of the editing team, as one of them is a Virgo and the other Aquarius,' the man said in all seriousness.

'Ah, well. Let me save you some time. I'm a Scorpio,' I replied, 'I'll see myself out.'

What a wanker! I thought as I took the tube back to my flat feeling mightily pissed off.

To cheer me up, a new friend called Sarah invited me to come with her to the Dominion Theatre to see Elvis Costello & The Attractions. We would only ever be 'just good friends' but this arrangement suited me, as she loved music as much as I did, so was the perfect person to go to concerts with. The warm up was the 'Punk Poet' John Cooper Clarke who treated us to some weird but wonderful poems all set to music, including *Beasley Street,* which features the brilliant lyric 'The rats have all got rickets. They spit through broken teeth.' Elvis' set included *Oliver's Army* from his latest album *Armed Forces* and his hit song *Pump it Up*, which the audience sang along to with gusto. Two days later we went to see Peter Gabriel at Hammersmith Odeon. The ex-Genesis singer sang many of his own songs including *On the Air*, *Not One of Us* and my favourite *Solsbury Hill* but he also did *The Lamb Lies Down on Broadway*, which went down well with his fans. The following night we went to Olympia see Rod Stewart on his *Blondes Have More Fun* tour. When the ex-Faces front man sang *Do You Think I'm Sexy*? It was a 'no from me', but it didn't really matter as I think it might have been a rhetorical question anyway. Rod the Mod included *Maggie May* in his set and ended with a terrific medley of *Twisting* and *You Wear it Well*, which brought the house down. It felt great to be going to live gigs again and sharing the experience with Sarah made them even more fun.

On Christmas Eve, I went home to spend some time with my parents and it felt surreal to think I had been at death's door only twelve months earlier.

On New Year's Eve, the road from Keyhaven to Milford on Sea was completely cut off so my old kindergarten friend Phil and I had to make our way across the fields, so we could meet up with our mutual mates Bruce, Bob and Nicol to participate in the Mummer's Play, which involved going on a pub crawl and performing a traditional play to the local revellers at each one. The characters included St George, the Turkish knight, the doctor and Beelzebub, which was the role I was asked to perform this year. If you can imagine the Cambridge Footlights Revue reserve team combined with a group of inebriated Morris Dancers, then you might get a rough idea of how the evening went but we had a lot of fun, and more importantly the drinks were free all night and I was allowed to partake, as long as I was 'sensible', which was never going to happen but at least I didn't become insensible.

With the money my parents gave me as a Christmas present, I bought *Playin' to Win*, the new album by The Outlaws. It wasn't as good as their previous three albums but there were still some great tracks on it including *Take It Any Way You Want It* and *You Are the Show* but the get down and dirty guitar jam by Billy Jones, Hughie Thomasson and Freddie Salem on the cover of the Sutherland Brothers & Quiver song *Dirty City* made the purchase more than worthwhile.

On the 16th of January 1979, *Life on Earth: A Natural History by David Attenborough* was shown on the BBC and I was transfixed by the magnificent images. If I ever became a documentary director in the future then making films about nature would be high on my list of priorities. I was also impressed with the score by Edward Williams, as he used a VCS3 synthesiser, which I first heard played by Brian Eno when he was with Roxy Music.

Two days later I sold some of the photographs from my American trip to *Vogue* magazine, which was a real feather in my cap as well as a few extra quid in my bank account.

At the end of the month, I went to see *The Rocky Horror Show* at the Comedy Theatre with Vicki and a group of her friends. The sweet transvestite was played by Daniel Abineri and Janet was played by a terrific young actress called Amanda Redman.

On the 2nd of February 1979 Sid Vicious died of a heroin overdose while on bail and awaiting trial for the murder of Nancy Spungen. Whether he actually committed the murder or not was never resolved.

My next job was as an assistant editor on a TV drama called *Kids* for London Weekend Television (LWT). The series was based around a fictional assessment centre for children who have been taken into care. My job was syncing the rushes, logging, edge numbering and track laying, which I knew how to do backwards by now so it was a fairly cushy job. Martin, the editor, had also worked in Australia so we got on really well from day one. John Frankau was very generous with his time and shared his knowledge on how to direct young actors, which I will always be grateful for. I learned a lot from him simply by keeping quiet and listening to him speak. When the gig was over, I asked his advice on how to become an assistant director and he told me the best thing I could do was to be patient and just keep doing my best at whatever I did, wherever I did it, and eventually someone in authority would notice my abilities, hard work and perseverance and give me the break I needed.

It wasn't quiet the answer I was looking for but it would prove to be the correct one.

I hadn't seen my friend Steve for ages so when I met up with him and his fiancée Karen in London. It was always going to be a fun evening. Steve had bought tickets for us to see Barry Humphries as *Dame Edna Everage* and had invited his ex-girlfriend Honor, who he was still good friends with, to make up a foursome. Having front row seats wasn't such a great idea, as Barry, whose first set was as the offensive ocker Sir Les Patterson, decided to pick on us all through his act. After he asked Honor her name and she told him, he pointed at me and said, 'I bet yer on 'er and off 'er all night eh mate?' After the intermission, Barry came on as Edna and pointed at me again but this time told the audience I looked just like *her* mother, 'except her moustache is grey!'

On the 29th of March, Supertramp released *Breakfast in America*, which had many memorable songs on the album, including *The Logical Song, Take the Long Way Home* and *Child of Vision*. I wondered how long it would take before the LP was being played in a tiny bar in Santiago Atitlán, Guatemala. I smiled at the thought.

In April, my mate Nicol and I took a hovercraft from Dover to Calais and continued onto Paris by coach. We thought it was time to get a bit of culture to broaden our minds so after a quick unguided tour of the Champs Elysees, Arc de Triomphe, Notre Dame, Sacre Coeur and Montmarte we decided to go to the Louvre. As we were walking into the art gallery, I recognised a well-known Aussie film director on his way out. He waved at me in recognition, which was amazing considering we had only met once or twice when I was in Sydney, 'G'day Jamie, I've just been to see the whinging Lisa, the saucy minx!' he joked, meaning the painting of the Mona Lisa, and then added, 'and you should take a look at the graffiti in the dunny. I don't understand the lingo of course but the images are in Australian!' As there is only so much culture you can take in a day, we decided to give his suggestion a miss and head straight for the Caravaggio's.

A week later, now back in London, I woke up with a really bad eye infection so took myself to Moorfields Eye Hospital. To my complete surprise I bumped into Bob Gavin in the waiting room who I hadn't seen since we worked together on *The Kids are Alright.*

'Well, you're a sight for sore eyes!' he joked as he shook my hand, 'Pun intended.'

While I was waiting for my turn to see the specialist, he filled me in on what had happened after I left the film, including the extra filming at Shepperton and of course Keith Moon's death, which he explained was an accidental overdose. Before he left, Bob gave me a number to call re a potential job with a director called Don Boyd. When I rang the number, the phone was answered by an Australian woman called Dee, who told me the position had already been filled but if I popped into the office in the morning, she would introduce me to everyone just in case other work cropped up in the near future. When I met Dee, she told me was working as Don's PA during the day but in the evenings, she was creating some stunning outfits for the Aussie rock band Midnight Oil whose music I really liked. Although they didn't have any work for me, one of the other staff members suggested I call a company called Platypus Films, so I did and they agreed to hire me for two weeks, syncing rushes and track laying the film inserts for a TV comedy they were making called *Bless Me Father* starring Arthur Lowe of *Dad's Army* fame.

We dubbed the inserts at Cine Lingual Sound Studios, which was the first time I met the amazing sound mixer Tony Anscombe, who told me his job was very 'rock'n'roll', which I thought was very funny but what he actually meant was that he used a system called rock'n'roll, which allowed him to rewind the mix and punch in so he could stop and start at will to make adjustments.

On the 4th of May 1979, Margaret Thatcher became the first woman to be appointed Prime Minister of the United Kingdom and five days later I went to see Status Quo at Wembley with my mate Nicol. When the band played *Is There a Better Way,* I did wonder at the choice of our new political leader but after the widespread strikes during what was known as the 'Winter of Discontent', I could appreciate the need for change. However, I don't think any of us could have foreseen Maggie would go on to reset the *status quo* of British politics forever.

On the 13th of May, I went to see Kate Bush perform the *Tour of Life* at Hammersmith Odeon. I had bought two tickets earlier in the year, as I had planned to go with Sarah but as she couldn't come, I decided to try to sell my spare seat at the gig. In the end I was lucky enough to find someone who was willing to exchange my two seats near the back for their single seat in the front row. The show was spellbinding, combining music, magic, mime, poetry and dancing, all brilliantly choreographed by Kate herself and included seventeen costume changes. She finished with *Oh England My Lionheart* and came back on stage to sing *Wuthering Heights* as an encore. Being so close to Kate as she performed her unique songs made it an unforgettable experience.

Having sold some of my photos and been to a few live gigs already this year, I was really enjoying life. I was just starting to think it can't get much better than this and then it did. I met lovey girl called Anne at a party and we began a relationship soon after. When I say soon, I mean about five minutes after we got back to my flat for a nightcap.

My new girlfriend lived in Brighton so we only got to see each other at weekends but this arrangement suited both of us at the time.

I never imagined I would ever work for the Post Office, but to my surprise they had their own Film Unit and offered me a job editing a short film for them. Once it the pictures were cut, I recorded a voice over at De Lane Lea Studios with actor Percy Herbert who had starred in some of my favourite war films including *The Guns of Navarone*, *Tobruk* and *Bridge Over the River Kwai*, which he told me had also worked on as a consultant.

The studios were in Dean Street in Soho and it felt good to be working in the same place The Who, Jimi Hendrix and Pink Floyd had once recorded in, even if only on a small budget film.

Anne and I went to see Roxy Music at Hammersmith Odeon on

their *Manifesto* tour and the support act were The Tourists. When they did a cover of *I Only Want to Be with You,* I thought the female singer sounded just like Dusty Springfield. Her name was Annie Lennox and the guitarists were Peet Coombes and Dave Stewart. (Annie and Dave would later become better known as the Eurythmics.)

Three weeks later, Sarah and I went to a Royal Gala Performance of *The King and I* at the Palladium, starring Yul Brynner and Virginia McKenna. When Anne found out, she got jealous and despite my attempts to assure her my relationship with Sarah was purely platonic, she decided to end ours.

Feeling a bit sad after the break up, I bought myself Dire Straits new album *Communiqué*, which was sublime especially the opening track *Once Upon a Time in the West.*

Although I had managed to keep my budding career going, and even progressed it by editing a couple of small films rather than just being an assistant I still hadn't worked out how to become an assistant director. John Frankau had told me it would take someone in authority would notice my abilities, hard work and perseverance. I just had to be patient, which wasn't one of greatest virtues at the time.

The next company to offer me a job was Roger Cherill Associates. There was a man called Harry Bruce in charge of the editing staff and he treated me as a professional from day one, which gave me a huge confidence boost. I was back to being an assistant editor again but as I would be working on a documentary series; I thought this was the perfect opportunity to learn how they were made. The series was about Middle East Peace, and there were two episodes, one about Mohamed Hasseinein Heikel and the other about Indira Ghandi. It was a fascinating series to work on and some of my photos of India were used as part of the graphic title sequence, which gave me some additional income.

On my last day at Cherrill's, Harry called me into his office and told me Gerry Hambling, the editor of Alan Parker's great movie *Midnight Express* was working in the same building and asked me if I would like to meet him, which of course I did. After I had been introduced, Gerry kindly showed me the TV commercial he was editing standing next to an old Moviola machine. I noticed he was wearing a white glove on one hand so as not to get his greasy fingerprints on the frames and held a Chinagraph grease pencil in the other to mark his cuts. While he continued working, he told me how he enjoyed cutting 'TVCs', as they were known as in the industry, between feature films and how directors like Alan Parker, Hugh Hudson and the Scott brothers, Ridley and Tony, had all directed TV commercials before making the leap from advertising into feature films. I took note and wondered whether it might be possible to get wok as an assistant director on TVCs, so when I said goodbye and thank you to Harry, I asked his advice.

'I have absolutely no idea', Harry said honestly, 'but I'll ask around.'

At the end of June, I flew to Los Angeles to attend my cousin Jamie's wedding to her fiancé Mark. I arrived a week before their big day and stayed with the lovebirds for a couple of nights at their home in San Clemente. They lived right by the beach so I got the opportunity to go surfing on a boogie board and play frisbee with them every day. In the evenings we listened to music and after hearing *Gator Country* by Molly Hatchet for the first time, I became a huge fan of the Southern Rock band.

As the wedding wasn't until the following Saturday, I had time to get a coach to Burbank and catch up with Dinty and Sally Moore, who I had met the previous year. This gave me the opportunity to go to Warner Brothers studio for the second time and while I was there Dinty introduced me to Fred Talmage, the head of editing and Stuart Baird who had edited the movie *Superman* the year before. Stuart had also edited the Ken Russell film *Tommy* based on The Who's rock opera, so I had a lot of questions for him, which he graciously answered. After a long languid liquid lunch, Dinty took me to meet the legendary Hollywood producer Irwin Allen, also known as the 'Master of Disaster' because he was responsible for movies like *The Poseidon Adventure* and *The Towering Inferno.* When we arrived at his plush

Penthouse, I was in need of a pee so excused myself for a moment. I had never seen such a swish looking loo. Everything was made of marble or gold, including the taps, towel heater and flush handle. I was careful not to pee on the floor, thus avoiding an unscripted disaster.

In the evening Dinty drove me to his new house, which was right on Malibu's Broad Beach and his wife Sally gave me a huge hug, which made me feel like the prodigal son. Although, rather than a fatted calf we had salmon and asparagus for dinner. While we ate, they told me stories about their neighbours Steve McQueen and Ali McGraw who had split up a year earlier but remained friends. They also told me some very funny stories about Keith Moon, including one which involved Moonie in full Nazi Uniform, which I found hard to believe but they swore was true.

In the morning, Dinty took me for a walk along the beach to see Keith's old house and I raised an imaginary glass of brandy to him one last time. I then rang Jeff Stein, the director of the *The Kids Are Alright* to let him know where I was and we had a good catch up over the phone. The movie had just been released so I was interested to know how it had been received but he said it was too early to tell as 'the numbers weren't in yet.'

When I got back to Long Beach, Elmar's son Ken took me to see The California Angels v New York Yankees at the Anaheim Stadium. I wasn't a baseball fan but seeing the Angels' right-handed pitcher Nolan Ryan, better known to his fans as the 'Ryan Express', throw pitches at around 100 mph was quite something. Reggie Jackson, another legend of the game, was playing for the Yankees, so I felt quite privileged to witness the historic event which took place on the 13th of July.

Jamie's wedding took place at a small church in St Clemente. The bride looked stunning, as all brides do and 'us menfolk' didn't look too shabby either in our suits and ties. The reception was held in the garden of their house, and this is where I met a beautiful girl with high cheek bones and long blonde hair called Emily who I was attracted to immediately.

When she left the reception, she gave me a big hug and as she did so, I felt her put something into my suit pocket. I discovered later it was her phone number.

The following day, I arranged to meet Emily at a nearby park, which is where and when I met her four-year old son Leo, who loved football so the three of us mucked about with a soccer ball a for a while. I pretended to miss the ball every time I should have trapped it, which made the young lad giggle and when it was time to leave, he gave me a big hug and said he didn't want me to, which made me wonder what it would be like to have a son of my own. I had never really thought about becoming a father before but even though I had only just met them both I wasn't averse to the idea. After dropping Leo off at her parents, Emily and I went out for dinner on our own and afterwards she took me to a romantic spot where we could get to know each other a bit more intimately.

I would have liked to have stayed in L.A longer and spent more time with Emily and Leo but I had to fly back to England, as the following Saturday I had agreed to act as my best mate Mike's best man at his wedding to his fiancé Kim. Thankfully. I didn't forget the rings on the day and my slightly risqué speech didn't offend too many people.

Over the next two weeks I went sailing with my parents on the Solent, played squash with Jon G and watched in awe as Nicol played boogie-woogie on his upright piano.

At the end of July AC/DC released *Highway to Hell* so I had plenty of new riffs to learn on my guitar and as Bon Scott's lyrics had a number of sexual references, they made me think about my latest love interest. However, as I hadn't had a reply to either of my letters to Emily, I presumed she wasn't as interested in me as I was in her, so decided the most sensible thing to do was to try to forget about her and move on. Fortunately, I didn't have to wait long.

I met Beverley at the bank where she was working as a teller. It was lust at first sight. We went out for dinner and afterwards drove to a secluded car park in the New Forest, placed a picnic rug on the ground and started to get amorous. I left the driver's door open so we could hear music playing on the radio, but this meant the interior light was on, which is why a passing police car noticed the abandoned vehicle and came to investigate what was going on. Beverley and I were happily enjoying each other's company, when we became aware of a torch beam getting closer and closer to us. As soon as we realised, we were no longer alone, we stopped our nocturnal dalliance and tried desperately to put our clothes back on before being confronted by the torch bearer. The young policeman knew exactly what we were up to but instead of moving us on, just warned us not to leave the car light on as it might make the battery go flat, and then we would be stuck there all night. After the considerate copper had gone, we decided the right thing to do would be to go straight home, so we turned off the radio, closed the door to save the battery and then decided to continue our alfresco frolics in the dark unabashed.

When I listened to my new AC/DC album the following day, I couldn't help but laugh when I heard *Beating Around the Bush*. The Acca Dacca song would have been an entirely appropriate soundtrack for our completely inappropriate behaviour the night before.

In August I bought Led Zeppelin's latest offering *In Through the Out Door*. It wasn't well received by some but I liked it and thought Jimmy Page's guitar solo on *I'm Gonna Crawl* was one of his very best he's done and John Bonham's drumming on *Fool in the Rain* was exceptional.

Later in the month, Beverley and I went to see the movie *Quadrophenia* in Bournemouth, which was based on The Who's Rock Opera set in 1964 when The Mods and The Rockers were always at each other's throats. I loved the soundtrack but found the film a bit depressing. Beverley found the whole film far too violent and made me promise to take her to see a comedy at the weekend but I wasn't able to fulfil it as I got a call out of the blue from Mary Evans, who was the producer at a film production company called Gillie Potter Productions, telling me our mutual acquaintance Harry Bruce had recommended me to them as they were looking for an assistant director on a film for the British Tourist Authority for the next two months, and the job started immediately, so was I interested? 'Yes please…and thank you.'

After ringing Harry to say thank you for the introduction, I made my way to the Gillie Potter office, which was in the basement of a huge building in Holborn, which they had converted into a film studio with an editing room and a tiny kitchen near the back entrance. There were no windows at all so it took me a while to get used to the lack of fresh air. Mary treated me like a younger brother from day one, which made me feel completely at ease. She said she had four sisters and two brothers, so adding another male to her family would even things up a bit.

Gillie Potter was considered one of the best special effects directors in the advertising industry and known as 'the man who could do the impossible'. I couldn't wait to meet him but Mary explained he was currently overseas directing a commercial, so they had hired an experienced freelancer called Richard Taylor to direct the film. Gillie co-owned the company with their in-house cameraman Ken Friswell, who was a proud cockney with the deepest voice I had ever heard. Their focus puller, Johnny Outred and camera assistant, Dave Ball were also cockneys and they had worked together for years, so had a wonderful rapport with each other, which made me laugh out loud. As soon as they heard my public-school voice, they gave me a hard time and told jokes, which were all at my expense. The title of the film was going to be *It's Good to be Here,* which was exactly how I was feeling.

The first thing Richard asked me to do was to help work out a shoot schedule. I had never made one before but having travelled so much I was more than able to read a map to work out the distances between our locations and the rest was just common sense.

As we would be filming all over England, Scotland and Wales over the next two months, I realised there was no point renting a flat in London, so asked a friend if he could put me up on his sofa for a few nights until we went on location. Thankfully he not only agreed to let me stay but also told me I didn't have to pay any rent, which was a godsend.

Day one of the shoot was by the swimming pool at the Chelsea Holiday Inn in London and on the second day we flew from Gatwick to Edinburgh with British Caledonian. On the way, we filmed a scene with Mary playing the part of 'happy customer 'being given a glass of champagne by one of the hostesses. For some unknown reason, she kept fluffing her line and we had to do three takes with a fresh glass of bubbly each time.

The Palace Hotel was a good choice location-wise as it was central to everything in Edinburgh, including a number of decent restaurants. In the morning, I got up early to organise breakfast for the crew but when I went into the kitchen it was empty so I asked the receptionist when it would open. She informed me their chef wasn't coming in, so I told the crew we would have to find a cafe in town. Our focus puller Johnny said, 'Sod that for a game of soldiers!' and after donning a chef's hat and apron made us all bacon and eggs. The wonderful smell emanating from the kitchen must have attracted the other hotel guests as one by one they came downstairs to the dining room demanding to be fed, so without batting an eyelid Johnny cooked breakfast for them as well.

After filming various scenes in Edinburgh, we drove to Crieff to film some special paperweights at the Caithness glass factory. Richard had the idea of filming through the handcrafted glass objects at some of our locations to create some unique images in-camera. When we shot it the first time at Lock Leven, they looked amazing, so we then filmed similar images at each location.

The miserable weather made it hard to get any good shots, as we ideally needed sunshine to film the Trossachs at their very best. Our first set up was in the tourist town of Callander, described in our travel guide as the 'Gateway to the Highlands'. We went to see the grave of the famous outlaw Rob Roy at Balquhidder Kirkyard before going to dinner. I had booked us into Loch Achray Hotel for the night but the menu didn't look very appealing, so we drove our van into Aberfoyle and ate at Trossachs Kitchen. This was a smart move as we all had one of the best meals any of us had ever eaten. I had venison loin with celeriac puree and roasted carrots, parsnips and roast potatoes. The taste was truly sensational.

As soon as the sun was up, we drove back to the Trossachs to get some scenic shots and I was amazed at how beautiful it looked now the heather had sunlight on it.

'Without understanding light, you can never become a good cameraman,' Ken said to no one in particular, 'and that applies to photographers too.', which he added looking at me.

We arrived in Wales just as it got dark. Ken and Mary treated us to a five-star meal at the Walnut Tree, a fabulous restaurant in Abergavenny. I had Royal sturgeon cooked in plum sauce, which was very tasty but quite rich, so I was grateful my liver had fully recovered.

Our next location was Portmeirion, a quirky mock Italian village which had been used as a location for a number of films and television shows, including *The Prisoner* starring Patrick McGoohan as 'Number Six'. I had the enviable job of driving a red Lotus Éclat through the village as part of one of the scenarios. It was a pretty special moment so I rang Beverley to tell her about it. She said she was envious but when I added I had to climb Mount Snowden in the morning, she was a bit less so.

In the end I had slightly exaggerated, as we only had to climb half a mile up the mountain to get the shot our director was after.

During the shoot, I discovered Ken had a few sayings which he would often repeat at the appropriate moment, which always made me laugh. When asked how long it would take him to set up the shot, he would say, 'Well... 'ow long's a piece of string?' And if our esteemed director asked him if he would prefer to film the scenic view looking to the left or the right, he would reply, 'Well, its six of one and 'alf a dozen of the other really.'

When our filming in Wales was over, we were given a few days off, so I went home to see my parents and to relax for a while as carrying heavy camera gear and tripods is tiring work. I also caught up with Beverley but sadly she wanted to split up and told me what she really wanted was a boyfriend who lived locally and not one who she might only get to see a couple of times each month. I was a bit upset but respected her honesty, which made the break up a bit easier.

The rest of the shoot would be in London, so I quickly needed to find somewhere to live. After a short search, I found somewhere to rent in Barnes. The house was owned by a woman called Susie who worked at the BBC. The room had a Queen-sized bed in which looked a lot comfier than my mate's sofa, so I moved in at the weekend.

Over the next couple of weeks, I organised shoots all over London and on the last day we filmed at the Dorchester Hotel. One of my jobs was to find some unpaid extras. Richard wanted two extras to stand by the reception counter pretending to check in and two others to stand near the lift next to a small table with an enormous vase full of flowers on it while we shot the scene. I had become used to asking strangers to do this everywhere else we had been filming but this time I managed to persuade a couple of 'extras' with a bit more experience than the others. Just as we were about to roll the camera, Roger Moore and Jack Nicholson walked into the hotel, so I went up to them and quickly explained how we were just about to shoot a scene for the British Tourist Authority, and would it be alright if we filmed them as they walked through the lobby. To my amazement they said yes and as they walk through the shot, they were grinning at each other like naughty schoolboys.

I rather suspected they had just come back from a languid liquid lunch.

To mark the end of the shoot, and getting paid, I bought myself *Damn the Torpedos* by Tom Petty and the Heartbreakers. It was an exceptional album with *Refugee* and *Here Comes My Girl* destined to become classics. I hoped I would get to see them play live one day as I had heard they put on a great show.

I went to see Leo Kottke the following evening with my new housemate Susie. Leo's fingerpicking style and unconventional tunings were out of this world. The song which stuck in my head after the gig was over was called *Vaseline Machine Gun.*

At the weekend, Nicol and I took ourselves to Amsterdam and had a great time full of laughs, windmills, canals and art galleries. We went to the Van Gogh Museum and then on to the Rijksmuseum to see the Dutch masters. After seeing the genius of Rembrandt, Vermeer and Brueghel, we took ourselves to the red-light district and flicked through a pile of dirty magazines with images in them I will never unsee. When we got back to our tiny hotel room, I washed my hands for 'a quarter of an hour' like Lady Macbeth lamenting 'will these hands ne'er be clean'.

A week later, I bought a second-hand Renault 5. It was a garish bright yellow but as it only had 30,000 miles on the clock it was too good a deal to miss out on.

I had achieved my goal of working as an assistant director just before turning 25, which I was quite proud of but I also appreciated I had a long way to go before I was likely to get regular work as one. However, it was a good enough start to treat myself to an early birthday present, so I bought *The Long Run* by the Eagles, as the title said it all for me.

I was now in the film industry for the long run.

I had my 25th birthday party at Susie's house, while she was away for the weekend, and invited a group of my friends, including Nicol, Bruce and my old concert cohort Mark and his wife Sarah. I also asked a young woman who I had met on one of our shoots the previous month.

Lorraine was brought up in the East-End of London and had a cockney accent, which having just worked with Ken, Johnny and Dave, I found endearing. I liked her because she was very down to earth and wasn't focused on her good looks, which were obvious for all to see. After handing her a glass of bubbly, she told me she was a legs model and had just done a shoot for Pretty Polly Nylons. The image of her long legs in sexy black stockings could currently be seen on billboards at nearly every underground station in London.

When I said I couldn't wait to see them, she cheekily said, 'Why wait?', so I arranged a private viewing.

The next night we went to Wembley together to see The Moody Blues on the *Out of this World* tour. Their classic songs were all given new life by Swiss musician Patrick Moraz who was now playing keyboards with the band.

For the next few days Lorraine and I got to know each other better and I had high hopes I might have finally found someone to have a long-term relationship with. One night we went to the Scarsdale pub in Kensington to meet Vicki and a few of our mutual friends. While I was at the bar getting the drinks in, Vicki asked Lorraine if my snoring drove her mad, which made them both laugh at my expense but I was pleased to see they were getting along. Just as I was handing them their drinks, Vicki then asked my new girlfriend if she had any bad nocturnal habits and her quick and honest reply made us all laugh out loud, 'On no, I'm good in bed!' I could certainly vouch for her veracity.

In mid-November, we went to see Monty Python's *Life of Brian*, which we loved of course and Eric Idle's song *Always Look on the Bright Side of Life* became our mantra.

When I got a job with Document Films, I had to take a step-backwards again to act as an assistant to Neil Thompson, but I was happy to do so as he who had a reputation for editing films which told fascinating stories, so I could learn from him.

*No Known Grave* was made for BBC's Inside Story. The film was about a Hurricane fighter which had crashed in WW2 and had recently been found with the skeleton of the English pilot still inside it. The investigators worked out it had been shot down in 1940 and eventually tracked down who the pilot was and informed the family, so they could give the poor young man a proper burial. It was a compelling story and while we were editing it Neil told me another.

Pink Floyd's bassist. Roger Waters, lost his father in WW2 when he was just 5 months old and when he was old enough to understand, he was told his father had been reported as 'missing presumed dead' at the Battle of Anzio in Italy in 1944. Pink, the protagonist in Pink Floyd's new double album *The Wall,* grows up longing for a father figure, which resonated with me and I completely understood how he must have felt, having lost my own father when I was only three. After hearing the album for the first time, I thought Roger's lyrics were quite brilliant but noticed the press were giving the album some rather unflattering reviews. The Guardian called it 'a bleak, manic and agonised album'. Needless to say, I didn't agree. The record had a number of great songs on it but *Comfortably Numb* was the stand out track for me and David Gilmour's guitar solo. He used so much sustain it seemed as though he could hold each note forever.

*No Known Grave* was screened at BBC TV in December and everyone there seemed very happy with it. While we were waiting for a taxi outside afterwards, there was a sudden commotion because the Queen had just arrived. When her Majesty got out of her limo, we were all told to stand stock still until she had left, which we did and a minute later our beloved monarch walked past me so closely I could have touched her. We then took a taxi back to the office. The cabbie had his radio on quite loud so I could hear John Graham Mellor, better known as Joe Strummer, singing *London Calling*, which had recently been released by The Clash and had become the latest earworm.

The next day I got a call from Gillie Potter himself to ask me if I would be interested to be his assistant director on a TV commercial the following week, as Ken and Mary had recommended me to him. The job was for Pye Televisions and would feature the wonderful comedian and magician Tommy Cooper, so I said yes, 'Just like that!'

Unfortunately, Tommy changed his mind at the last minute and was replaced by another magician called Paul Daniels. We were all a bit disappointed to start with, as Tommy was such a legend, but when Paul performed some impressive close up magic tricks for us during the lunch break, he won us all over. He took my signet ring and one of Mary's rings and put a pencil through the middle of them both. After placing his left hand over the rings so we could no longer see them but could still see the pencil either side of his hand, he said his irritating catchphrase, 'You'll like this...not a lot, but you'll like it!'

Paul then pulled the pencil out of his left hand with his right hand to reveal both rings were now interlocked despite both being completely solid with no breaks in them. It was impossible of course but thankfully he then did the impossible again and reversed the trick so we could have our rings back. I still have no idea how he did it.

Working with Gillie was a great fun and I dearly hoped I would get another chance to assist him again in the new year.

Christmas was quiet affair this year as it was just me and my parents. The rest of the family were busy doing their own thing but New Year's Eve was a different kettle of fish, as Bruce and his brother Bob, Nicol and a couple of our other mates performed the Mummers play again, and this time I was Saint George. We repeated our performance at seven different pubs in a row, and as free drinks were provided at each one, our inebriated impromptu innuendos got ruder as the evening wore on. However, they also created much laughter everywhere we went. Despite our unprofessional antics, our intentions were honourable, and we managed to raise a decent amount of money for charity.

What better way to end the 1970s.

*Perseverance is not a long race; it is many short races one after the other.*

Walter Elliot

## CHAPTER 17: COMFORTABLY NUMB

On the 1st of January 1980, I received a phone call from Lorraine to let me know she had met someone else over the Christmas break and hoped I would understand. I was really upset as I hoped our relationship would last. Listening to Pink Floyd's *The Wall* helped for a while until I got to *Comfortably Numb*, which was when I began to feel a bit sorry for myself, so to 'ease the pain and get back on my feet again', I went to the pub to drown my sorrows with my mates.

The following weekend, my godmother Puck invited me to a smart drinks party at their house about an hour's drive outside of London. 'Make sure you wear a suit and a tie please!' she ordered. I adored Puck and her husband George, who knew my father during the war. Their daughter called Liz, whose nickname was Mops, was a year younger than me. We got on so well we were more like siblings.

At the party, Mops introduced me to some of her parent's friends who had a young American girl staying with them for the weekend. Cheryl was petite, pretty and polite, studying law at Bologna University and heading back to Italy in the morning. When I asked her what she was doing later in the evening, she told me she was going to a classical concert at the Royal Albert Hall with her hosts and showed me her ticket, which is when I memorised the seat number and came up with a ridiculous, but hopefully rather romantic idea.

As soon as Cheryl and her friends left the party to head to the concert, I waited a couple of minutes, said my goodbyes and drove back to London as fast as I could. All I needed now was a bunch of flowers but half way back I realised had no cash on me, so it was time for Plan B.

Having filmed at the Dorchester Hotel quite recently, I remembered there was always a huge bunch of flowers on the table near the lift, so I drove straight there, double parked illegally and said to the doorman as I went into the hotel, 'Good to see you again Tom!' before walking across the lobby to the table by the lift. I lifted the flowers out of the vase, and I use the word advisedly, and calmly walked back to my car. I think the only reason I wasn't challenged by anyone was because I was still wearing my suit and tie, so looked as if I belonged there.

When I got to the Royal Albert Hall, I wrote a short message telling Cheryl how much I enjoyed meeting her and asking her to call me before she left for Italy and then persuaded one of the stewards to put the flowers and the note on Cheryl's seat for me. I just hoped I had memorised the correct seat number. I suffered a mild panic-attack on the way home, wondering if instead of finding it romantic, she might think I was a stalker, but it was far too late now.

I was just about to turn in for the night when the phone rang. It was Cheryl. Thankfully she loved the flowers and invited me to come to Italy at the end of her next term and go travelling together.

'Sì, grazie mille!' I said, which were the first three words I ever spoke in Italian.

As I had a whole month before going to Italy, I had time for a couple more concerts. The first was Blondie at the Hammersmith Odeon. The band were on top form and their set included *Heart of Glass* and *Hanging on the Telephone*. The delectable Debbie Harry sang a great cover version of the Randy and the Rainbows song *Denise* and towards the end they did a cover of Bowie's *Heroes,* so one way and another it was a pretty special night.

A month later I saw Wishbone Ash at the same venue with Andy Powell and Laurie Wisefield on lead guitars. They played a few songs from their new album *Just Testing* but it was material from their older albums which really got the crowd going, especially midway through *Blowin' Free* when everyone screamed '1-2-3-4' at the top of their lungs to cue the band back in after a gentle instrumental passage.

On the 19th of February Bon Scott the singer with AC/DC died while he was in London, which upset me a lot. I was sad I hadn't been able to see him perform live while I was in Australia and hoped the band would find a way to continue without him.

Three days later, I flew from Luton Airport to Bologna and Cheryl met me off the plane. We had a quick drink together and then took the crowded night train to Naples, spending most of the night sitting on the dirty corridor floor. When we arrived the next morning, it was still so early all the cafes were still shut, so we took a taxi to the Palace of Capodimonte and walked through the park until we found a secluded spot to lie down and rest. When the museum opened, we looked at all the masterpieces on display including paintings by Michelangelo, Titian, Botticelli and Raphael. I enjoyed Cheryl's company and her interest in a different culture to her own reminded me of why I like travelling to foreign countries so much.

We stayed the night at the equivalent of an Italian YMCA and slept in the same dormitory but in separate beds, as Cheryl made it clear she only wanted us to be friends. Although I was a bit disappointed initially, as she was so attractive as well as highly intelligent, I respected her wishes and was genuinely happy to have a new female friend who shared my passion for travel, music and art.

The ferry ride to the Isle of Capri took about an hour. When we got there we then got into a small wooden boat and were taken to a sea cave known as the Blue Grotto. When we arrived, our guide rowed us inside where the sea was a bright crystalline blue, which looked like it had been artificially lit from underneath rather than by passing sunlight. It was an unforgettable moment made even better by being shared with such a lovely woman.

The next morning, we took a train to Pozzuoli. This was the place where Caligula ordered a floating bridge to be constructed across the sea when he became Emperor, so he could cross from the town to nearby Baiae on his horse, just so he could defy an astrologer who made the prediction he had 'no more chance of becoming Emperor than of riding a horse across the gulf of Baiae.' Afterwards we took a coach to Pompeii to see the remains of the Roman city which were destroyed when Mount Vesuvius erupted in 79 AD. It was hard to imagine the absolute terror the citizens must have felt as tons of volcanic ash engulfed them. Seeing the preserved bodies of a couple of the victims was enough to make us weep. Just as we were leaving, we saw a large group of Nuns wearing black habits and veils with white caps and wimples, carefully walking over the cobbled stones in a long line one behind the other. It was an amusing sight. Cheryl asked me if I knew the correct term for a collective of nuns. I hadn't a clue, but told her I did know a group of penguins was called a waddle and a herd of zebras known as a dazzle, but this was the limit of my knowledge of collective names for groups of black and white creatures.

For future reference and reverence, it's a superfluity of nuns.

I wish we had spent more time in Sorrento, as it was a stunning little town. We had lunch in the Piazza Tasso and I enjoyed taking a stroll through the old streets. The peaceful atmosphere was broken for a moment when we heard the piercing sound of a siren getting closer to us but after a police car came into view and drove right past us at speed, it all went quiet again. Hearing a siren wail here was rather apt as Sorrento is thought to be the home of the mythological sirens who lured sailors onto the rocks with their beautiful voices.

While Cheryl did some shopping, I wandered into a record store and looked at the latest albums on sale. American singer-songwriter Christopher Cross had just released a self-titled album, which contained the song *Ride like the Wind*, featuring backing vocals by part-time Doobie Brother Michael McDonald. There was a fabulous guitar solo by Chris at the end, which blew me away. I did a bit of research on him at a later date and discovered he had once been asked to fill in for legendary guitarist Richie Blackmore. On the 28th of August 1970, Deep Purple were about to perform at the Jam Factory in San Antonio, Texas, when Richie became unwell, so as it was Chris' hometown and Joe Miller, the promoter knew what a great guitarist he was he asked him to step in. Luckily, Chris was a huge fan of the band and knew how to play some of the songs already and for the rest of the gig they played some blues jams and covers of The Rolling Stones' *Paint It Black* and Little Richard's *Lucille*. Finding out fun 'alleged' facts like this fills me with joy.

Meanwhile back in Italy…We all know Rome wasn't built in a day but as we discovered it can't be thoroughly explored in just one either, so Cheryl and I allowed ourselves three and still didn't see everything we had on our wish list. We started at the Pantheon and walked to the Trevi Fountain where I threw a coin over my left shoulder, using my right hand just as they had done in the movie *Three Coins in the Fountain*, made in 1954, the same year I was born. When we got to The Spanish Steps, I remembered Audrey Hepburn had eaten an ice-cream there in the film *Roman Holiday*, so we did the same.

The Colosseum, the Forum and Palatine Hill were all full of interesting history and I loved going back in time trying to imagine what it must have been like when Rome was in its heyday and everybody spoke in Latin. Once we were inside the ancient amphitheatre, which could hold up to 50,000 spectators when it was still in use, I could almost hear the roar of the crowds in my head as they watched the gladiators fight each other to death in the arena below.

Cheryl suggested we get up at the crack of dawn, so we would be first in line to see the Sistine chapel and it proved to be a wise decision, as although we arrived at 8am, some other early birds had already beaten us to it and within another twenty minutes the queue behind us was as far as we could see.

As soon as the Vatican doors opened everyone rushed in. Fortunately, most tourists usually start in the rooms closest to the entrance, so Cheryl and I did the opposite and walked as fast as we could through the empty galleries to get to the chapel before anyone else. As soon as we were inside the room, I lay on the floor on my back, took a deep breath to steady myself and took a photograph of Michelangelo's wonderful fresco on the chapel ceiling. I then swopped lenses so I could get a close up of God reaching out to touch Adam. Less than two minutes later the chapel was completely full, so we decided to take a quick look at The Last Supper, but not the one we were taught about at school. There are actually quite a few works of art with the same title, but the one I was interested to see was a fresco by Italian Renaissance artists Cosimo Rosselli and Biagio d'Antonio. What they did differently to the other artists who portrayed the same scene was to put Judas on the viewer's side of the table to show we are also sinners. But what I wanted to see was how they painted the table in a U shape, as it demonstrated they understood how to create perspective, like taking a photo with a wide-angle lens. Learning about all the different lenses had become my latest project as I constantly wanted to improve my knowledge about all the tools available for making movies.

In the afternoon we took a coach to Villa D'Este in Tivoli, about an hour from Rome. The 16th Century villa was breathtakingly beautiful and the terraced gardens were magnificent. I don't think I have ever seen so many fountains in one place. 500 of them in all or thereabouts.

When we arrived in Florence, the first thing I took a photo of was the Cathedral of Santa Maria del Fore. Filippo Brunelleschi's Dome is the largest masonry vault in the world. It was hard to believe it was built without a supporting structure. Michelangelo's David was next on our list and the statue was even more impressive than I expected. The fact he was only 26 when he started this marble masterpiece made me re-think my own achievements, as I would be the same age on my next birthday.

The Uffizi must rank as one of the best art galleries anywhere. Their collections of paintings, statues and busts were outstanding. Seeing 'The Birth of Venus' by Botticelli in the flesh, so to speak, was a bit special but having seen Monty Python's animated sketch 'The Venus Painting Dance', I was half expecting Venus to start dancing and fall out of the shell into the water. I loved Caravaggio's 'Medusa' and I also admired Titian's erotic nude painting 'Venus of Urbino. It looked quite tasteful to me but it had once been considered pornographic.

The Ponte Vecchio was looking very picturesque so I took a few photos before we head off to the Boboli Gardens to have a picnic with some of Cheryl's friends. The view of the Duomo from there was lovely and the perfect place to end our short Florentine sojourn.

The next part of our mini-adventure was a bit quick but we decided it would better to try to see as much as we could of Pisa and Sienna in the short time we had left, just in case we never got the chance to go back. After making sure The Leaning Tower of Pisa was still leaning by nearly four degrees due to its unstable foundation and discovering Pisa and Pizza are not connected in any way, we became temporary experts on Pisa's famous gelato. The best flavour was rose and pistachio. It was filled with only natural ingredients and had no artificial colouring, or so we were told.

Having a second one 'sulla casa' was an offer we couldn't refuse.

When we got to Siena, we climbed the Torre del Mangia so we could look down at the Piazza del Campo where they hold the famous Palio horse race. From the top of the bell tower, we could also admire the medieval architecture of this beautiful city.

In Venice, we stayed at a hotel near the Rialto Bridge, which was a bit more expensive than the cheap ones we had previously slept in but the central location was worth the extra cost, as we could walk over the Grand Canal and get to San Marco Square in under ten minutes. From there we walked to and through the Giardini Reali, a park on the waterfront, to get to the Doges Palace and Saint Mark's Basilica, which housed the Pala d'Oro, an incredibly ornate mural behind the high altar. As we wanted to know more about it we hired some headsets but it was too hard to understand what the narrator was saying as he was speaking English with such a strong Italian accent it made certain words unintelligible. The narrator told us there were 250 animals in the mural but however hard I looked I could only see 4 birds and 2 lions. The man's voice then told us these animals were 'zemi pressure us, which confused us even more. It was only after I borrowed another tourist's pamphlet written in English, I realised what he had been trying to say was there were 250 enamels in the mural and they were semi-precious. We laughed so loudly we had to leave the church before we got thrown out by one of the nuns.

After taking the train back to Bologna, Cheryl insisted I accompany her to the Teatro Comunale di Bologna in the evening to see *Otello*. I am not a fan of opera but I must admit watching one from the gallery in this magnificent opera house was a real privilege.

Two days after I got back to England, I went to see Peter Gabriel at the Hammersmith Odeon. This time his setlist included quite a few songs from his third album, including *Intruder, Family Snapshot, Not One of Us* and *Biko*. His talented band were extremely tight and I loved every minute of the show. I still had the uplifting *Solsbury Hill* playing in my head the next morning when I got a call from Harry Bruce offering me some more work as an assistant editor but this time it be on a feature film called *Maya*. Although it was a short job it paid well and was just what I needed to help recoup some of the money I had spent on my Roman holiday.

When I got a call from Mary Evans at Gillie Potter Productions asking me if I would like to edit the British Tourist Authority film, which we had shot the year before, I was thrilled, as apart from getting a decent film to edit it also gave me the chance to work with Ken and Mary again.

Editing the images for *Its Good to be Here* was quite straightforward as having been there when it was filmed, I knew all the shots off by heart, but tracklaying the sound was much harder as we had filmed everything mute to save costs, so it was down to me to re-create the right background atmosphere for each scene and also choose the music. I was in my element as this was just the sort of challenge I thrive on.

On the 10th of April Vicki and I went to see Jethro Tull at the Hammersmith Odeon and they played a few songs from their *Stormwatch* album. The live versions of *Dark Ages, Dun Ringill* and *Something's On The Move* sounded even better than on the record. The rest of the setlist was peppered with old favourites like *Aqualung, Heavy Horses, Songs from the Wood, Thick as a Brick* and *Minstrel in the Gallery*. As a longstanding Tull fan, it couldn't have been better.

A couple of days later, Ken asked me to help out on a small visual effects sequence for the movie *Superman 2*, which was a bit of a thrill. He had done the same in-camera effect a couple of years earlier for the original *Superman* but as the aspect ratio for the sequel was going to be different, they were going to have to start from scratch this time.

*Superman* was shot in 35mm in the widest aspect ratio; known as anamorphic widescreen format but the follow up was going to be screened in 70mm, so a different ratio was needed. It was all a bit technical for me so Ken explained, 'Aspect ratio is how the width and height of the screened image is described.'

'Right got it... I think,' I replied not really getting it at all.

The scene we worked on was where General Zod, played by Terence Stamp, and his followers Non and Ursa, were all banished to the Phantom Zone as punishment for trying to take over the planet Krypton. The action involved a 2D mirror prison floating through space before capturing the prisoners inside it. This would have been an easy task with today's computer-generated imagery (CGI) but in those days we had to achieve it the old-fashioned way, which involved using a single-frame projector to screen the footage onto an eight-inch square piece of white cardboard which had been firmly mounted onto a stand we could rotate 360 degrees by hand one frame at a time.

The idea was to film the empty mirror prison flying towards and away from camera and then do almost identical shots with the criminals now trapped inside it, to and away from camera. To make this happen 'in-camera', we rotated a zoom lens from one extreme to the other to make the square smaller or larger at the same time as sliding our large heavy but solid Mitchell camera backwards, or forwards as the shot demanded, on a handmade dolly, which was made by Dave and Johnny re-utilising some discarded scaffolding. Although it all looked rather unsophisticated it was remarkably smooth and did its job perfectly.

Because we were filming in stop-motion, meaning only one frame at a time, we had to calibrate every single move of every frame of the projected image onto the cardboard square, as well as the zoom rotation and the camera moves in tiny increments, all marked up on white camera tape with a pencil.

Ken and Dave took charge of the camera moves, Johnny was in charge of the zoom and I was given the task of aligning every frame of the live action footage projected onto the cardboard square so it fitted correctly every time it was moved. It was extremely complicated and took many hours to get it right but the end result worked rather well.

After we finished our shots, they were sent to the optical printing department at Pinewood Studios and they combined what we had shot with the relevant backgrounds to create the composite shots which would then be edited into the movie.

Working as an assistant director on a cinema commercial for Dewar's Scotch Whisky was a doddle. Paddy Carpenter was the director and as he had loads of experience it went very smoothly and was a really enjoyable shoot. Dewar's distillery is based in Aberfeldy, so when I told the client it was the town where I was born, he insisted I have my photo taken with the Dewar's Pipe Major who we had filmed earlier in the day. Thankfully he was a true gentleman, meaning although he knew how to play the bagpipes… he didn't.

Paddy asked me if I would like to edit the commercial, so I said yes straightaway but when I had a quick look in the edit room, I discovered to my horror instead of a flatbed Steenbeck, which I was used to editing with, they had an old-fashioned Moviola machine and I had absolutely no idea how to use it.

Luckily for me, Harry Bruce came to the rescue. After giving him a call to explain my problem, he told me to come to Cherill's after work and he would see what he could do to help. When I got there, he told me to have a word with Gerry Hambling, who I had already met and watched cutting a commercial. I had forgotten he loved working on a Moviola, even insisting on using one when asked to work on more modern systems. I was a bit nervous to start with but he was a very patient teacher. I stood in front of his editing machine and looked down at a small viewing screen, which allowed me to view each individual shot very closely. I then had to determine precisely where to make my cut, which took me a while to get right but once I had done it a few times, I felt confident I could manage on my own the following day. Before I left, Gerry told me the Moviola would teach me to appreciate the value of each and every frame. He was absolutely right and I have never forgotten his words or his kindness to me.

Editing the Dewar's TVC went to plan and after getting the fine cut approved by the client, I decided it was time to have a few beers, so I asked Mary's brother Jim, who composed the music for the spot, and his brother Bill who was also a muso, to come out with me to celebrate. We ended up at the Half Moon in Putney and just as we arrived the music started.

The band was led by Ronnie Lane, the bassist from The Faces and his band featured Henry McCulloch on guitar and Ian 'Stu' Stewart on piano. Henry had been the guitarist for Paul McCartney's Wings and Stu had played with Led Zeppelin and The Rolling Stones.

A fun night was had by all and I got home very late but my housemate Susie was still up and chatting with an old friend of hers, Spike Milligan, the creative force and main writer of The Goon Show. I couldn't help but notice his eyes were red, as if he had been crying but he smiled at me when he shook my hand vigorously and said, 'I'm sorry but I am having a bad case of the shakes today!'

When Susie offered to make us a cup of coffee, Spike told me she had mentioned I lived in Australia for a while, which he found interesting as he had been there quite a few times. In fact, his parents emigrated there in the 1950s.

'They lived in Woy Woy. The world's only above-ground cemetery!' Spike joked. It was obvious this wasn't the first time he had said it but we both laughed as if it was.

When I told him I was thinking about going back he said, 'You should... and soon!'

I took his comment as my cue and went to bed, so they could continue talking in private.

In the morning, Susie told me how Spike often came to her flat for a late-night chat as he suffered from bipolar disorder and knew she would be understanding as well as be discreet. It had been an honour to meet the comic genius, albeit briefly, but I was sad to find out he had such crippling anxiety and depression. However, it was good to know he had such a kind friend who had his back and would always be there for him.

On the 16th April Eric Clapton's double album *Just One Night* was released and it soon became one of my favourite live albums of all time. His guitar solos were superb especially on the cover versions of *Tulsa Time* (Danny Flowers), *After Midnight* (J.J. Cale) and *Setting Me Up* (Mark Knopfler) but the best tracks for me were *Blues Power* because of Chris Stainton's boogie woogie piano and Eric's Wah-Wah solo, which must rank as one of his best of all time, and the encore *Further on Up the Road,* which features a sublime solo by second guitarist Albert Lee.

A week later, I got another call from Gillie Potter, as he had been asked to direct a TVC for Braun and wondered if I would be interested in co-directing it with him. I was very flattered until he told me what the product was. A cleaning system for false teeth!

I met the German client at the studio and the first thing he told me was Braun was pronounced 'Brown' in Germany but pronounced 'Brawn' in England. When I asked him why, he told me their UK offices were based in Staines and after hearing their cockney receptionist answering the phone by saying, 'Good morning, Brown Staines here!' they decided it might be a good idea to change it.

While I was editing the commercial, I was able to talk to Gillie about how he achieved some of his in-camera tricks. He knew more about film optical effects than anyone I had ever met before, so it was like having my own private masterclass.

On the 20th of May, Mary and Ken decided to have a lunch party to celebrate the success of the British Tourist Authority film and asked me if I would like to invite my mother. Mum was thrilled to be asked and interested to see who I had been working with on and off for so long. Mary's sister Cath, did the catering and Johnny told some rather close-to-the-bone jokes, which thankfully weren't too rude for my mother to hear and she thoroughly enjoyed herself.

In the evening, I took Mum to see SKY at Hammersmith Odeon. The band comprised of Australian classical guitarist John Williams and Kevin Peek on guitars, Herbie Flowers on bass, Tristan Fry on drums and Francis Monkman, ex-Curved Air, on Keyboards. I had no idea what my mother would make of their music but to my surprise, and perhaps hers too, she loved them.

After the concert finished, Mum asked me if she could meet John Williams, so we went to the stage door and asked if this was possible. It was, so we both got to meet the guitar virtuoso whose *Theme from The Deer Hunter – Cavatina* my mother liked so much. Mum chatted with him while I talked to Kevin Peek, who told me he lived in Western Australia, so if I was ever there to look him up. 'Kev' then introduced me to the legendary Herbie Flowers who had played bass for George Harrison, Elton John and David Bowie and had created the memorable bass line on Lou Reed's *Walk on the Wild Side*. It was a truly memorable night and to have shared it with my mother made it pretty special.

At the weekend, Ken's son, Andy, drove down to Keyhaven to stay with me at my parent's house. He had the same cockney accent as his father and was just as much fun. I took him to our local pub The Gun and while we were there, we met three young women who were standing next to us ordering their drinks at the bar. Two of them said they were from Kuala Lumpur and the other one was from Hong Kong. Jackie, as her name turned out to be, was very attractive and had a laugh like a snorting warthog, which made us all laugh. She told me her parents owned a house in Lymington but also had homes in Hong Kong and Australia, dividing their time between the three. Now there's a lifestyle to aspire to I thought.

The following weekend, Andy and I headed up to Oxford to stay at his girlfriend Linda's house as they were having a party. It ended up being a very boozy couple of days but enormous fun as Linda had a wicked sense of humour.

When Linda told me she was going to Australia at the end of the year on a working holiday, I told her what it was like there and what to expect.

A week after I got back to London, I got a call from Vicki to let me know her friend Nick had asked her if she knew anyone who might like to rent his spare room in Earls Court, so she had thought of me.

As it would be much easier to get to work from there than from Barnes, I left Susie's two weeks later and moved into Nick's flat in Old Brompton Road.

I wasn't particularly interested to see *The Rocky Horror Show* yet again but thought it might be a good way to bond with my new flatmate, and I was glad I did as Tim McInnerny's comic timing as Frank'N'Furter was superb. A young comedian called Adrian Edmondson played Brad and Janet was played by the hilarious and glamorous Gina Bellman.

At the end of June, my kindergarten friend Mark and his wife Sarah told me they were emigrating to Australia. Part of me would have liked to have gone with them but for now I was happy where I was.

I got a job a week later, directing a two-minute title sequence for a new TV series called *Something in Disguise.* I was very excited as this was exactly the kind of work, which I had hoped to get one day after I attending the lecture by Saul Bass when I was still at Film school. I only got the break as Gillie was busy elsewhere and didn't have time to do it himself. The graphic designer was a talented concept artist called Rob and his idea was to get the main actors faces to appear in the clouds above a miniature model of a stately home which featured in the series. Rob and his team painted various images of the actor's faces in the clouds in different positions on large sheets of celluloid for Ken, Johnny, Dave and I to film in sequence, so when the images were played back at normal speed it would look like the clouds were moving naturally across the sky. It worked brilliantly and although it was all Rob's idea and Ken's lighting, I was given my first credit as a director.

In July, I went to see ex-Genesis guitarist Steve Hackett on his *Defector* tour at Hammersmith Odeon. Steve's unique guitar style wows the audience every time. *The Steppes* from his new album and *Spectral Mornings* from his last one got the biggest cheers of the night.

I had read *The Hitchhikers Guide to the Galaxy* the year before and loved it, so I was really looking forward to seeing how they would perform the book live at the Rainbow Theatre. Unfortunately, it wasn't done very well and went on, and on for an uncomfortable three hours. I thought it was a very disappointing performance but I did enjoy seeing David Lerner as Marvin the Paranoid Android, as he really milked the robot's lines for all his worth.

'Life! Don't talk to me about life!' and 'I think you ought to know I'm feeling very depressed.'

'Say Cheese!' Mary said as I walked into their office, so I looked for a camera there were none to be found. Ken then explained how they had just been asked to produce a TVC for Roquefort Cheese for a French client and, as Gillie was still away, they wanted me to direct it. Roquefort is a blue cheese made from ewe's milk, which smells disgusting, as we soon discovered when twenty large cylindrical wheels of cheese known as truckles were delivered to our small underground and windowless studio later the following day. The brief was to make it look like a sheep and her baby lamb were walking across frame from right to left using truckles as the body, a slice of the cheese as the head and animation to create the animal's legs.

The set was quite simple and consisted of a large sheet of white Perspex which was lit from underneath and a piece of polystyrene was then placed three feet above it to bounce the light back onto the top of the cheese. However, as cheese and hot lights don't really mix well, the smell soon became quite impossible and we had to rent an industrial size freezer to keep the product cool. Ken was the cameraman and his usual team of Johnny and Dave were also on hand. It was a painstaking shoot but we got it done and once the cheese pieces had been shot, we handed our footage over to an animator who drew red knives and forks in place of the sheep's legs, which was a rather quirky idea but worked très bien. The leftover truckles of cheese were offered to anyone who wanted one to take one home. But despite being a rather splendid, if somewhat smelly fromage, there were no takers. Even our French client said waving his hands animatedly in the air, 'Non merci…Bon Dieu non!'

Nicol's old school chum Randle, lived in Walton-on-Thames and I was invited to stay with them one weekend. Randle had two sisters and a brother who immediately made me feel like part of their family. Their mother was a retired-history teacher and I loved chatting to her as she knew so much and taught me more historical facts than I ever learned at school.

When one of Randle's friends announced she was having a 1960s party, we were all invited but only on one condition. Fancy-dress was compulsory. I was a bit unsure about how to do this but Randle's sisters had an idea. One of them found an old black dress and the other padded a bra with old newspapers. After they put mascara and lipstick on my face, they placed a wig on my head and when I saw myself in the mirror, I was looking back at a rather dodgy version of 60's *Ready, Steady, Go* presenter Cathy McGowan!

My sister would have laughed if she had seen me as she was a guest on the show once; talking about her fashion designs and afterwards Sandie Shaw sang *Puppet on a String*.

Luckily, I wasn't the only one who looked a prat as both Nicol and Randle had made a similar effort and when we looked in the mirror we couldn't stop laughing. As soon as we arrived at the party, which was already in full swing, I lost confidence as I felt such a dick being cross-dressed, if that isn't a contradiction in terms, but Nicol quickly put my mind at rest by comparing our costumes to the Mummer's plays we had both been in on New Year's Eve.

The only way to overcome my shyness, shame and fear of ridicule was to start drinking as soon as and for as long as possible. I got increasingly drunk as the night progressed. Just before midnight a lovely looking blonde called Annette told me she was not only amused by my amateur attempt at female impersonation but also weirdly aroused. Things then got a lot weirder when she told me she had been a nurse for the last seven years, so knew her anatomy and now wanted to get to know mine.

As Kenneth Williams said in the film *Carry On Doctor,* 'Oooh Matron!'*Rank Organisation 1967

I woke up feeling hungover but happy. Life got even better when

Aussie rock band AC/DC released *Back in Black*. They now had Brian Johnson as their new singer who was previously in a band called Geordie. The album was sensational and I played it as loud as possible whenever possible. When Nicol rang me to talk about it we agreed the best tracks were. *Hells Bells, Let Me Put My Love into You, Back in Black* and *Rock and Roll Ain't Noise Pollution.*

As Di and Julie were the ones who introduced me to the group when I was in Melbourne, I wrote to tell them I was thinking of them while listening to the album and was surprised, when I got their reply, to hear the record hadn't been released in Australia yet, but they would both buy a copy as soon as it was available. I suddenly missed Australia terribly, especially the friends I made when I was there and wondered whether I would ever see them again. I really hoped so but at the moment I was having too much fun. I had a couple of credits under my belt as a director, I had attended some great gigs and I now had a new girlfriend.

1980 was proving to be rather productive year... and it was still only August.

*'Take care of all your memories.' Said my friend Nick. 'For you cannot relive them.'*
Bob Dylan

## CHAPTER 18: TUNNEL OF LOVE

Taking charge of a 30-foot yacht is a very special experience and I felt blessed whenever I was given the opportunity. Having sailed down to Cornwall numerous times and across to France once or twice, my parents were more than happy to have a break and let me take the helm. I made sure we never went above 4 knots but it always felt like we were going much faster. The Solent was beautiful at this time of year and seeing my folks looking so happy made me feel grateful to have them in my life, as they always believed in me and encouraged me to be myself.

Half an hour after we got back to my parent's house in Keyhaven, I received a call from Mary to let me know the Roquefort commercial had been approved by the client, so I could send them my invoice, which was good to know as I had a few outstanding bills to pay.

My next directing job started less than a week later. This time the commercial was for a Belgian company and the product was a margarine made of corn oil called Natura. Our brief was to film a single corn on the cob, as it revolved 45 degrees anti-clockwise, while its leaves peeled off by themselves just as the sun was rising, revealing the rest of the field of corn in the background now bathed in the early morning light. We achieved it by making a life-size model of a corn on the cob with mock leaves and husk which could be animated in tiny increments as we turned the cob on a miniature turntable. The dawn sun was created by covering a small light with an orange gel and by using a dimmer switch we could also move frame by frame using stop-motion, which took about fourteen hours and needed a lot of patience. It was a bit tricky but we were happy with the end results and more importantly, so was the client.

A week later I was asked to supervise some voice-overs at John Wood studios in Soho. The first one was with Michael Jayston, who played Tsar Nicholas 11 in the movie *Nicholas and Alexandra* and the next one was with Hannah Gordon, the actress who was in the TV series *Upstairs, Downstairs.* She also appeared on the *Morecambe & Wise 1973 Christmas Special*, so after we finished, I asked her what it was like to work with Eric and Ernie when they made her sing *Windmills of Your Mind* while doing their comedic antics behind her back on a large prop windmill. She said it was almost impossible to keep a straight face, as the pair were so funny. I got to do another one a few days later. This time it was with BBC Breakfast radio host Terry Wogan, who was absolutely charming, but he also enjoyed telling some rather vulgar jokes which you might describe as more 'In your-end-o' than innuendo. The last voice-over session was with Patrick Allen, who had appeared in many films, including *Dial M for Murder, The Eagle Has Landed* and *Force 10 from Navarone.* Patrick had a very distinctive voice and as he got so much narration work, he set up his own recording studio. After we finished the job, he suggested I should consider doing voice-overs. When I told my friends what he said they all laughed and said, 'Why not! You've got the perfect face for radio!'

On the 25th of September, John Bonham, the drummer for Led Zeppelin, died after drinking 40 shots of vodka before choking on his own vomit in his sleep. He was only 32. As I thought the track *Fool in the Rain* demonstrated Bonzo's incredible talent at its very best, I played it three times in a row and drank a shot of vodka each time in his honour.

When Ken and Mary asked me if I would take the Gillie Potter Productions showreel to a few advertising agencies in Paris to try and get them some work, I said, 'Oui s'il te plaît et merci.' I stayed in a tiny hotel with an even tinier room but I didn't mind one bit as this was my first work overseas trip where everything was paid for by someone else. After a breakfast of strong black coffee and a croissant while looking up a few new words in my Berlitz French for Travellers, I was ready for action. I saw six different agencies on the first day. All the creative directors had great names like Thierry, Jacques, Dominique, Franco and Chantal but the one who was impressed most by the showreel and promised he would give us a job was called...

Paddy.

The following weekend, I moved into my friend James' house in Turnham Green. We had known each other for years and had mutual friends in the New Forest, but he had a different set of friends in London so whenever he went to a dinner party, I also got invited. James really enjoyed a glass of red wine as soon as he got home from work and encouraged me to share this rather civilised habit with him. It soon became a ritual with the words 'Chin, chin!' said before each glass was consumed. I thought the toast was Italian but James corrected me and said it was actually derived from an ancient Chinese greeting 'qǐng' made popular by European merchants and later adopted by the Italians. Not a lot of people know that!

One evening after polishing off a particularly good bottle of Napa Valley red, we discussed our individual experiences of going to boarding school and being bullied. It brought back some painful memories but after James told me about some of the awful goings on at his school, I felt my experiences were minor by comparison. While topping up my glass, my friend asked me if I had ever told my mother about it, as he had been reluctant to tell his parents because he had been told it was a normal rite of passage. I told him I had felt much the same at the time and didn't want to tell her now in case she thought I was blaming her for sending me away to such a ghastly institution. We had both survived boarding school and felt this deserved a toast.

'Chin chin!' we said in unison.

As I had been busy directing commercials recently, I hadn't had much time to take any photos, so I bought myself a second-hand Nikon FE with a Nikkor 28mm lens with the intention of doing some photography as soon as possible. My new purchase coincided with an invitation from my sister to visit her in Mallorca for a few days. When I arrived at her house in Establiments, Nicci's four children all rushed out to greet me and after a huge hug-fest they took me to see the latest addition to the family, a beautiful horse called Bonnie. This was the perfect opportunity to try out my camera and after taking a group photo I then got them to all jump into the pool at the same time so I could take an action shot, capturing them in mid-air.

While I was on the island, we did a day trip to Pueblo Español to see a mock Spanish village which featured reproductions of some of the most famous houses in Spain. I quite enjoyed seeing the different styles of architecture but as the children had been there before, it didn't take them long to get bored and demand to be taken to the beach. Feeling the sun on my skin was bliss and the ocean was incredibly clear so I had a swim in the shallows while my nieces and nephew did their dolphin impersonations further out to sea.

When I got back to London, I was pleasantly surprised to find a message from Jackie, telling me she was back in London and asking me to give her a call. We met up the following evening and she made me laugh with stories about growing up in Hong Kong and it didn't take long before I was completely under her spell. Fortunately, she felt the same way about me and we spent the next 24 hours together getting better acquainted. Over the next few weeks, we saw each other as often as we could and one night, she treated me to dinner at a posh restaurant and told me she loved me. I felt the same about her but as she was about to go back to Hong Kong fairly soon and we had no idea when we would see each other again, I didn't think this was the right time to make any long-term commitment. Jackie agreed, or at least said she did, and a week later she left the country but with the promise she would stay in touch.

On the 17th of October, Dire Straits released *Making Movies.* Mark Knopfler's guitar playing on this album was remarkable and his storytelling skills were his best to date. The opening track *Tunnel of Love* told the story of a boy falling for a girl about not wanting to spoil the relationship by getting in too deep, so it resonated with my feelings for Jackie, who I was missing a lot. I loved *Romeo and Juliet* of course as it was so beautiful but the track which really triggered my imagination was *Skateaway.* This song told the story of a girl who listens to a rock'n'roll station on her headphones, as she roller-skates around the city 'making movies on location' in her head. I can still see her now! Toro! Toro! Taxi!

The next TV commercial I directed was for Danone. The food company had recently replaced the preformed plastic yoghurt pot with what they called the Erca pot, which was cylindrical with a paper flap on top. The brief was to see the old pot floating in space like a satellite, with the Earth as seen from space, floating behind it. As the sun came up over the Earth's horizon, the silhouette of the old pot had to change into the shape of the new pot and when it floated nearer to the camera, we would see the Danone name on it for the first time.

To make this vison a reality, we mounted a 3-foot circumference globe, painted with wispy clouds to look like the images of Earth from space, onto a small mechanical rig which allowed us to spin the globe one frame at a time. A starry background was created by hanging a large black backdrop between two stands and making hundreds of tiny holes in it with a set of darts which were lying around the office. After hanging long silver ribbons made from torn rolls of aluminium kitchen foil from a cross bar, the same height as the top of our backdrop, we pointed a light onto the shredded curtain and aimed a small fan on them. When the ribbons moved, they shone the reflected light through the black backdrop and voila. Twinkle, Twinkle Little Stars!

After Ken, Dave and Johnny patiently listened to me explain how I wanted to set up the shots, Ken asked. 'Is that it?'

'Yes, that's it.' I replied feeling rather pleased with myself.

'Right then my old China,' Ken said with a grin, 'In that case, as you are now the only one not busy setting up the shot, you can go and make us all a nice cup of tea', so I did.

Ken was very good at keeping my feet firmly on the ground and he never let me get above myself, which I will always be grateful for. I once heard him say, 'There's no room for egos if you want to be part of a successful team.' Thankfully he wasn't talking about me at the time.

On the 12th of November, Nicol and I went to see AC/DC at the Hammersmith Odeon and it was a truly memorable gig right from the first chime of the enormous bell hanging from the stage ceiling. As soon as new frontman Brian Johnson started singing *Hells Bells* the crowd went wild. The band were in fine form and Angus Young played his guitar like a man possessed, especially on *Highway to Hell* and *Whole Lotta Rosie.* They finished their extremely loud set with *Let There Be Rock*, by which time our ears were almost bleeding but this was a small price to pay to finally see Acca Dacca perform live.

When Nicol and I went to see Bob Seger and the Silver Bullet Band at Wembley Arena a week later we felt extremely lucky to get seats so near to the stage as the venue was packed. Sitting behind us was none other than one of my heroes, Bob Harris the DJ from *The Old Grey Whistle Test*, who seemed to be enjoying the show just as much as we were. It was a long set so we got our money's worth. Bob performed a few songs off his most recent album *Against the Wind,* including *Her Strut, Horizontal Bop* and *Betty Lou's Getting Out Tonight* but my favourite song of the night was *Katmandu.* He also did two encores. The second was a medley which started with *Let it Rock* followed by *Shake It Baby/Little Queenie/Do You like to Rock* and finally back to *Let It Rock*. The standing ovation afterwards said it all.

The following night I went to see Jethro Tull yet again but this time at The Royal Albert Hall. To say it was a disappointment would be an understatement. The band played well enough and Ian Anderson's flute playing was as flawless as ever but for some reason, he didn't communicate with the audience in the light-hearted way he normally did and it felt like he just wanted to get the show over and done with as quickly as possible, which was how we started to feel halfway through the set. Part of the problem may have been the decision to play so many songs from their recent album *A*, which didn't go down too well with the audience despite the best efforts of Eddie Jobson on keyboards and violin to bring them to life.

I directed a couple of other TV commercials over the next few weeks and with the proceeds I ought myself an All-in-One Music Centre with stereo speakers, so I could listen to the radio, play a cassette or put an LP on the turntable whenever I wanted. As soon as I got back to James' house, I set up my Music Centre and was just about to change the mode from radio to turntable, so I could listen to

John Lennon's *Double Fantasy,* when I heard on the news the former Beatle had been shot dead in New York. After listening to the report of when and how it happened, I turned the radio off and cried like a baby. It just didn't make sense. I then carefully placed the needle onto the vinyl and listened to his last album from start to finish.

I was much happier the following day after receiving a letter from Jackie. She sounded happy to be back in Hong Kong but also said she was missing me. I missed her too but couldn't see the point of having a long-distance relationship. Also in the mail was an invite to spend Christmas with my American cousins in California, which I accepted straight away.

On the flight to L.A, I sat next to Professor Benjamin Volcani who was a microbiologist and had discovered life in the Dead Sea, which was previously thought to be far too salty to sustain life. He also pioneered biological silicon research at Scripps Institution of Oceanography. While we flew over America, he told me silicon was thought to be biologically inert but he had proved it was not only active but was required for many biochemical pathways in diatoms. I didn't understand a word of course but nodded in encouragement to keep talking in the hope I might eventually grasp what he was saying, but it was all far too scientific for my simple mind to understand. As we disembarked, he handed me his card and invited me to come and see his laboratory when I was next in San Diego.

My Uncle Elmar met me at the airport and took me back to their new house in Huntington Beach where his wife Jeanne was preparing dinner. In the morning, I caught up with their daughter Jamie and her husband Mark and saw them again on Christmas Day, when her brother Ken and wife Jodi and their son Sean joined the family gathering. After a fabulous lunch with all the trimmings, Mark told me Emily had recently got married. I was a bit surprised at first but it explained why she hadn't replied to any of my letters. A couple of days later, the Baxter clan met up with their other cousins, the Binford and Box families, so I got to see my second cousins Tony and Robin again. I also got to meet their younger brother Mike for the first time. He was really into movies and music so had a lot in common. In the evening, I decided to give Emily a quick call to congratulate her and I was glad I did because I discovered the reason why she hadn't replied to my letters was that never received them. She sounded so upset, I realised she was telling the truth, so when she asked me what I had said in my letters, I told her about the feelings I'd had for her and Leo after meeting them, and this was when she started to cry.

I took a coach to San Diego in the morning and went to the Scripps Institute for a couple of hours to visit Professor Volcani. He was pleased I had made the effort to come and showed me around his lab while explaining why silicon was so important and would become more so as computer technology advanced. I found it hard to understand most of what he said but I did remember one fact. Silicon makes up around 27% of the Earth's crust.

On New Year's Day 1981, Emily rang to tell me her sister-in-law had thrown my letters away as soon as they arrived, as she hadn't wanted her to get involved with someone she had only met once and who lived in another country. She apologised and asked me if I would like her new address but I wasn't sure if I should write to her again as she was now married so I gave her my address instead and left it to her to decide if she wanted to stay in touch with me or not.

I stayed with Jamie and Mark in San Clemente the next night and we listened to the latest albums by two of my favourite Southern Rock bands. *Ghost Riders* by The Outlaws and *Beatin' the Odds* by Molly Hatchet. The first record had a song on it called *I Can't Stop Loving You* and the other had one called *Get Her Back*, but perhaps *You Can't Always Get What You Want* by The Rolling Stones would have been more appropriate as to how I was feeling at the time.

I had a short stopover in New York in the first week of January to see Cheryl, who had kept in touch with me regularly since our Italian adventure. The Big Apple was freezing compared to L.A. There was thick snow on the ground and the 'wind chill factor' was a whole new experience for me. This is the term used to describe what the air temperature feels like when it is already cold outside but then combines with the wind blowing at about 20 mph. The wind chill factor makes it feel as though it is much, much colder.

In the morning, we went to an exhibition at the Metropolitan Museum and afterwards we had a lovely lunch before Cheryl went back to her parent's house in New Jersey and I went to see Mark, the younger brother of my kindergarten friend Richard, who was in New York studying photography at Parsons School of Design and his fiancé Suzanne was studying opera at the Juilliard School. The couple had a fabulous apartment close to Central Park and it was interesting to see a part of Manhattan I hadn't seen before. In the evening we went to Broadway to see *Death Trap* a play starring John Wood as Sidney Bruhl the murderous playwright and it was excellent. I stayed with Mark and Suzanne for the night and then flew back to the UK the next day.

On the 22nd of January, I attended another play but this time I was at the Queen's Theatre in London. *Moving* starred Penelope Keith from the BBC sitcom *The Good Life* and she was wonderful. A month later I saw *Rowan Atkinson in Revue* at the Globe Theatre, which included 'The Schoolmaster' sketch where he reads out the names of the boys one by one as if taking the morning register. Starting with Ainsley. Babcock. Bland. Carthorse and so on and finishing with Zob. Absent. His show was a master class in comic timing.

When Gillie Potter announced he was retiring and closing the company down, it was a big surprise but he said he wanted to spend more time with his family. Although Ken and Mary would keep the business going, they would have to start again under a different name so there would be no more work for me with them until they were up and running again, which might take a while. They suggested I put all the stop-motion spots I directed for them on a showreel and look for work elsewhere...but as to who would employ me next, I had no idea.

In the end, I decided to ask Harry Bruce for advice as he always had his finger on the pulse of who was doing what in the film industry but when I got to Roger Cherill's it was like a Ghost town.

'Where is everybody?' I asked Harry as I walked into his office.

'The film industry is in a slump' he replied, 'there are fewer films being made this year than any since 1914! That's why we're virtually empty at the moment.'

Harry then explained how most of the bigger companies who made movies like EMI and Rank were pulling out of production in the UK. This was bleak news indeed. However, he thought TV commercial making was still alive and after showing him my showreel, he suggested I hire myself out as a freelancer and let me use his phone to make a few calls. There were only a few other special effects companies in London at the time, so I started with them but they already had directors with much more experience than me.

The only other option I could think of was to go to the ACCTT notice board to see if there were any editing jobs available but having had a taste of directing, I wanted more.

I had no idea what to do next, so went to my parents for a few days to have a long hard think.

On the 7th of March, Jon G and I went to watch our beloved Saints play Manchester United at The Dell and we won 1-0 with a great goal by Kevin Keegan. As we walked back to the station to get our train home, I told my old friend about my current situation and he asked me if I had thought about the possibility of going back to Australia. I hadn't, but the more I thought about it the more it made sense. When I saw my mate Nicol the following week at the Status Quo concert at Hammersmith Odeon, he told me he thought it was a great idea and suggested I contact everyone I had worked with when I was there the first time and ask them what they thought my chances were for getting work as a director down under.

I got a reply from Mike Reed, who I had worked with in Melbourne, telling me there weren't many other director's he knew of doing the kind of work I was doing like stop-motion and other in-camera special effects, so I might be able to fill the gap in the advertising industry. I then got a letter from Edwin telling me he was still busy making 'docos' and he would let me direct one if I did come back to South Australia one day.

This was just the encouragement I needed.

After thinking about all my options, I decided my best course of action was to return to Australia on a six-month working holiday visa, if I was allowed another one, and try my luck as a TV commercials director there and if it went well, I could then apply to stay longer and if not, at least I had given it a go and could come back to the UK and start again. Ken and Mary would hopefully be back in business by then and might be in a position to hire me by then.

I thought my mother would have a fit when I told her my plan but she thought it was a wonderful idea and said how pleased my Aussie friends would be to see me again. Typical Mum, always seeing the best in every situation. Her only demand was for me to write home more often than I had the last time I was there. I would miss my Mum terribly but the call to adventure was getting louder by the day.

After I told James I was planning to go back to Australia to try my luck once more so he would need to find a new flatmate, he opened a bottle of red, poured us both a glass and said, 'Hope to see you there one-day old boy. Chin, chin!'

My Australian visa was approved far quicker than I had thought it would take, so I decided to leave a bit sooner than originally planned. When I let Jackie know what I was up to, she asked me if I could stop off to see her on the way to Australia, so of course I said yes. Before I left home, I asked my mother what advice she thought my father might have given me if he had still been alive, and she said he would have just wanted me to be kind to everyone I met and try not to judge other people but be curious about them instead.

I took this advice on board, gave her a huge hug and then after saying a tearful goodbye made my way to Heathrow and on the evening of the 22$^{nd}$ of April 1981 I flew to Hong Kong.

As soon as we saw each other it was pretty obvious we still felt the same way about each other so we rekindled our romance as soon we got back to her parent's house in Tai Tam, which is in the Southern district of the city. Jackie's folks were currently in Australia so we had the place to ourselves for the next ten days. After walking hand in hand on the beach at Repulse Bay, the most expensive residential area on the island, we had a quick swim and then went on a day trip to Victoria Peak where there was an amazing view of the city below. For lunch we had stir fry crabs with scallions at the Royal Hong Kong Yacht Club and after getting a taxi home we resumed what we had been up to when we first woke up in the morning.

The next day, we took a ferry to Cheung Chau Island, as the annual Bun Festival was in progress. The first thing I saw was three huge towers covered with hundreds of buns. Jackie told me in the past men had raced up the towers, which were constructed with bamboo, to snatch a bun and bring it back down. The higher up the bun was the better the fortune they would get. However, in 1978 one of the towers collapsed and injured over a hundred people so now they only allowed one climber on each tower to perform this traditional Chinese ritual.

Jackie told me to bring my passport for our next adventure but didn't tell me where we were going until we boarded a Hydrofoil, which would take us to Macau.

It was fascinating to see how the autonomous territory had managed to blend both Chinese and Portuguese cultures with old temples and colonial buildings standing side by side. Macau was also becoming a gambler's paradise but as going to a casino and throwing away our money wasn't really our scene we took the coach across the border into China instead and wandered through the old streets of Zhongshan until we found the local food market, which had been running since the 11th Century and looking around I suspect it hadn't changed much in all since then. When I saw some monkeys in a cage, Jackie told me monkey meat was considered a delicacy in Chinese cuisine, which is when I decided I'd had enough and was ready to go back to Hong Kong.

Saying goodbye to Jackie was really hard. We had become very close during the last couple of weeks but after talking it through we agreed we were far too young to settle down right now and should follow our own dreams and focus on our careers, at least for now. Who knew what the future might bring? After a tearful farewell at the airport, and the promise to stay in touch, I continued my journey to Australia... the land of opportunity, or so I hoped.

As we took off, I looked out of the plane's window and could see it was raining but there was also a rainbow in the sky, a symbol of hope, which is when I remembered what Miss Le May, my prep school art teacher, had once told me, 'Hope is the will and the way to success.'

I tried to hold on to this positive thought all the way to Sydney but at the same time I was more than a little anxious as to what might happen when I got there. I had left England because of the lack of opportunities in my chosen career but there were no guarantees I would fare any better in Australia. However, by the time we were told to fasten our seat belts for landing at Sydney Airport, I was so excited, any doubts and fears were temporarily pushed aside and I felt a sudden surge of optimism caused by the adrenaline pumping though my body.

I was ready for a brand-new adventure.

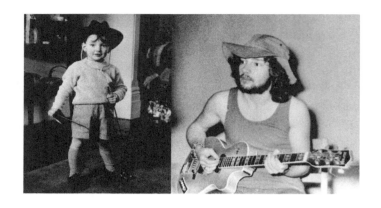

Jamie '*Boomerang*' Robertson

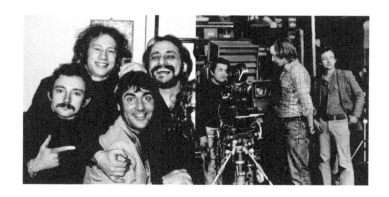

# Volume Two: 1981-1997

*Hope lies in dreams, in imagination,*
*and in the courage of those who dare to make dreams into reality.*

Jonas Salk

## CHAPTER 1: HISTORY NEVER REPEATS

'G'day folks! Hope you had a pleasant flight. For those of you coming here for the first time, welcome to Australia and for the rest of youse, welcome home, we've missed you!' our cheerful pilot announced as we landed in Sydney on the 17$^{th}$ of May 1981.

The reason I had come back to Australia was because the British film industry was currently going through a lull and I felt I had a better chance of furthering my career in the land down under. The passport queue was reasonably short, my working holiday visa was stamped without any hassle and my suitcase was one of the first to come off the baggage carousel, so it felt like getting three green traffic lights in a row.

'You always were a jammy bugger!' my old friend Mark remarked as he greeted me inside the airport's arrival area.

'You are welcome to use our spare room until you get yourself sorted,' his lovely wife Sarah added while giving me one of her famous hugs, 'Our flat is in Mosman, not far from your favourite beach!'

When I woke up the next morning the sun was shining, so I walked down the steep hill to Balmoral Beach where the water was crystal clear and inviting. Having an early morning dip in the sea, followed by a 'proper' cup of coffee and Vegemite on toast for my brekkie was the ideal way to start the day. It felt good to be back in Oz.

Over the café's loudspeakers, I could hear the song *History Never Repeats* by Split Enz off their album *Corroboree*. Carl, the Kiwi café owner, said it was called *Waiata* in New Zealand but both were names for singing and dancing, the first an Aboriginal term and the second a Māori one. I couldn't help but smile when I heard the lyrics, 'Better to jump than hesitate. I need a change and I can't wait,' as this was exactly what I had just done.

With my energy levels now boosted by the intake of caffeine and some decent music, I went for a brisk walk along the esplanade from one end of the picturesque beach to the other and then had another swim in the calm clean ocean. After having a shower next to the steps to wash the salt off my body, I headed to the heritage-listed Bather's Pavilion to have lunch with Jenny, the receptionist at my first-ever job in the British film industry. It was great to see her smiling face again and to meet her new boyfriend, Tony. They were both so sun-tanned I looked like a pale waning moon in comparison, but spending time with such positive people was infectious and by the time I got back to Mark and Sarah's flat, I was feeling proactive and started looking for work straight away. I called five different film production companies to ask whether they would be interested in hiring me as a director, and arranged to meet three of them the next day.

Although everyone I saw was friendly and made complimentary comments after viewing my showreel of TV commercials and title sequences, nobody offered to take me on as a director, but at the last company, one of the female producers suggested I talk to a woman called Liz Hynard who had recently started a booking business called Technicians Answering and Booking Service (TABS), as they thought she might be able to help me. After giving Liz a bit of background about myself, she promised she would do all she could and a few days later, was true to her word and set up a meeting for me with a well-respected producer-director called Alastair Macdonald.

When I first met Alastair, I was a bit intimidated as he was well over six foot tall, built like a rugby prop forward and had a huge black beard the infamous pirate Edward Teach would have been proud of, but he immediately put me at ease by showing genuine interest and asking me about my ambitions in life. After he had looked at my showreel, he said he liked my work but couldn't afford to give me a full-time job but was willing to offer me a small retainer, if I was happy for him to represent me. He also promised to mentor me and help me become a better director. I thought about it for about 30 seconds and then said, 'Yes please…and thank you.'

I started working at Alastair Macdonald Productions on the 25th of

June. My new boss warned me it would take a while to find me some work but the retainer should cover my accommodation and food needs so at least I wouldn't starve.

Now I had sorted out my work situation I could satisfy my desire to see some live local music. Alastair told me there were quite a few new Aussie bands on the scene since I had last been in Sydney and as luck would have it, I was able to see three in one go when I went to a gig one night at the Capitol Theatre. The headliners were called Flowers and the support acts were The Numbers and Men at Work. This was the last time Flowers ever played under this name as they were forced to change it for legal reasons and decided to use the same name as the title of their last album. Icehouse. Their singer-songwriter, Iva Davies, had a very distinctive voice and the songs I enjoyed the most were *Can't Help Myself* and *We Can Get Together.*

As I was now receiving a small retainer, I decided I could afford to fly down to Melbourne for the weekend to see Mike Reed, my old boss from 1976 on my first visit to Australia. After showing him my reel, he said, 'Your work is quite different to any other director's reels I've seen, which is good and bad. If one of the advertising agencies wants a new look then you have a good chance but I have to warn you they tend to go with directors they already know and trust so you will just have to be patient and persevere. In other words, you need a lucky break!'

The break happened on the 7th of July when Alastair asked me to be his co-director on a Television commercial (TVC) for Nescafe. One of my tasks was to make the instant coffee look better than it did in reality. To get the perfect-looking cup of coffee we watered-down some soy sauce and added a tiny bit of gelatine, which made the 'coffee' look much smoother than it did normally and as the client wanted to emphasize the curls of rising steam above the rim, we placed a back item behind the cup and used a tiny mirror to bounce light onto the back of the steam, which worked well. It was simple but effective and all created by smoke and mirrors. Well, one anyway.

Over dinner, Alastair told me an American film director called

Nancy was looking for someone to rent her house in Queenscliff for the next three months and thought it might suit me, so I grabbed the opportunity and went to see it as soon as possible. Nancy explained she spent half of the year in Australia and the other half in the USA, which is why she was looking for a tenant who was willing to move out when she came back. Her home was on Pavilion Street, which overlooked Freshwater Beach. After we had agreed on the cost of the rent, Nancy said I could also hire her Mini-Moke for an additional fee, which was a real godsend.

In the evening, I met up with Linda, an English girl I had met in Oxford the year before, and who was now in Australia on a working holiday. When I told her I was about to move into a two-bedroom house right next to the ocean, she asked me if I would be willing to share it with her if she paid half the rent.

Finding somewhere so spectacular to live, a set of cool wheels and an attractive housemate all in one day felt quite extraordinary. Australia was proving to be the lucky country for me once again.

As soon as Linda and I moved in we got into a nightly routine of opening a bottle of Aussie red and listening to music while gazing out to sea and searching for ships on the horizon. The first album we played was *Sirocco* by Australian Crawl. The song I liked the most was *Things Don't Seem* partly because I was impressed with the complex guitar solo played by Simon Binks but Linda's favourite track was *Errol*, a song about the legendary Tasmanian actor Errol Leslie Thomson Flynn, who had a 74-foot ketch named Sirocco, hence the title of the album.

Living by the ocean gave me the perfect opportunity to use my camera, so now my passions for music, photography and film were all being indulged in equal measure. Life doesn't get much better than this, I thought as I topped up my glass…again.

Our little home by the sea was the ideal spot for a BBQ, or a barbie as the Australians call it, so Linda and I hosted one over the weekend and invited Mark and Sarah as a thank-you for having me stay when I first arrived. I also invited David and Tricia, another couple of my friends from the New Forest, who were living in Sydney at the time. Everybody was suitably impressed with our uninterrupted view of the ocean and after cooking a few snags on the barbie and downing a few cold ones, we could have almost been mistaken for locals. Almost. Our British accents were a bit of a giveaway.

The barbie was such a success we had another one the following weekend but this time we invited Sue, the sister of an old friend and her husband David Bagnall. With the sound of the barbecue sizzling in the background, Sue told us her brother called her husband 'Baggers' and he called her sibling 'Twiggsy', so we should do the same from now on.

Baggers was as big a Tommy Cooper fan as I was and knew many of his jokes off by heart, such as, 'Last night I dreamed I ate a ten-pound marshmallow, and when I woke up the pillow was gone,' which made us giggle but I think we all thought his impersonation of the great comedian was even funnier than the jokes.

After Alastair and I had gone to half a dozen advertising agencies in Sydney and shown them my director's reel with the hope of impressing them enough to give me some work, I asked him how long he thought it might take before we had any success.

'All human wisdom is summed up in two words; wait and hope,' Alastair replied.

'Wow! That's profound. Did you make that up?' I asked.

'Actually no, it's a quote by Alexandre Dumas,' my new boss admitted and then told me the film industry had their own saying for times like these called 'Hurry Up and Wait!'

The more time I spent with Alastair, the more wisdom he passed on to me. It was like suddenly having a father figure in my life, which made me think of my real father who had died when I was only three and how much I missed having him in my childhood. There had been so many times I could have done with his advice and guidance along the way, so to find someone willing to give me both now was a real godsend. As Alastair also loved music, we had plenty to talk about when we weren't discussing work. He taught me how important music was in the movie business as it could add a whole new depth of meaning to a scene. To illustrate what he was trying to convey, he showed me a ¾" video tape of a TV commercial, which had shots of a smiling grandfather picking up his grandson from school and then walking him home hand in hand. It was a heart-warming scene and the music was played in a major key to emphasize the joy. Alastair then turned the sound down on the video monitor and as we watched the TVC for the second time, he played some rather menacing music in a minor key, which gave exactly the same images a completely different meaning. Instead of seeing a trustworthy grandpa picking up his grandson, I now saw an evil predator abducting a child.

'Music is a powerful form of storytelling,' my mentor explained to me, 'it has the power to take your imagination on an adventure.'

I learned so much from Alastair while I was at the office but also enjoyed his company after work once or twice a week when he and his girlfriend Annie invited me for dinner. Afterwards he would play his congas while playing records by Santana, which was an absolute joy to witness. It was a good feeling to have a new mentor in my life but I hadn't forgotten my old ones, so when I got a call from Edwin Scragg, the owner of Scope Films who I had worked with in South Australia in 1977, to ask me if I would be his assistant cameraman on a documentary to be filmed the following week in Queensland, I was excited but didn't accept the job until I had spoken to Alastair first, as having just signed an exclusive contract with him, I didn't want to start on the wrong foot, but I needn't have worried as he assured me our agreement was for TV commercials only.

Our first location was in Mackay, one of the most prolific sugar cane growing and milling areas in Australia. Edwin and I met our client, John Hare, at the local sugar mill, which was owned by CSR to get fully briefed and then shoot the refining process from start to finish. It didn't take long before our lungs filled with the thick smell of molasses, which made me feel a bit nauseous, so I was glad when the day's filming was over.

The next morning, we flew up to Townsville to film the same

process inside their mill and then on to Cairns the day after to get some exterior images of a mechanical harvester as it moved slowly along the rows of cane removing the tops and cutting the stalks into short pieces, which were then loaded into bins before being taken by a small train specifically designed for this job to the sugar mill. We also had to film a controlled burn, which was done to eliminate excess organic material before they started the harvesting.

Over dinner, Edwin explained the reason we were having to film everything out of sequence was because of the farmer's availability at each location, but he wasn't fussed as he would edit it all later to look like the whole process was shot in chronological order, once he got back to South Australia. I was lucky to have two such experienced and generous filmmakers hand down their knowledge to me and soaked up every new bit of information like a sponge.

When I got back to Sydney, Alastair told me there was a Melbourne advertising agency who wanted to hire me to direct a TVC for Kitten car polish, so two days later I flew down to Victoria. Lighting automobiles in a studio is a very specific skill, so I was extremely lucky to have Keith Wagstaff as my Director of Photography (DOP), as he had shot several car commercials before and I hadn't shot any, especially as the car in question was a rather expensive looking bright red Porsche. Eliminating all the reflections in the car's windows was always going to be difficult but to make matters worse, the creative team had briefed us to, 'pepper the car with tiny drops of rain all strategically placed to look artistic.'

The script called for the plastic container of Kitten car polish to look as if it had just popped out of one of the minuscule drops of rainwater as if by magic. If we had been able to use computer generated-imagery (CGI), which is how most visual effects are created today, it would have been a doddle, but as this was 1981, we had to shoot everything in-camera and then combine our film elements using an optical printer. Unfortunately, the result wasn't as good as it could or should have been and Mike Reed, who had been hired by the agency to edit the commercial wasn't backwards in telling me his honest opinion, 'Well, you've made a right dog's breakfast of this one, haven't you young Jamie?'

Luckily for me, my old boss managed to work out a clever and cost-effective way of resolving the problem in post-production, saving my posterior in the process. Phew!

When I was back in Sydney and explained what had happened to Alastair, instead of berating me, he simply said, 'Hey man, we all make mistakes, so just learn from it and move on, man!' He then apologised for not looking at the script himself before sending me down to Melbourne, 'If I had, then I might have suggested a different way of approaching the job, so from now on I will mentor you a bit more closely. Don't worry too much. There are much more important things in life to be good at than your profession.'

I felt terrible but took his wise words on board and then tried my best to forget my recent experience as quickly as possible.

Thankfully my next TVC, which was for Trans Australia Airlines (TAA) went much better as instead of doing the visual effects on an optical printer at a film laboratory as we had done in Melbourne, we used the latest cutting-edge post-production technology at a post house in Sydney. When the client saw the end result, they were happy, and therefore the agency was happy and more importantly for me, so was Alastair. I had learned from my mistake, moved on and now had a new commercial to add to my showreel.

In the evening, I asked my flatmate Linda if she would like to go out to dinner with me to celebrate. We walked along Manly Promenade until we found a restaurant which we liked the look of and then sat down at a table overlooking the ocean, which was very romantic. We both ordered red snapper with salad and drank two bottles of white wine between us, so by the time we got home we were more than a little tipsy and ended up in the same bed. Living in such a delightful beach house right next to the ocean and waking up to beautiful sunrises every morning was like being on holiday every day. Sharing this blissful existence with someone as special as Linda was like living in a dream. We both knew it couldn't last forever so we made the most of every moment.

In September, I flew down to Adelaide to be best man at my buddy Hugh's wedding. It was good to see him again and to meet his fiancée Debbie for the first time. Hugh had sensibly decided not to have a traditional stag do, so he wouldn't be hung-over on the big day, so we strolled down to the local bottle-o to buy a few stubbies and then went back to his place to listen to some music before having an early night. But when the groom-to-be turned the radio on The Divinyls' new single *Boys in Town* was being played, and as it seemed highly appropriate with us 'boys' catching up after so long, we abandoned the sensible option and took a taxi into town to find some action. Thankfully, the wedding went ahead without a hitch, but as they say, every picture tells a story and in the photos I took, I must admit Hugh does look a bit green around the gills.

My passion for new music was still as important to me as it ever was and when I saw INXS at the San Miguel Inn in Cammeray the following week, I was completely blown away. Not only were they a talented band but they also had a good-looking frontman with a great voice called Michael Hutchence, who had the charisma of Jim Morrison and the animalistic dance moves of Mick Jagger. It was pretty evident they would go on to bigger and better things, so I was glad to have seen them when they were still at an embryonic stage. I wasn't familiar with many of their songs at the time but enjoyed *Stay Young*, which would become their first single from their second album *Underneath the Colours.*

Linda and I went to the Cambridge University Footlights Revue the following weekend to see *Botham (The Musical),* which had absolutely nothing to do with the great English cricket legend at all. The cast included a young woman called Emma Thompson, whose acting abilities were rather impressive, Tony Slattery who was a very funny man and made us laugh out loud and a couple of up-and-coming young comedians called Stephen Fry and Hugh Laurie.

After three blissful months at our intimate little beach dwelling, we had to move out as Nancy would soon be coming home. Linda decided to go backpacking around Australia before returning to England and I rented a tiny granny flat in Cremorne on a short-term basis, while looking for something more suitable long-term. After saying goodbye and good luck, we both promised to stay in touch and then suddenly she was gone and I wondered if we would ever see each other again.

Two weeks later, I was invited to a fancy dress party with the theme 'Come as someone famous from history', which was hosted by a stunning Russian woman called Veruschka. She was dressed as the 'alleged' nymphomaniac Catherine the Great and I had come as the French nobleman, part-time erotic writer and 'alleged' sexual deviant, the Marquis de Sade, so we couldn't have been better matched. Wild Bill Hickock and Calamity Jane were also in attendance, although after a quick introduction, I discovered they went by the names Rich and Marcia when they weren't in disguise. I liked the American couple immediately, as they were great fun to talk to and loved many of the same bands as me.

Just after midnight, the Russian Empress informed me she had taken a bit of a fancy to the Marquis and wanted to know more about his perverse sexual preferences in private, so staying in character…and costumes, we then discussed it thoroughly until dawn.

I moved into a spacious two-bedroom flat in Cammeray at the end of November but as the rent was too expensive to pay on my own, I decided to advertise for a flatmate but before I had a chance to put the ad in the paper, Jackie rang to ask if she could stay with me for a few nights before heading back to Hong Kong. As soon as we saw each other, it was obvious we still cared about each other but as both of us were doing well in our chosen careers, the timing still wasn't right to make any long-term plans to be together, so we agreed to keep doing our own thing in Australia and Hong Kong respectively.

A few days after Jackie had gone home, Alastair asked me if I would like to co-direct a commercial for Dettol with him. He would direct the actors and I would direct the visual effects, which included the iconic Dettol sword flying through the air. We couldn't have hired a better DOP, as Don McAlpine was already a legend in the film industry and his assistant Andrew Lesnie was also well respected, so it was a very enjoyable shoot and we all worked well as a team. The production design was done by Peter Avery and the edit by Paul Maxwell. I made friends with both of them on the shoot and got to meet their other halves when we all went to see singer-songwriter Jon English at the San Miguel Hotel in Cammeray, which was just across the road from my flat. Jon had a raspy voice and an amazing stage presence a bit like Alice Cooper with only slightly less mascara, which is most probably why he had been chosen to play Judas Iscariot in the musical *Jesus Christ Superstar* back in 1972. Halfway through his set he said he needed to have a break and grab a beer so we might like to get another one too, and then added, 'The more you drink the better we sound!'

On the 7th of November AC/DC released *For Those About To Rock (We Salute You)* in Australia so a few days later, I bought the cassette as a belated birthday present to myself. While I was in the record shop, I heard a fantastic song being played over the store's speakers called *Don't Wanna Be the One* by Midnight Oil, so I got their album *Place without a Postcard* as well and became a fan of 'The Oils' forever.

In mid-December, Alastair and I went on a helicopter trip to Kangaroo Valley, in the southern highlands of New South Wales, to recce potential locations for a series of TV commercials for St. George Bank, which we would shoot the following year. My job was to take photos of each location, which would be shown to the client along with a storyboard to give them a better idea of what to expect when the shoot commenced.

As it was my first time in a chopper Alastair asked the pilot on the return trip to fly right over the top of the Sydney Harbour Bridge and the Sydney Opera House. It was a breathtaking experience and I loved every minute of it.

To top off an already fabulous day, I was then invited to the Spectrum Films Christmas party, which was held at the same place where I had worked as an assistant editor on the movie *The Irishman* in 1977. As soon as I arrived, I knocked back a couple of drinks to help me relax and then introduced myself to a group of people who seemed as interested in meeting me as I was them, which was a relief and gave me a sense of belonging. I had just been accepted as part of the local film industry.

As I only had another month left on my current visa, I decided to apply for a temporary resident visa, which would allow me to travel in and out of Australia without having to re-apply to enter the country every time I left, so the next day I sent off my application along with references from Alastair and my previous employers, Mike Reed and Edwin Scragg, all recommending the government should allow me to become an Australian resident as they believed I was an asset to the Australian film industry.

Now all I had to do was wait and hope.

I flew to Adelaide on Christmas Eve to spend a few days with my buddy Hugh and his wife Debbie and while I was in South Australia, I borrowed his motorbike to visit Edwin and his family in Gumeracha. It felt strange to be back at Scragg End, almost as though I had never been away except for the fact the girls, Emma and Sarah, had grown so much since I had last seen them but they were still young enough to call me 'Uncle Jamie', which made me miss my real nephews and nieces who lived in the UK and Mallorca.

Since returning to Australia, I had been sending more aerogrammes to my mother as promised but I really wanted to hear her voice, so when I got back to Hugh's I gave my folks a call to wish them Happy Christmas and pass on my love to the rest of my family.

I got back to Sydney on the morning of the 3$^{rd}$ of January 1982, and in the afternoon, I received a call from Di and Julie to say they were in town, having just sailed from Melbourne on a huge yacht as part of the crew, and wanted to know if they could have a hot bath at my place as they'd only had a tiny handheld shower on the yacht and were desperate for a decent soak. When I said yes, they took a taxi to my flat and as soon as the front door was closed, they stripped off right in front of me and got in the bath together. While I was in the kitchen opening a bottle of wine, I could hear them giggling away like naughty schoolgirls. Di then called out for me to join them. When I asked why, she replied, 'Because you're a dirty-dirty boy!' I couldn't argue with her comment, so stripped off and got into the bath, now full of soapy bubbles, purely in the interest of science you understand... and to disprove the theory two's company, three's a crowd.

A week later, my visa was approved, which meant I could now stay in Australia for at least another year and it would also allow me to go in and out of the country whenever I wanted, so the world was my oyster.

I kept hearing Devo's catchy song *Whip It* on the radio, so when the American band came to Sydney two days later, I decided to go and see them perform at the Hordern Pavilion. They wore bright red 'energy dome hats', which looked a bit weird but they were a lot better musically than I expected and their cover version of the Allen Toussaint song *Working in the Coalmine* made it worth the price of the ticket on its own.

Alastair and I finally got the go-ahead to produce the commercials for St. George Bank in mid-February. The shoot involved two separate crews driving down to Kangaroo Valley to the locations we had found on the helicopter trip in December. Alastair directed all the shots featuring popular entertainer Julie Anthony while she sang to a playback of a song specially written for the spot called *St. George has got it!* and I went off with the second unit to direct the shots of the St. George mascot, which was a large Green Dragon costume worn by the agency producer. It was straightforward but great fun and allowed me to see some wonderful scenery at someone else's expense once again.

After the agency saw my still photos of their mascot at each location, they paid me a bit extra for using them in their publicity campaign, so I treated myself to Cold Chisel's latest album *Circus Animals*, which had two of the best songs ever recorded by an Australian band on it. *You've Got Nothing I Want* and *Bow River* with Jimmy Barnes screaming for all his worth on the first track and Ian Moss's more soulful voice on the second. I also bought *The Number of the Beast* by Iron Maiden, which was their first album to feature another great high-pitch screamer Bruce Dickinson. The record was considered controversial partly because of the lyrics of the title track but also for its cover art, which depicted their mascot 'Eddie' controlling Satan like a puppet who in turn is manipulating a smaller puppet of Eddie, raising the question…who is controlling who?

Having enjoyed 'some kind of hell', musically, I was then hired to make some motor oil glow in a 'heavenly manner' for a TV commercial in Melbourne. The spot was for Mobil Oil and the brief was to film a young vicar coming out of an old church carrying a container of the product with him and then film him pouring the oil into his old Holden's engine. The oil itself had to look celestial, so Keith Wagstaff our DOP, suggested we shoot the close-up of the oil in slow motion and backlit it using a miniature dimmer switch, which would allow him to turn the level of brightness up from hellish darkness to heavenly light at will. It worked perfectly…thank God!

On the 12th of July, the Australian Music Industry put on a very special event at the Sydney Entertainment Centre. *OZ For Africa* was broadcast as part of *Live Aid* to help raise money for famine relief in Africa. The event was hosted by 'Molly' Meldrum and all 17 bands donated their services and did short sets. Mental as Anything opened the show followed by Machinations, The Models, D-Re-Mi, Electric Pandas, Dragon, Men at Work, Australian Crawl, Party Girls, Uncanny X-Men, Goanna, The Little River Band, Mondo Rock, The Angels, Renee Geyer and INXS. It was quite an occasion and my dream to see more Aussie bands was now well and truly satisfied.

The next morning Alastair came into my office and said, 'Hey man, I think it's time you had a company car,' which made me quite excited until he walked up to my desk and pushed a miniature toy car across the desktop towards me.

'Ha fucking ha!' I said picking up the tiny replica of a Peugeot to give it a closer look. As Alastair left my office, he turned around at the doorway, threw a set of car keys in my direction and said, 'Oh, I nearly forgot. The real one's downstairs!'

When I walked down to the garage in the basement of our offices a couple of minutes later, I could see Alastair's old Peugeot 504 sitting there waiting for its new owner. Me.

I really benefitted from having Alastair as my mentor and he was becoming more like a father figure to me every day, giving me pieces of advice taken from his own experience of life. He taught me to trust my artistic judgements and not to worry what others thought, as 'it's all subjective man!' and most importantly to never *ever* give up.

While Alastair was away in the Cook Islands shooting a cinema commercial for Air New Zealand, I got a call from Edwin asking me to fly to Singapore to help him on a documentary for Singapore Tourism called *Moods and Images*, which he was co-producing with his friend Jon Noble. I wouldn't have been able to go if I hadn't already got my temporary resident visa so I was glad to have got it all sorted earlier in the year.

As soon as I arrived at the Raffles Hotel, Edwin explained how we would be filming everyday life scenes in Singapore all shot 'fly on the wall' style, and then we would intercut the images of an orchestra playing a few selected pieces of classical music, which they had already shot the week before.

'I need you to act as my assistant cameraman on the shoot and as Edwin's assistant editor once we have shot all the material. Think you can handle that mate?' Jon asked but didn't wait for an answer as presumably Edwin had already said yes on my behalf. I liked Jon straightaway as he had a sharp mind but spoke bluntly, so I knew what I needed to do and when without question. Over the next week, we filmed people doing their morning exercises and playing a variety of sports, locals selling fresh produce at the markets, and tourists visiting the city's landmarks, including several temples as well as the zoo.

We stayed at the Raffles Hotel for the duration of our stay, but unfortunately their budget didn't allow me my own suite with a double bed so I slept on a fold-up Z-Bed in a tiny airless editing room, which they had commandeered near the hotel's kitchen. After filming all day, we worked on the edit in the evenings until it was time for bed. Although, my sleeping arrangements were 'cost effective', I was allowed to eat my meals in the hotel's fancy restaurant and have a nightly Singapore Sling at the famous Long Bar, all of which was covered by expenses. It was a lot of fun and I got to see everything Singapore had to offer at the time.

When I showed my new visa at passport control at Sydney Airport, I was waved through without any trouble, which was just as well because three days later, after receiving a call from Jon Noble to tell me a local agency called Batey Ads wanted me to direct a commercial for them, I was on my way back to Singapore. Sitting next to me on the plane was the distinguished actor Ron Haddrick and winging his way to Singapore direct from Melbourne on the same day was our DOP Keith Wagstaff. The job was for Carrier Air Conditioners and featured Ron as The Devil, sitting in his favourite armchair in a temperature-controlled living room, talking to camera about why he preferred this particular brand of air conditioning to keep him cool in Hell. As there were no film studios available, we built the set in a large room at a conference centre in one of Singapore's many high-rise buildings. 'Hell' was currently just a blue screen placed behind the flimsy set seen through a window frame directly behind The Devil, but the chromakey blue would eventually be replaced by some Dante's Inferno-like 'fiery flames' shot in a controlled situation at a later date and inserted in post-production.

After discovering there was a lecture for Christians going on in the room next to ours with the theme 'Hell: Suppose it's true after all?', Ron and I decided to do a prank on them. Dressed as The Devil in a smart red three-piece suit with a set of horns on his head, a goatee beard fixed to his chin, a forked tail hanging down at the back and carrying a huge pitchfork, Ron suddenly burst into the meeting and yelled using his most dramatic Shakespearean voice, 'What do you mean, *suppose* it's true?' We only intended it to be a childish prank but the terrified screams running for the exits still haunt me to this day.

When I got back to Sydney, Alastair was excited as he had just been hired to direct a series of TV commercials for New South Wales Tourism and an advertising agency in New Zealand had contacted him about hiring me to direct an orange juice commercial for them, so it looked like we were both going to be busy for a while.

Thank goodness I had made the decision to return to Australia the previous year, I thought to myself. Everything had worked out just as I had hoped with my career and with Alastair's gentle guidance things could only get better.

A week later, Alastair started his shoot and I flew to New Zealand to have a production meeting with the agency in Auckland. As soon as I got back, Paul Maxwell, our editor, showed me the rushes from Alastair's shoot, which looked beautiful as they had been shot by Gary Hansen, one of the best DOPs in the country. I thought about trying to give Alastair a quick call to let him know how good everything looked but decided it could wait until the next day, so went home with the plan of having an early night. I was just about to get into the shower when I received a phone call which changed my life forever.

Alastair, Gary, and his camera assistant John, had all been killed in a helicopter crash.

I may have been too young to know what real grief felt like when my father died but I was old enough now to experience its full might and my heart was completely shattered. My dear friend, mentor and father figure was dead. I felt completely and utterly numb.

*Only time and tears take away grief; that is what they are for.*

Terry Pratchett

## CHAPTER 2: GREAT SOUTHERN LAND

The fatal accident happened while Alastair was filming a group of horse-riders on a trail ride, along a ridge line, back-lit by the late afternoon sun. The production team had done a ground survey of the area about ten weeks earlier, as well as an aerial survey in the helicopter on the actual shoot day before doing any filming runs to make sure it was safe to fly at heights between 10 and 100 feet above ground level, but at the last minute, Gary fitted a wooden platform to the landing skids underneath the helicopter to carry himself and his camera gear, so he could get clearer shots. During the last filming run, the skids struck the two cables of a spur, which ran from the main power line and the chopper then pitched nose down and struck the ground. A fire broke out on impact and only the pilot survived. When I heard the news, I was completely devastated. It felt like someone had suddenly pulled the rug from under my feet and I was falling into a bottomless pit.

When someone close to you dies, it's not just the person you love who isn't there anymore but also any future plans you had hoped to have with them are now gone. The grief never leaves you and you can only cope one day at a time. Alastair had been an unassuming gentle giant who was not only well-respected for his talent as a film director but also loved for his passion for life, his generosity to others and his natural charm.

I was really going to miss him.

Paul and I, with help from Alastair's partner Annie, organised the funeral and provided refreshments for everyone afterwards. Well over a hundred people from the film industry attended the service, as well as members of his family and close friends. I managed to put on a brave face until I got home and then I cried like a baby.

The following day, Paul rang to tell me we were contractually obliged to complete the commercial Alastair had been filming, and suggested we split the directing duties, so I could focus my energy on the New Zealand commercial, which also had to be shot before the end of the month. Neither shoot went particularly well but we fulfilled the contracts, got paid and eventually closed Alastair's company down.

I had never felt so sad and on top of the natural grief I also felt irritable and didn't want to see my friends, despite their kind calls to see how I was coping. In fact, I did all I could to avoid seeing them as I just wanted to be on my own. In the end, I decided to take myself on a short holiday to Bali to get over the shock and to grieve for Alastair in my own way.

Rather than a cheap Losmen, I stayed in a 4-star hotel this time, as I wanted privacy and was willing to pay for it. I went for long walks along the beach in the mornings, slept in my hotel room in the afternoons and went from bar to bar in the evenings having a drink or three at each one. After a week of doing much the same thing every day, I walked into a bar in Kuta one evening and asked the local singer-guitarist if I could jam with him. He kindly agreed to let me play his electric guitar while he played his acoustic. We played a few blues songs like *Stormy Monday* and *Sweet Home Chicago*, which seemed to go down well with the tourists who kindly bought us both drinks for the rest of the night. Playing improvised blues with a complete stranger was a freeing experience as it allowed me total self-expression, which in turn enabled me to grieve in a way I felt comfortable with.

Music and grief for me are entwined like hope and joy. I have always found listening to music or playing my guitar very healing when I am feeling sad as it acts like a time-machine and enables me to travel right back to a specific happy memory. Music allows me to access my deepest emotions and gives me a safe place to grieve.

In the morning I set off in search of some new music and discovered a shop which sold 'unofficial' Indonesian cassettes. The C90 tapes consisted of reasonably recent releases by various popular artists on one side of the cassette with extra tracks by the same artist but from completely different albums on the other side. After a long browse I bought *El Loco* by ZZ Top, which had their latest album on side one and a compilation of songs from all their previous records on side two, so was more like a 'best of' mix tape. I now had 90 minutes of bad-ass-blues-boogie to listen to so I was one very happy hombre.

On my last night, I had a magic mushroom omelette and then went to Kuta beach to watch the sunset. It was one of the most colourful I had ever seen, which made me feel like crying, as I remembered how much Alastair loved sunsets but would never get to see another. I then heard his deep voice as clearly as if he was standing right next to me say, 'Hey man, you should see the view from this side!'

I couldn't help but smile, as this was exactly the sort of thing he would have said. I will never forget Alastair but it was time to go back to Australia and continue living my life.

On the 6<sup>th</sup> of September 1982, Icehouse released their second album called *Primitive Man*, which ironically was what I was starting to look like because I hadn't cut my hair or trimmed my beard in weeks. There were some great tracks on the album, including *Hey Little Girl* but the song that meant the most to me was *Great Southern Land*. I would associate this track with my mentor Alastair Macdonald for the rest of my life.

Scottish band Simple Minds new album *New Gold Dream (81-82-83-84)* was released a couple of weeks later. *Someone Somewhere in Summertime* was my favourite track and while listening to the song for the umpteenth time my simple mind started to drift and I began wondering what titles I could come up with containing the word 'somewhere' if I was recording an album about my life and each song had to reflect a different period in my career. The opening track was obvious. It would have to be *We All Have to Start Somewhere* followed by *Always Somewhere Else* to represent my transient lifestyle and then perhaps *Somewhere Over the Rainbow* to suggest hope for the future. In theory, *Finally Getting Somewhere* should be next on the list but as I no longer had an office to work from or a retainer to pay off my bills, I would have to come up with a new plan… *Somehow*.

The following month I rang every production company in the telephone book and let them know I was available as a freelance film director specialising in TV commercials.

Thankfully a couple of other exceptional albums were released while I was 'in between' jobs, so instead of getting anxious or depressed as I might have done in the past, I was able to go to my 'safe place' inside my head and relax while listening to them both. The first was *Love Over Gold* by Dire Straits, which had the 14-minute epic track *Telegraph Road* on it and *Private Investigations*, a song which made me remember all the Film Noir movies I had so enjoyed when I was still at film school. The other album was *Famous Last Words* by Supertramp, which included the excellent song *Waiting So Long*, although the title didn't bode well as far as when my next gig might happen, and *Don't Leave Me Now,* which was one of the saddest songs I had ever heard. Roger Hodgson's wailing guitar on the closing track brought a tear to my eye.

The next two gigs I went to helped me feel much more positive as they were both held at the beautiful Capitol Theatre, one of my favourite venues anywhere in the world.

The Motels were at their peak the night I saw them and I loved watching Martha Davis sing *Total Control, Dressing Up* and *Celia.* Meanwhile, Madness did their utmost to live up to their name and Suggs, their charismatic cockney singer, had us all in the palm of his hand the moment they played *Baggy Trousers* and before the show was over the British Ska band had turned the Capitol into *The House of Fun.*

The next day I got a call out of the blue from a Sydney production company to ask me whether I would like to direct a commercial for them. The spot was for Jacob's Creek wine, who up until then had only been known to make red wine but were now about to sell white wine as well. The script called for a full glass of red wine to be twisted clockwise to reveal the glass now contained half a glass of red and half of white divided equally by a vertical line. To ensure the spot was lit well we hired a brilliant stills photographer called Billy Wrencher, as his lighting for food and beverages was quite extraordinary. Billy was from the East End of London and had worked as a gravedigger before getting an interest in cameras. When he was a bit younger, he was

David Bailey's assistant for a while and learned a lot of his lighting skills from the famous fashion photographer before becoming a much sought-after photographer himself. The shoot went smoothly but combining all the film elements afterwards in post-production proved to be an absolute nightmare. Thanks to the help of Mirage VFX, we ended up with a great-looking commercial… plus two cases of wine as a thank you from the client, one with bottles of red the other white.

In December, I went to see The Divinyls at the San Miguel Hotel in Cammeray. I was entranced by their singer Chrissy Amphlett as she wore a school uniform and fishnet stockings and waved an illuminated neon tube around like a whirling dervish while singing *Boys in Town* and *Elsie* off their album *Monkey Grip*. Their raw energy was infectious and I danced in front of the stage all night until a pretty girl who was as equally drunk as I was yelled in my ear, 'Get me out of here!'…so I did.

I directed two more commercials before Christmas. The first was a live-action spot for NatWest Bank, which we shot in a studio in Sydney and was easy to do or a 'piece of piss' as one of the crew declared once it was in the can. The other was for Kraft Cheese, which Michael Elphick, a director in Melbourne, asked me to help him with as it required some special effects, including an 'in-camera' logo shot which revealed the name of the product to look like the word was carved in relief from a block of cheese just after a knife cut the first slice. The popular brand Coon Cheese got its name from American pioneering cheese maker Edward William Coon who patented a ripening process in the 1920s. But historically the word 'coon' has been used as a racist slur so I suspected it would only be a matter of time before the company would be forced to change the name.

The unexpected windfall of two well-paid gigs in a row meant I could now look for some better accommodation, so I moved into a townhouse in West Street, North Sydney with two female friends from the UK called Debbie and Eleanor. Madness ensued all through Christmas and it soon became known as The House of Fun.

Wild Bill Hickok and Calamity Jane now going by their real names,

Rich and Marcia, invited me to dinner on New Year's Eve at their harbourside flat in Kirribilli, which was right opposite the Opera House so the view was spectacular. They had also invited another couple called Geof and Jana, who were from San Francisco, and a stunning woman called Gai who flirted with me outrageously all evening. At midnight we went outside to watch the fireworks over Sydney Harbour, which were out of this world. When Gai offered me a lift home, I gladly accepted as I had drunk a bit more than was good for me. When we arrived at my place, she told me she wanted to make 'mad passionate love' to me, so as it would have been rude not to, I acquiesced to her perfectly reasonable request.

The first gig of 1983 was on the 22nd of January when Gai and I went to see Gold Rush at the San Miguel Hotel in Cammeray. The band featured some of Australia's finest musicians who played a mix of boogie, country and western, bluegrass and funk. The reason I was keen to see them was because their guitarist Phil Emmanuel was known in the music industry as The Wiz, and as soon as he started to play, I could understand why. His brother Tommy was on drums to start with but towards the end of the set the two Emmanuel brothers played guitars together on a couple of songs, which had us all spellbound.

A couple of weeks later, Gai and I along with our mutual American friends Rich, Marcia, Geof and Jana, went to see Simon and Garfunkel at the Sydney Sportsground. Hearing *Bridge Over Troubled Water, The Sound of Silence* and *The Boxer* sung live by these two extraordinarily talented singers was magical. Rich told us on the way home, the duo began recording together at high school under the names of the cartoon characters Tom and Jerry. My friend was always full of fun facts but I had rarely seen him look so animated.

Having had a fairly quiet start to the year, everything changed dramatically in February. On the 4th Melbourne had a huge dust storm caused by high winds carrying red soil and sand from Central Australia through Victoria to the city and on the 16th a series of intense bushfires fanned by winds of up to 68mph (110km/h) occurred in South

Australia and caused widespread destruction. 75 people died, more than 2500 people lost their homes and over 3000 buildings were destroyed. Ash Wednesday was the most destructive bushfire event in Australian history at the time.

When I rang Edwin to make sure he and his family were safe, his wife Jane told me she and the girls were fine but her husband was 'out there somewhere' filming the brave firefighters and volunteers who were doing their utmost to save lives and property, so she was more than a little concerned for his welfare. After an anxious few hours worrying about him, Edwin rang me to let me know he was back home safe and sound, which was a relief as I couldn't bear the thought of losing another friend and mentor.

A week later, I went to the Australian Film Commission to pitch a couple of concepts in the hope of obtaining a grant from them. The first idea was to set up an Australian School of Special Effects Technicians (ASSET) for film students wanting to learn how to learn this exciting craft from technicians currently working in the industry. The other idea was to make a short film using a combination of holograms and 3D photography. I got a grant to do both and it was a privilege to meet some of the best special effects technicians in the business as well as some of the pioneers of holography. One of the people we interviewed had a girlfriend called Marisa Fitzgerald, with whom I became good friends and after a while we were like brother and sister. When I told her I was going to Melbourne to do an interview with a holographic artist, she insisted I go and see her family who lived in a rather posh part of the city. When I met them a week later, I thought they were rather posh too.

Marisa's father Paul was an acclaimed artist who had been commissioned to paint portraits of the Queen, Prince Philip and Prince Charles, as well as a Pope and a couple of Australian Prime Ministers. Her mother Mary had once been an actress appearing on stage in London's West End as well as in a couple of movies starring Douglas Fairbanks Junior and Boris Karloff. As Mary's brother Michael was currently visiting the family, I got to meet him too. He told me he was

Prince Philip's private secretary and equerry-waiting to the Queen, so I made sure I was on my best behaviour.

The Fitzgeralds had six children, including Marisa. Three other girls, Emma, Maria and Fran, and two boys, Fabian and Ted. Fabian, or 'Fabes' as the rest of the family called him, had the same passion for music as I did so we soon became 'brothers from another mother.' Before I left Melbourne, Mary told me I would always be welcome at their home and to consider them as my 'Aussie Family', which was one of the loveliest things anyone has ever said to me. It also made me miss my own family in England, so I decided I would fly back and see them the following month but rather than buying a return ticket to London, I decided to buy an around-the-world ticket instead, flying to the UK via Japan and returning to Australia via the USA, which would allow me to see my cousins on the way back.

After I had told Gai I was going overseas for a while, she suggested we break up before I left and just be friends from now on, so there would be no unrealistic expectations from either of us of whether we would continue our relationship or not when I got back. I thought this was very mature of her, but when I got home, I wondered whether her decision might simply have been because she had already found a new boyfriend.

The first thing I noticed when I got to Tokyo was all the skyscrapers and the neon lights. They made the city look like a scene from an old Science Fiction movie. The Imperial Palace did the exact opposite and made me think of all the successive Emperors who had lived there since 1868. As I watched hundreds of people walking across the busy Shibuya Crossing all at the same time, it was almost impossible to imagine this huge metropolis had once been a tiny fishing village called Edo.

The Shinkansen or bullet train as it's more commonly called, took just over two hours to get from Tokyo to Kyoto, but it was a very smooth ride. Kyoto had once been the capital of Japan and the day I arrived the cherry trees were just beginning to blossom, making my view of Nijo Castle look like a traditional painting, or Nihonga as the locals call them. When I got to the Golden Pavilion I sat beside the peaceful lake and took several photos of the temple. I tried 'thinking about not thinking' but I couldn't clear my mind enough to meditate the Zen way. A skill I still haven't fully mastered.

On the way back to Tokyo, I stopped off in Nara to see the Todai-ji Temple because I wanted to see the giant bronze statue of the seated Buddha before going to Nara Park to take some photos of the free-roaming Shika. The deer looked like they were bowing at the tourists, but when I saw a stall selling shika senbei, which means deer crackers, I realised they were just lowering their heads to get fed in the same way dogs do tricks for treats.

After checking in at my hotel, I went in search of a Japanese restaurant where only local people go to eat, as I wanted to taste some authentic national cuisine. It didn't take long before I got lost in a labyrinth of dark alleys. Thankfully my nose came to the rescue. The smell of recently grilled chicken led me to a small but interesting-looking restaurant. When I peered through the window, I liked what I saw, so went in. A waiter witnessing my entrance, said something to me in Japanese but as soon as he realised my grasp of his language was somewhat limited, he handed me a menu. However, as everything was written in Japanese it wasn't quite as useful as either of us had hoped, so I attempted to mime what I wanted to eat by pointing at the wonderful-looking food on the table to my left, hoping he would see I wanted to order the same food they were eating.

This is where it all started to go horribly wrong. My hand gestures had been interpreted in an entirely different way to how I had intended and before I had time to point out 'his' mistake, the waiter had forced the customers, who were sitting at the table I had just pointed at, to squeeze up so I could join them at their table. These poor innocent victims were either too polite, too confused or still in shock to say anything about the sudden appearance of the strange looking foreigner who had just gate-crashed their dinner party and kindly made a space for me at their table, accepting my unintentional intrusion with grace. As I sat down, I smiled at my dinner companions and luckily, they smiled back. After I had pointed at my chest and told them my name, they each did the same, one by one, around the table. The waiter then asked me if I would like some saké but as I was having enough trouble sober, I thought I'd better not drink any alcohol and make the situation worse, so I waved my hand shooing the waiter away as politely as possible hoping he would understand my hand gesture so when he looked at me and said, 'Go?' I nodded and replied, 'Yes please. Go!' When the waiter returned a couple of minutes later with five small cups of saké on a tray and placed them in front of me, everyone at the table suddenly stopped talking. It was a bit like one of those scenes in a cowboy movie, where the mean looking gunslinger pushes through the swing doors and as everyone turns to look at him, the bar falls silent, including the piano player, knowing a fight is about to ensue. This was when I realised my mistake. Ichi, Nee, San, Shi and Go are the numbers 1-5 in Japanese, so when I waved my hand and said 'Go' the waiter had put 2 and 2 together and made 5. Well, obviously there was only one course of action I could possibly take, so I lifted the first cup of saké to my lips and said to my companions 'Ichi' and downed it in one. You can most probably guess what happened next. 'Nee' and 'San' were dispatched in similar fashion and by the time I got to 'Shi' I was starting to think this might not have been such a great idea after all. Swallowing 'Go' in one go was a feat of shear willpower but I managed and placed the cup back on the table with a loud thump.

To my surprise and relief, instead of being thrown out into the street, my companions burst out clapping and then one of the men ordered another round of saké for all of us, which in hindsight is perhaps what I should have done in the first place. When the cups arrived, I made a toast to my new acquaintances and they all knocked back their saké like true professionals. Thankfully, some 'interesting' looking food was then placed on the table and silence ensued while we ate it. When it came time to leave, my new friends insisted on paying for everything and after we left the restaurant, they took me to a birthday party at one of their homes but how I got back to my hotel remains a mystery to this day.

When I woke up the next morning, I had a terrible hangover, so while I was checking out, I asked the hotel receptionist if he had any Paracetamol. He then said in perfect English, 'Sir, please understand the alcohol content of saké is much higher than in wine or beer.'

'Really! Tell me something I don't know!' I said rather ungraciously.

'Chintsū-zai!' He replied with a cheeky grin.

'Ah,' I sighed, 'OK, you've got me there.'

After explaining Chintsū-zai was the Japanese word for painkiller, he then kindly gave me a couple of pills and a glass of water, exactly what I needed before going on the long-haul flight to London.

*We must be willing to get rid of the life we've planned,*
*so as to have the life that is waiting for us.*

Joseph Campbell

## CHAPTER 3: RECKLESS (DON'T BE SO)

Feeling restless and like a lost soul without a sense of direction, I made my way to Hampshire and as my train rattled along the tracks, I had the strangest feeling of being a stranger in my own country. I no longer belonged, or at least this is how I felt when I got off at New Milton, the station where my mother and step-father were waiting to pick me up. There is nothing quite like a hug from your Mum, however old you are, as it gives you a feeling of security, so when we finally arrived at my parent's house and my mother put her arms around me, I immediately started to relax and unwind.

After catching up on the latest family news, I told her how upset I had been about Alastair's death, how he had been like a father to me and how he had made me feel I belonged in the Australian film industry but now he was gone I felt lost and alone.

'Grief is a personal thing, 'my mother said taking my hand in hers, 'Nobody else can tell you when it's time to move on, so just be patient, be kind to yourself and if you want to have the sense of belonging again then it's up to you to make the effort to engage with like-minded people. You don't need to wait for an invitation!'

When I started asking her questions about my real father, my mother suggested we drive up to Scotland together to see where our family had lived when he was alive. As we drove north, she told me how she had met my father during WW2 when she was testing the pilots for night vision and about the life they had shared before he had died. It was a bitter-sweet conversation.

Once we were across the Scottish border we stopped off in Aberfeldy, so I could see where I was born and then we drove to Pitlochry to look at our old family house. We ended the day at Faskally Wood, which had a wide range of tree species, some more than 200 years old. As we walked through the ancient woodland, Mum told me how Dad had taught her the names of all the trees and flowers while he was working for the Scottish Forestry Commission. She remembered him telling her how connecting with nature is important for our well-being and noticing beauty around us is essential to our happiness. I had no idea my father was such a forward thinker and vowed to become more aware of my natural surroundings.

As my sister and brother both had four children now, my mother was in constant demand for Granny duty, which she loved and to my surprise my stepfather also seemed to enjoy his role as Grandpa. 'It's much easier being a grandparent than a parent,' he told me, 'as when you've had enough you can hand them back!'

On the 14th of April 1983, David Bowie released *Let's* Dance, so I bought a copy of the album, produced by Chic's Nile Rodgers, to listen to on the plane to L.A where I had arranged to meet my American cousins Jamie and Mark before going on a short holiday with them to Mexico. I liked the upbeat opening track *Modern Love* as I could identify with the idea of someone who is always looking for a meaningful relationship but never quite manages to achieve it. I also enjoyed *China Girl,* which was co-written with Iggy Pop but my favourite track was *Let's Dance.* Stevie Ray Vaughan's sublime and subtle guitar solo still gives me the chills every time I hear it.

When I got to Los Angeles, my cousin Elmar was there to meet me at the airport and took me straight back to his house where the rest of the family were busy helping his wife Jeanne prepare dinner. After a lovely meal, Jamie, Mark and I discussed what we wanted to do while we were in Mexico and then I gave Emily, whom I had first met at my cousin's wedding in 1979, a quick call to see how she and her son Leo were doing. She told me she was still with her husband but it wasn't going well at the moment, so I told her if things didn't work out, perhaps she might consider coming to Australia.

'I might just do that!' she replied with a laugh, 'be careful what you wish for Jamie.'

Our flight to Mexico only took four hours and when we arrived, we took a taxi straight to our hotel on the Zócalo, which is what they call the city's main square. As soon as we had unpacked, we headed out to look for some street food. Mark ate Tamales, which were full of chicken and chillies and Jamie and I had fresh corn Tacos al pastor, which was sliced meat similar to a kebab topped with pineapple, salsa and cilantro. Delicioso!

On our first full day in Mexico, we took ourselves to the Frida Kahlo Museum. The cobalt blue house was where she was born and lived with her artist husband Diego Riviera until she died, which I discovered was the same year I was born. The museum was full of wonderful works of art painted by both artists but it was the personal items dotted around the house, which made me feel their presence was somehow still present.

When I first saw the Teotihuacan Pyramids in 1978, I never imagined I would be walking down the Avenue of the Dead again a few years later, but here I was with my cousin and her partner exploring the ancient city once more. I climbed the Pyramid of the Sun just as I had done before but this time felt one pyramid was more than enough. The Pyramid of the Moon and the Temple of Quetzalcoatl would have to wait for another day.

In the evening, I phoned Rocio and her sister Sandy, the sisters I had met on my previous trip to Mexico, who suggested we meet at their parent's house, so I wrote down their address on a tiny scrap of paper. Our taxi driver, after swiftly glancing at the address assured us he knew exactly where it was, but after only driving a quarter of a mile, he stopped the car and showed my paper scrap to another taxi driver to ask for directions. This performance was then repeated every couple of minutes without getting any nearer to our destination but then I had another problem and this one was more to do with digestion than direction. The spicy food I had eaten earlier in the day was starting to disagree with me and I needed to find *un baño rápido*.

Suddenly, the driver jammed on his brakes and then reversed at speed down a one-way street before stopping outside a large house with ornate gates at the front. We were there.

Although I was very happy to see Rocio and Sandy again, I was in desperate need of the loo, so after a quick introduction I left Jamie and

Mark to get to know the girls while I went in search of their *baño* to relieve myself. When I had finished my business, I realised there was no toilet paper to be seen and the only alternative I could think of was to use an old edition of National Geographic on the far side of the bathroom. 'Sorry amigos but needs must!' I said to myself as I ripped a few pages from the magazine. Not wanting to defecate on, deface or destroy the delightful photos taken by some of the most respected photographers in the world, I left the glossy pages intact and only tore out the pages with advertising on them. A moment later, I managed to get myself into some sort of respectable shape but then disaster struck. The toilet wouldn't flush. After several failed attempts, I sat down on the loo and tried to come up with a plan, as there was no way I was going to leave behind what had recently… come out of my behind. The only viable option I could think of was to fill one of my boots with water from the sink tap and fill the cistern one boot full at a time until there was enough water to attempt another flush. There was no guarantee it would work but as Anon once said 'When you only have one option, you have yourself a plan', so I proceeded with caution. After filling the cistern with five boots worth of water, I thought it must be full enough by now to try the flush again and thankfully it worked. With a slightly soggy foot and a rather sore bottom but a much-relieved stomach, I finally joined the others. While I had been at my wit's end, the girls had decided they wanted to take us to a restaurant which specialised in really hot chilli dishes. ¡Qué coño!

The in-house Mariachi band must have played *La Cucaracha* at least half a dozen times while we ate our spicy food and I can assure you once is quite enough. Between courses Rocio told me the song was about a cockroach who can't walk because it has no legs. As I resumed my meal, I bit into something crunchy, so I think I knew where they ended up.

It took just over six hours to get to Oaxaca, pronounced *wah-hah-ka*. We loved the small city as soon as we got off the coach. The pace felt much slower than it had in Mexico City and everyone seemed to be extremely friendly, although they may have just been drunk from the effect of mezcal, their local signature drink made from agave, a local plant. We decided the best thing to do was to try a glass for ourselves. I found it a bit too smoky for my taste but Jamie and Mark loved it and ordered another glass. After wandering the streets looking at the local handicrafts for a while, I bought a piece of 'Barro Negro' pottery, which is what the area is famed for. The black clay pottery dates back to Monte Alban, once home to the Zapotec culture, and some of the ruins are open to the public, so we took a short bus trip there to explore them. When we arrived, we were surprised to have the place all to ourselves, which was great for me as I was able to get some photos without any other tourists milling around. After a few days relaxing in this beautiful city, eating and drinking too much while enjoying each other's company, we returned to Mexico City and from there Jamie and Mark flew back to L.A and I took a plane to San Francisco because I had a wedding to attend.

My old kindergarten friend Mark and his fiancé Suzanne, whom I had met in New York, had decided to tie the knot in style. Mark's brothers Richard, Bill and Charlie were acting as ushers but as they needed four, they asked me to be an honorary brother on the day. Vicki, who I had travelled around North America with in 1978, had also been invited so there was quite a contingent there from the UK.

Our dear friends had a lovely pre-wedding party at a vineyard in the Napa Valley, which was great fun and the quality of the wine was quite exceptional as you might expect. After a boozy dinner we danced to music provided by a local DJ and when he played Billy Idol's *White Wedding,* we all did our best to imitate Billy's famous snarl lip while singing the chorus in a rowdy and raunchy fashion. It was great fun.

The wedding took place in a small forest under some giant redwood trees, which was a really romantic setting. There were rows of white chairs on either side of an aisle and as a token gesture to Australia, Mark had scattered some fresh eucalyptus leaves on the forest floor, so when the happy couple walked down the aisle together for the first time, the distinct smell reached our olfactory systems immediately. As the nuptials commenced, I noticed Suzanne's attractive maid of honour was crying, presumably from the emotion of such a beautiful service, so in an attempt to be a gentleman, I tried to comfort her by putting my arm through hers for the rest of the ceremony. After the knot was tied and the happy couple and their guests were making their way to the reception, I tried to disengage my arm and follow everyone else but my tearful new friend had other ideas. After guiding me through the forest to an empty log cabin, we went inside and the maid of honour asked me to comfort her again but this time in a slightly less honourable way.

I had a quick stop-over in Hawaii to refresh my batteries sunbathing on Waikiki beach and then flew back to Australia. While listening to the rather appropriately titled album *Here, There, and Back* by The Allen Collins Band on my headphones, I felt grateful to have been able to catch up with my family and friends on this trip. Even though I had decided to make a life for myself in Australia, they would always be important to me and in an ideal world I would like to see them every year, so I would just have to find a way to fulfil this ambitious notion and then I could have the best of both worlds.

When I got back to Sydney, I kept hearing a catchy song on the radio by The Police called *Every Breath You Take*. Apparently, the lead singer wrote the lyrics in Jamaica while sitting at Ian Fleming's desk, the same one where the author had written many of the James Bond novels. I tried to imagine him standing at a bar introducing himself to a beautiful woman while trying to sound like Sean Connery.

'Hi, my name's Sumner... Gordon Sumner.... on second thoughts ...just call me Sting!'

In late June I flew to Adelaide as Edwin was about to produce a film for the South Australian government about the local mangrove swamps and had asked me to direct it, so he could concentrate on the camerawork. The film was called *No Man's Land* and told the story of how mangroves are ecologically important ecosystems, which link the land and the sea and provide a habitat for migratory shorebirds, as well as many fish species, crustaceans and molluscs.

While we were filming some scenic shots one morning, a helicopter suddenly flew overhead and landed quite close to us. Before I had time to take it all in, I was bundled on board and less than a minute later we were high above the ground looking down at the mangroves below. As Edwin leant out of the chopper to get some aerial shots, he yelled at me to hold onto his belt so he didn't fall to his death. Not much in the way of health and safety in those days but my old friend was always taking risks to get the perfect shot. When we landed, he told me he had organised the helicopter to arrive when and where it did without telling me on purpose thinking I might be too nervous to go up in a chopper again after Alastair died in one, but surprisingly I wasn't scared at all and loved seeing the beauty of the mangroves from such a wonderful vantage point.

It was during the making of this film I first met a couple of wildlife filmmakers who would change the way I saw nature forever. Over a strong pot of tea, Jim Frazier and Densey Clyne told me they had once made a film about spiders called *Aliens Among Us*, which the BBC liked so much they had then been asked to supply a few shots for David Attenborough's *Life on Earth* series and this is when they had formed a company together called Mantis Wildlife Films. Densey was a naturalist, writer and photographer who had won a Hasselblad Masters award, and Jim was a cameraman specialising in macro and micro photography, which is why Edwin wanted me to meet them. The mangrove ecosystem has a diverse range of microorganisms and we needed a few shots of microalgae to explain this section of our story. I had brought a specimen with me from Adelaide, so Jim was able to film the tiny microphytes for us using his specially adapted micro lens. I remember telling Edwin. 'I think I might have just met my first genius!' Thankfully he was very humble and didn't take offence I hadn't meant him.

In July, I was lucky enough to fly over the Whitsunday Islands and the Great Barrier Reef in a 1947 Grumman G-73 Mallard, with Ann, the girl I had stayed with in Moree who was now living and working in Airlie Beach in Queensland.

Seeing the reef from the air for the first time was a sensational experience. The Seaplane landed in the lagoon at Hardy Reef and floated towards a permanently anchored semi-submersible glass bottom boat. There were hundreds of colourful fish and coral and I could see them so clearly it felt like I was wearing 3D glasses. Ann went snorkelling but as I wouldn't be able to see anything without my prescription glasses, I just swam close to the boat, wearing a T-shirt so I didn't get sunburnt.

A week later I moved into a three-bedroom flat in Cremorne, which was walking distance to The Oaks, the most popular watering hole on the Lower North Shore, partly because it had a BBQ in the garden where you could buy a steak for a reasonable price and cook it yourself. My flatmate was an old friend from the New Forest called Jerry who was in Australia on a working holiday and had found a job as a sales rep for Castlemaine Tooheys. Our third bedroom was used to store all Jerry's boxes of wine and cartons of beer, which he used as samples when he went on his rep trips around New South Wales. Our new pad was on the eighth floor and it had a great view from our balcony, ironically looking towards a suburb called Crows Nest.

One afternoon, Jerry told me to come to the balcony to see the view. When I looked at the skyline he said, 'No mate, not there... down there!'

Lying next to the swimming pool below were two stunning girls sunbathing.

'Let's invite them for a drink,' he said with one of his trademark cheeky grins.

'Ok!' I replied, easily led.

'Hang on a minute, I've got a better idea.' Jerry said, his grin getting even wider.

'Oh dear,' I replied, slightly concerned, as Jerry's spontaneous ideas usually meant one or other of us would get into trouble if not both, 'Is this something we will regret later?'

'Nah mate, this is something we'll regret if we don't do it!' With those words of wisdom still ringing in my ears, my unpredictable flatmate grabbed some chilled champagne out of the fridge, secured a fishing line around the neck of the bottle and, after testing it could take the strain on his fishing rod, lowered the bottle a few feet at a time until it landed right next to the girls lying beside the pool. I was just thinking about what might have happened if the line had broken and the bottle had fallen on top of them from eight floors, when one of the girls yelled, 'Well, are you going to join us or what?'

As Jerry grabbed four champagne flutes, he said, 'I think we should wear our dinner jackets,' and then by way of explanation added, 'They look a bit out of our league.'

As the girls were only wearing bikinis, I am not entirely sure what he based his assessment on but wasn't about to ask so simply suggested we put on our swimming trunks. A compromise was agreed. DJs with swimming togs underneath …and bow ties!

Thankfully the girls thought we looked hilarious and laughed with us not at us, which is always a promising sign. After a couple of glasses of champagne, they explained they had only just moved into the flat above us the night before and had managed to lock themselves out after leaving their keys in the flat when they came down for a dip, which is why they were waiting by the pool for the caretaker to arrive with a spare set of keys.

'No need to wait for him, I've got a better idea,' Jerry said to our new neighbours.

Having ascertained they had left their balcony doors open, Jerry took the lift up to our flat on the eighth floor, climbed onto the ledge of our balcony, hauled himself up and over onto their balcony on the ninth floor, entered their flat, grabbed the keys and then got the lift back down to the pool before calmly handing the keys to the girls, as though he did this sort of thing every day. The girls gave Jerry the full hero treatment for the noble deed he had just done but I just felt a bit sick, as the chances of my macho mate falling to his death from one of the balconies was a gamble, I would never have risked sober, let alone with a couple of glasses of champagne on an empty stomach inside me. The hero of the hour however was cool as a cucumber and simply said, 'Sorted!'

On the 11$^{th}$ of November Yes released *90125,* which I was interested to hear as their original keyboardist Tony Kaye was back in the band and Trevor Rabin had replaced Steve Howe on guitar. The opening track *Owner of a Lonely Heart* became a huge hit and gave new life to Yes at a time when progressive rock wasn't as popular as it had been in the 70s. It also introduced them to a whole new set of younger fans. Many years later Trevor admitted he wrote the song while sitting on the loo. Another of his songs is called *Leave It*, which I assume he wrote immediately afterwards and the full title originally included the words '*for at least five minutes'*.

On the 19$^{th}$ of November, Jerry and I went to see the return of 'The Thin White Duke' on his *Serious Moonlight* tour at the Sydney Showground. As soon as David Bowie ran onto the stage and started singing *Look Back In Anger,* the crowd went wild and surged forward like a mini-tsunami crushing the poor people standing right in front of the stage. *Heroes, Let's Dance, Life on Mars?, Cat People, China Girl* and *Space Oddity* were the songs I was looking forward to seeing performed the most and I wasn't disappointed. Earl Slick's energetic and exceptional solos were first class and I felt blessed to have witnessed one of the most underrated axemen in the music industry at his very best. Carlos Alomar also played some great licks and Carmine Rojas was outstanding on bass. There were four encores. *Rock 'n' Roll Star, Stay, Jean Genie* and *Modern Love.*

On Christmas Eve, we decided to have a barbie at our place with our upstairs neighbours, which went well until I slipped over on our alcohol-soaked balcony floor and sprained my ankle rather badly. When it swelled up to twice its normal size and a nasty bruise appeared, Jerry decided it might be a good idea to take me to the nearest hospital. It was a good decision, as after they had taken an X-Ray I was told I had a transverse fracture and would have to have a plaster cast for a while.

On Christmas Day, I hobbled from my bedroom on the crutches the hospital had lent me to the kitchen to look for some painkillers. I was surprised to see Jerry was already up and had started to prepare a traditional Christmas lunch for us. After handing me 'a nice little Mosel' to start the festivities off in the right way, my flatmate gave me my Christmas present, which was a cassette of the new Australian Crawl live album *Phalanx*. This was the perfect gift, as I loved the band. The record included the songs *Errol* and *The Boys Light Up,* but the track I will always associate with my dear friend Jerry, especially after his recent Spiderman antics was *Reckless (Don't Be So).*

As Jerry had invited the 'pool girls' for lunch as well as a bunch of his workmates, it was quite a raucous party and the booze flowed constantly and consistently all day. The women drank Buck's fizz out of cheap plastic picnic glasses and the men drank bottles of beer placed in stubby holders. We had fresh prawns with chilli and lime as our first course followed by Jerry's turkey, which he had cooked to perfection.

After lunch, everyone went for a swim, except for me of course. Unfortunately, I wouldn't be able to swim again until my cast had been removed, so I went to my bedroom to have a quick rest but I wasn't alone for long as Debbie, one of Jerry's female friends from work knocked on my door and asked me if I would like some company.

The first thing I noticed was how attractive she was. The second was how quickly she was able to get undressed. There may have also been a third thing, but by then Debbie had climbed on top of me and was kissing me passionately, so I can't remember whether it was important or not. She then began divesting me of my clothes, starting with my shirt, which she unbuttoned… very slowly, and then after pulling my shorts over my plaster cast… very carefully, she whispered in my ear what she was about to do to me.

'Please be gentle with me!' I said as a joke but meaning it, as having already got one fracture, I didn't want another one if she decided to 'jump my bones' a little too enthusiastically. In the background I could hear our party guests singing the chorus to Australia's current Number One single *All Night Long (All Night)* by Lionel Ritchie, which would have put a big smile on my face if I hadn't already got one.

In the morning, Debbie signed my plaster cast and then wrote her phone number next to it, which was in such an awkward place I had to ask Jerry to read it out to me after she had left so I could put it in my address book. As I still needed crutches, I wasn't able to do very much for the first few weeks of 1984 but on the 26th of January I took myself to Circular Quay to watch the Australia Day Ferrython on Sydney Harbour. The only reason the race got a mention in my diary was because it nearly ended in disaster. On its way back to the finish line 'Karrabbee' started to take on water and the old ferry only just managed to get back in time to let the passengers disembark before it sank. The next noteworthy date was the 1st of February, as it was the day Medicare came into effect in Australia, establishing basic health care for everyone in the country, which was, and would remain a great help to me and thousands of others over the years. It was also the day my cast was finally removed and I no longer needed crutches.

Two days later, Jerry and I went to see Robert Plant, the ex-Led Zeppelin vocalist, at the Sydney Entertainment Centre. He started his set with *In the Mood* from his second solo album *The Principle of Moments* and then he played a mixture of songs from his first two albums but the highlight was when Elton John joined him on stage to play some brilliant boogie woogie piano on *Treat Her Right*, which brought the house down.

Inspired by the recent ferry incident we decided to hold a fancy dress party at our flat with the nautical theme 'What you were wearing when the ship went down'. Our guests were a motley crew consisting of a pipe-smoking Ship's Captain, a Catholic priest wearing a life vest and a Pirate wearing a false beard but with a real-parrot on his shoulder. They were then joined by three women wearing fabulous ballgowns but one of them was still wearing curlers, which I thought was a clever idea. Jerry wore his dinner jacket over a pair of stripey pyjamas so looked very smart and ready for action and I was dressed as Robinson Crusoe with Debbie as my 'Girl Friday', which wasn't entirely accurate but 'Girl twice a week and every other weekend' seemed a bit of a mouthful.

Scottish rock band Simple Minds released *Sparkle in the Rain* on the 6$^{th}$ of February. The repetitive and throbbing bass line on *Waterfront* created by Derek Forbes using a Dynacord bass amp was truly sensational. I thought Jim Kerr's voice was very powerful and his lyrics 'So far, so good, so close, yet still so far,' resonated with me long after the song had finished.

A week later I got a call from a production company called The Film Business, asking asked me if I would co-direct a commercial with one of their directors for Phillips as they had just brought out a new laser disc. The visual effect they wanted to achieve was to make it look like a hologram of a rock band magically appeared above the disc player as soon as it was turned on. Although it would have been easy to produce in today's digital effects world, back then it was quite a challenge. The first step was to film a mock rock band in the studio performing against a cyclorama painted chromakey blue, so they could then be superimposed in the edit. After we had got the shot of the talent, my animator friend Peter Luschwitz rotoscoped each frame of the take I had selected to create 2D animated characters doing exactly the same movements as the musicians. We then graded the animation the same shade of eerie green most holograms were at this time, and superimposed the 'second wavefront' images at 50% transparency over the live action, which was also graded with a green tint and added at 50%, thereby creating a mock interference pattern. The 'holographic band' were then added over the top of the disc player in post-production and intercut with the other live-action which had been directed on a different day. The client was happy, the director was happy and I was... relieved, as I needed the money.

We finished the job on Valentine's Day and when I got home, I heard on the news Elton John had just got married to his 'close friend' Renate Blauel at an Anglican church in Darling Point. I presumed my invitation must have got lost in the post.

On the 2$^{nd}$ of March, The Police brought their *Synchronicity* tour to Sydney, so Jerry and I went to see them at the Sydney Showground. Bryan Adams was the support act but we had really only come along to sing along with Sting, Andy and Stewart. They started their set with

*Synchronicity* and then did a few of their better-known songs like *Message in a Bottle, Walking on the Moon* and *Every Breath You Take.* The biggest cheer of the night was saved for *Roxanne*, the song inspired by a group of prostitutes Sting had seen near the band's hotel in Paris back in 1977.

As SKY were performing at the Sydney Opera House later in the month, I went to see them again and their show was just as entertaining as the London concert. Watching John Williams and Kevin Peek breaking boundaries with their different guitar styles on stage together was a real privilege. The obvious pleasure they got from playing together was written all over their smiling faces and the appreciation they had for each other's extraordinary talent was there for all to see. Afterwards I went backstage to catch up with Kevin Peek and discuss the possibility of working together in the future. I also had a quick chat with Herbie Flowers who told me how much he had enjoyed being part of T. Rex in the 70's. He thought Marc Bolan was 'a nice player' who knew exactly what he was doing. I still regretted not seeing them when I had the chance.

On the 19th of April, Australia changed its National Anthem from *God Save the Queen* to *Advance Australia Fair*, written and composed by Peter Dodds McCormick in 1878. I found it quite a stirring song and at the time thought it was the right choice but if it had been an option, I would have voted for Peter Allen's song *I Still Call Australia Home*, which still brings a tear to my eye every time I hear it, as it does for many Aussies.

A week later, Jim Frazier invited me back to the Mantis Wildlife Films office in Dural. When I arrived, Densey was standing at the top of her drive and greeted me like an old friend, 'I always speak kindly to my plants as it helps them grow,' she said as she showed me around her magnificent garden, 'If only we did the same to each other the world would be a much happier place.' She then led me to the garage, which had been converted into a studio. Jim's 16mm camera was set up next to a glass tank. Inside the glass prison was a miniature set which looked like a desert landscape complete with a mound of red sand and a few tufts of spinifex. After closer examination, I saw what Jim and his camera assistant were filming. A huge spider about the size of my hand.

'Selenocosmia stirlingi!' Jim said noticing my presence for the first time.

'It's a species of Tarantula, also known as a Barking spider!' His assistant said before firmly shaking my hand, 'I'm Glen by the way.'

'Hello Glen-by-the-way,' I said, retrieving my hand from his vice-like grip, 'Good to meet you.' I was just thinking they must be barking mad to be working so close to a Tarantula when Densey said, 'They don't have any teeth so they liquefy their prey with venom to help them digest their meals. However, we haven't asked you here to see our lovely spider. Jim why don't you tell Jamie what you have been up to.'

'I have just discovered a completely new form of art, quite by accident.' Jim said modestly as he turned on a lightbox and placed some medium format transparencies on it. On each of the frames was a stunning multi-coloured abstract design, some of them looked like alien landscapes to me and others had very distinctive faces with eyes looking back at me, 'I created these images by manipulating tiny crystals dissolved in solution as they grew on pieces of glass and then using fine brushes and small tools, I coerced the growing crystals into forming these incredible formations,' Jim explained, clearly proud of his achievements, 'I then had to develop a lighting and colouring process to enhance the finished art, which I did by lighting the translucent crystals from behind. I can alter them to any colour or colour combination you like just by using various colour filters.'

'They are absolutely stunning,' I said truthfully, 'I have never seen anything like it before.' This is when Jim told me he had invited me to see his crystal art and wanted to know if I would be willing to take a dozen of his framed photographs and a folder of transparencies to America in May on his behalf and exhibit his work at three trade shows, one in San Francisco, one in New York and another in Dallas. He then told me he couldn't afford to pay me but he had received a grant which would cover all my travel expenses, including accommodation, food and drinks. As I had no other work on the horizon, this sudden and unexpected opportunity to go back to America at someone else's expense was an offer I couldn't refuse, so I said 'Yes please… and thank you.'

*A little more persistence, a little more effort,*
*and what seemed hopeless failure may turn to glorious success.*

Elbert Hubbard

## CHAPTER 4: ALL LOVERS ARE DERANGED

A 6.2 magnitude earthquake occurred on the 24$^{th}$ of April 1984 in Morgan Hill in the Santa Clara Valley, and was felt throughout Central California. Its epicentre was only an hour south of San Francisco, so when I took a flight to the Golden City the next day and the talkative woman sitting next to me declared, 'San Fran is due for a big one soon,' I wondered if it would happen while I was there. To take my over-active imaginative mind off the potentially scary scenario, I put my headphones on and listened to *About Face,* the second solo album by Pink Floyd's guitarist David Gilmour. The two songs I liked the most were both written by The Who's guitarist Pete Townshend. The powerful rocker *All Lovers are Deranged* and the thoughtful track *Love on the Air* contained the whimsical lyrics, 'I was looking for love in wandering eyes like a ship trying to fix on a beacon.'

Although Jim's crystal images drew large crowds at the San Francisco trade show, when any potential customers realised his otherworldly images were photographs rather than paintings they lost interest, which was a pity as they were unique. In the evening, I had dinner with Cynthia, the maid of honour I had 'met' at my friend's wedding the previous year, who told me she was doing well with her career and had recently met 'someone special', which was good to hear as I thought she was pretty special herself.

In New York, the trade show had a completely different vibe to it, everyone was moving around much faster and sales were being done left, right and centre but unfortunately nobody wanted Jim's art hanging on their wall. One potential buyer did like them but wanted to know if we could print them on fabric, as they thought they could sell them as shirts and blouses and scarves. It wasn't a bad idea but the technology to print photos on material to a high quality hadn't been invented yet, so nothing came of it.

While I was on the East Coast, I caught up with Mark and Suzanne, the couple who had got married in San Francisco the year before. Instead of staying in Manhattan, they took me to their cottage in The Hamptons on Long Island for the weekend. It was right by the ocean so we went for long walks on the beach both days, which was wonderful.

The trade show in Dallas was completely different to the other two. Everyone loved Jim's crystal art but wanted them printed in 3D on coasters and placemats and asked if Jim could enhance the colours somehow, so they were more *garish*. Only in America, would this ever be considered an improvement. Although I was disappointed, I hadn't managed to get any sales on the trip, at least I had done some research and gathered some useful information, so once the show was over, I flew to LA to see my cousin Jamie and her husband Mark and while I was there, I also had time to catch up with Emily. Although I was still attracted to this beautiful and intelligent woman, I was genuinely happy when she told me her marriage was finally working out and how well her son Leo was doing at school. I wished her the best of luck with her life and then headed to the airport.

Having listened to David Gilmour on the way to America, I decided it was only fair to hear what Roger Waters had to offer on his debut solo album *The Pros and Cons of Hitch Hiking* on the way home to Australia. The co-founder of Pink Floyd had written the concepts for both this album and *The Wall* at much the same time and asked the band which one they would prefer to record together telling them the other would be a solo effort. *Bricks in the Wall*, as it was originally called, won the day and the rest is rock music history.

I liked the album musically, especially Eric Clapton's tasteful contribution on guitar and just wished I had a better set of headphones to appreciate the subtle production values.

The day after I got back to Sydney, still feeling a little jetlagged, I drove up to Dural to hand in my report to Jim. I thought he might be a bit disappointed not to have got any sales but when I arrived, he had a big smile on his face. After Densey made us a pot of coffee, Jim told me how one of the people I had met in New York had called him to offer to act as his agent in the USA promising she would put on a 'showing' at one of Manhattan's top art galleries, so thankfully it looked like the trip hadn't been a total waste of time after all. Over the next few weeks, Jim got several calls from her asking him to send original prints, each personally signed by him, for her to pass on to her wealthy clients, including Oprah Winfrey and Hilary Clinton. Jim was 'as happy as Larry', as they say in Australia.

By the way, the reason Larry was happy was because he never lost a fight. Laurence 'Larry' Foley was an Australian middle-weight boxer in the 1870s who was paid a huge amount of money every time he won, hence the oft-used term.

In May, I got a phone call from the legendary producer John Heyer OBE, who had directed the award-winning Australian feature-length documentary *Back of Beyond* in 1954, the year I was born. He was considered the father of Australian documentaries having spent his whole career making sponsored films, so when he asked me if I would like to direct a one-hour documentary about the Great Barrier Reef for him, I was completely taken aback. Apparently, I had been recommended to him but I never found out who it was who had convinced him to give me such a big break, so was never able to thank them.

John's only stipulations were for me to call the film *The Reef Builders* and to use the trims of archive 35mm underwater footage, which had been shot on one of his previous films by world-renowned Australian underwater cameraman Ron Taylor. Ron and his wife Valerie were famous for being the first people to film great white sharks without a protection cage, so I was very excited to meet them. As we viewed their deep-sea footage together, they told me the names of each species of fish and coral and where they had filmed them. I made copious notes but soon realised I was out of my depth and needed to talk to someone who knew the Great Barrier Reef like the back of their flipper, so after asking the Taylor's advice I made a call to Dr. John Veron, who was the principal research scientist at the Australian Institute of Marine Science (AIMS) in Townsville. After talking to him for a few minutes, I discovered he was not only a biologist and taxonomist but also a specialist in the study of corals and reefs. When he mentioned he had personally discovered more than 20% of the world's coral species, I knew I was also in safe hands. Despite being someone who obviously 'knew his stuff' and must have been well aware I didn't, he kindly put me at ease by insisting I call him Charlie, so having always believed honesty is the best policy, I was totally up front with him and admitted I was just a filmmaker and not a biologist, so would need to rely on him for all the facts. I then explained how my role was simply to turn his scientific jargon into layman's terms, without sounding too patronising, so the story of how the reef was built would be understood by a general audience. Charlie not only agreed to present the film but also suggested I film interviews with two research scientists from James Cook University, as Peter Harrison was an authority on coral spawning and Dr Vicki Harriott was an expert on the Crown of Thorns Starfish and its devastating effects on reef-building corals.

Although I had to use the Taylor's archive images of fish and corals, I also needed to get shots of Charlie when he was underwater and a few additional shots of specific corals which we didn't already have in our collection. As Ron was too busy to work on this film, he suggested I try a man called Walt Deas as he had been diving for over 30 years and was very experienced, so I gave him a call. Walt's Scottish accent was so strong I found it hard to understand anything he said to start with. His voice reminded me of my friend Alan who had been at film school with me, but after meeting him and seeing some of his terrific underwater images I knew he was the right man for the job. As the 'talking-heads' of Charlie, Vicki and Peter would all have to be shot above water, I asked Edwin Scragg if he would shoot them for me and then called Jim Frazier to see if he would like to film all the macro shots. Luckily for me, all three cameramen agreed to work with me and we started production on the 21$^{st}$ of May. It was a very exciting moment as this was my first full-length documentary and if I did a good job might open new doors which had previously been closed to me. I was determined to do my best, so put all my other interests to one side for the duration of the shoot and tried to just focus on the job at hand.

The Great Barrier Reef is composed of 2,900 individual reefs and 900 islands, so you only get an idea of just how huge an area it is from the air, as I discovered on my first flight over the world's largest coral reef system. To get the best possible shots I was advised to hire a seaplane and fly over Hook and Hardy Reefs. As the seaplanes flew from Hamilton Island, Edwin and I decided to base ourselves there for a few nights. The island was owned by entrepreneur Keith Williams and the construction had only started two years earlier, so the resort was still in an in-between phase.

On the first day of the shoot, we flew a Sea Air Beaver seaplane over 'The River' between Hook and Hardy reefs off the Whitsunday Islands and got all the aerial shots we needed. The Reef looked even more stunning than on my first scenic flight. It was a pity we had to shoot through the plane's window but Edwin made sure there were no reflections on the lens by using a polarising filter. I wish I had done the same with my still photographs.

The Great Barrier Reef formed on a coastal plain which was flooded during rapid sea-level rise, so to illustrate this fact, I decided we should film a timelapse shot of the sea-level rising above some exposed coral. To achieve it, we flew back to Hardy Reef the next day and as the aircraft had floats, we were able to land close to an accessible section of the reef at low tide and drift the plane towards the edge so we could walk directly onto the coral. Although we wore tough shoes to protect us from the sharp coral, carrying our heavy equipment over the uneven coral without scratching our ankles was quite a challenge. After I had carefully set up the Miller wooden tripod, Edwin placed his 16mm Aaton camera onto the fluid head and then programmed the timelapse system, which he had invented himself, and even though it looked like a Heath Robinson contraption, it worked brilliantly. As soon as we gave the pilot the thumbs up to let him know we were set up, he took off leaving the two of us completely alone in

334 *All Lovers Are Deranged*

the middle of the Reef with the ocean around us as far as the eye could see in every direction. We had no life jackets, no food or water and no satellite phone to call for help. It was sheer madness of course but this was how things were done in those days with no thought for health or safety. I have to admit I was more than a little scared.

While we filmed the timelapse shot, the sea level began to rise and cover the exposed coral far quicker than we had anticipated and I started to get a little nervous, especially since we had no way of communicating with anyone so we just had to trust the pilot would return at the agreed time to pick us up.

'I hope the pilot remembers where he left us.' Edwin said.

'What do we do if he doesn't come back?' I replied.

'Swim!'

'That's not funny Edwin,' although it was... sort of. Despite the tense situation we were in, we started to get the giggles. The simple act of laughing at our situation took away any fear I had previously felt and a sudden calm came over me.

Five minutes later we spotted the seaplane and more importantly, he saw us and an hour after being picked up we were back on the mainland with a cold beer in our hands.

After dinner, Edwin and I had a nightcap with some of the marine biology students at James Cook University and one of them played us a rather bizarre song on his portable cassette player called *Thorn of Crowns* by Echo & The Bunnymen, who I had never heard of before. The student told us he had only bought the English Punk band's album *Ocean Rain* because of the play on words of the title of this one track. The lyrics made little sense but were great fun and made me laugh out loud.

'You set my teeth on edge. You think you're a vegetable. Never come out of the fridge. C-c-c-cucumber. C-c-c-cabbage. C-c-c-cauliflower. Men on mars. April Showers'.

It wasn't really my kind of music but I always enjoy hearing something new and a bit different, which this band certainly were, so I borrowed the cassette and listened to the rest of the album on my headphones when I went for my evening stroll. The best track by far was *The Killing Moon*, which was far more sophisticated and a really good song. I loved Ian McCulloch's deep voice as it reminded me a little of a young Jim Morrison, although there were definitely elements of David Bowie at play here too.

The next part of the shoot was at Lodestone Reef, which was the closest of all the outer reefs to Townsville. The depth at this particular reef ranged from 1-20 metres, which made it ideal for us to film above and below water. The first set-up was of Charlie as he popped up from underwater, removed his snorkel and said his lines to camera, holding a piece of coral to tell the story of how the reef was made by millions if not trillions of tiny animals called coral polyps. Charlie and I had worked out a rough script before the shoot, so in theory, all he had to do was remember what we had agreed to say. He got nearly every take right without any mistakes, which made my job very easy. I have yet to meet anyone who knows more about the Great Barrier Reef than this humble and generous man.

Vicki did a sterling job when it was her turn in front of the camera but as I still had the quirky song *Thorn of Crowns* in my head, I got a little confused when she started to talk about the Crown of Thorns and nearly yelled 'Cut' thinking she had said the wrong words but thankfully managed to keep my dyslexic mind quiet before making a complete fool of myself. When it came to Peter's big moment, he delivered his lines to camera like a true pro and although it was a long day, we got everything we needed from our three 'talking heads' above the surface and Walt got some great underwater images of Charlie scuba diving and looking at various types of coral, as well as hundreds of colourful reef fish.

I now had enough wide shots of coral but still needed to get some close-ups but to do this underwater in those days wasn't possible. Fortunately for me, James Cook University had a large saltwater aquarium where they kept all kinds of coral for the students to study, so Jim Frazier and I filmed them there using his macro lens. The coral polyps are tiny, soft-bodied organisms but at their base is a hard, protective limestone skeleton called a calicle and these are what form the structure of a coral reef. When I asked Peter to explain on camera how coral mass spawning happens every year and multiple species of corals release their sperm and eggs at the same time following a full moon. These synchronized swimmers then headed for the ocean surface.

This phenomenon had never been filmed before and the technology to film such an event at night wasn't available yet but after Peter showed us a video of one polyp releasing itself and floating up through the frame, I had an idea of how we might be able to re-create or at least cheat a shot which looked how we imagined a mass coral spawning would 'most probably' look if it was possible to do it in a controlled situation. I shared the idea with Jim and Peter and they agreed it was worth giving it a go. The first step was to mount the camera upside down on the tripod using one of Jim's specialised mounts and point the lens at the side of a mid-sized aquarium where we had attached a dead piece of coral to the top but facing downwards. We then filled the tank with water and after placing some black velvet behind the aquarium to act as a background we side-lit the coral so the shot became monochromatic. Using a small packet of white polystyrene beads similar to the ones you stuff cushions with, we then pumped as many as possible into the bottom of the aquarium through a tube that went through a drilled hole which had been sealed on the outside so it wouldn't leak, and the poly-mock-polyps floated up to the piece of fixed coral at the top one after the other.

When we got the film back from the labs, we played the shot back in reverse and it looked like the mock coral polyps were all floating up and away from the piece of coral just as they would have done if they had been real. Peter said it was exactly what he imagined the mass spawning would look like, so Jim and I went out to dinner to celebrate.

While we were eating our meal, a young couple sat down at the table next to ours and asked us what the food was like. I was convinced I had seen them somewhere before but couldn't put names to their faces but Jim knew who they were straightaway. It was Jayne Torvill and Christopher Dean who had won Gold at the Sarajevo Winter Olympics earlier in the year for figure skating, receiving twelve perfect 6.0s and six 5.9s, becoming instant celebrities after skating so beautifully to Ravel's *Boléro.* After they had finished their dinner, they joined us at our table for coffee and a chat. When Jim asked them if they were an item, I thought he might be skating on thin-ice but Jayne just laughed and told him everybody asked the same question. The answer was no ...they were just good friends.

While I was away filming, I hadn't had the chance to listen to much new music, so I was interested to see what albums had been released recently. High in the Australian charts was *Body and the Beat* by the New Zealand rock band Dragon. Two songs stood out from the rest for me. *Rain* and *Magic:* both had catchy choruses and were almost as good as their 1977 hit single *April Sun in Cuba*, one of my favourite driving songs of all time.

Once I was back in Sydney, I hired Paul Maxwell, my editor friend from my time with Alastair Macdonald, to edit the documentary for me. As we worked on the film, we talked about our old boss who we were both still missing terribly. Swopping amusing anecdotes and singing Alastair's praises helped the healing process for both of us.

Once a week Paul invited me for dinner to enjoy his wife's wonderful cooking. She was a big fan of Cold Chisel, so the background music was always spot on. Chisel's last album *Twentieth Century* had a beautiful song on it called *Flame Trees* written by their drummer Steve Prestwich and keyboardist Don Walker. It is based on Don's memories of living in Grafton as a young lad and the regrets of 'the one who got away'. It is one of the most Australian songs I have ever heard and conjures up images of Rainbow lorikeets perching on the branches of the bright red Illawarra flame trees when they are in full flower in late spring on the east coast of Australia. A sight to behold and remember forever.

When we had a fine cut of *The Reef Builders,* I showed it to John Heyer and he was really happy with what we had achieved on such a small budget and asked us if we could edit a slightly shorter version as

Discovery Channel were interested in buying it. This was great news as apart from giving John a return on his investment, the sale would also give me my first credit as a director on an international documentary.

At the beginning of August, I got a phone call from Emily to say she was leaving her husband and asked if she could visit me in Australia and bring her son Leo with her. I was completely dumbfounded, as when I had last seen her it sounded as though everything was going well with her marriage, but of course I said yes straight away without really thinking it through. It was a classic case of thinking with my heart and not my head and making a quick decision based on romantic feelings rather than rational thought.

When I asked my flatmate Jerry if he minded Emily and Leo staying with us for a while, he told me it couldn't have been better timing as he was about to go on a ballooning trip so would be away for the next two or three weeks.

As soon as they came through customs, Leo rushed up to me and gave me a big hug. Although, I hadn't seen him for a long time he clearly hadn't forgotten me. Emily looked a bit nervous, so I just gave her a gentle kiss on the cheek and a reassuring hug, so she knew I understood this hadn't been an easy decision for her. When we got to the flat, Emily went straight to the balcony to see the view. Leo was more impressed by the pool and couldn't wait to swim. While Emily unpacked her case in my room, I showed Leo his bedroom, which he loved and called for his *Mom* to come and look. I had bought a matching duvet cover and pillowcases with a colourful design on them which I hoped might appeal to a nine-year-old boy. Thankfully, they did. I had also bought him a model of a pirate galleon, which he thought was *cool,* and a soccer ball as Emily had told me he had just *gotten* into this sport. I then took them to Balmoral Beach for a walk along the esplanade and while Leo had a swim in the sea, Emily told me about why she had separated from her husband and explained although she had come to Australia, she wasn't sure whether she could ever live here. I could quite understand her point of view so suggested she just enjoy her time here and take it day by day.

The longer they stayed with me the more I fell in love with Emily and the fonder I became of Leo. One morning, I took him to Mosman to play soccer with some kids of his own age, so his mother could have a sleep-in, and when someone asked me if he was my son, I felt like saying yes as he was such a good lad, but the reality was I wasn't his father. Emily had told me his real dad wasn't interested in getting to know him at all and I had no idea what his stepfather felt about him but suspected he would care for Leo as if he was his own just as I would if I was in the same situation. This random thought hit me like a tsunami. I suddenly felt a wave of compassion for this poor man and wondered how he must be feeling right now. After Leo was tucked up in bed and Emily and I were alone, I asked her if she had left her husband for me or if I was just a safe haven while she thought things through. She admitted it was the latter and after a series of long phone calls to her husband, Emily eventually decided to go back to him.

Despite knowing this was the right decision, I was still upset when the time came for them to return to America. Thankfully, Jerry got back from his trip on the same day they were due to fly back to L.A and offered to drive them to the airport, which saved me the agony of having to say goodbye to them inside the terminal. After giving them both a final hug, Leo clung to me for dear life and didn't want to let go, which was traumatising for all of us. In the end, Emily had to physically pry him away from me and as she did so she asked me not to contact her again so it would make it easier for them to move on with their lives. I could still hear Leo crying in the hallway as they got into the lift and left my life forever.

*The end of one thing is only the beginning of another.*

Laura Ingalls Wilder

## CHAPTER 5: GIVE ME LOVE, GIVE ME LIFE

After a short period of emotional distress, minor depression and feeling sorry for myself, Jerry suggested we drive his old Toyota Land Rover down to Adelaide to see our mutual friend Hugh for a few days. It was a good idea, as a mini-adventure was just what I needed and would allow me to re-focus my energies on the future, so we loaded up the car and set off on a road trip to South Australia. We stopped off for a glass of sherry in Wagga Wagga, resting the bottle on the bonnet of the car, and another by the side of the road in Hay, which kept us going while we drove across the Hay Plains, one of the flattest places on earth and where you get a 360-degree view of the horizon. While looking at this unique and unvarying landscape Jerry gave me his personal opinion on my situation with Emily, 'Never mind mate, better to have loved and lost than never having loved at all...or some such bollocks! Time to move on now.' I wasn't sure whether he meant with my life or with our road trip but before I had time to ask, we were on our way again.

After leaving New South Wales we drove into Victoria passing through Boinka and Cowangie, which weren't as interesting as their names suggested but were ideal spots for a couple more essential sherry stops, before crossing the border into South Australia. From there it was just a hop, skip and jump to our final destination, Mount Barker in the Adelaide Hills. By the time we got there, I was starting to feel more like my old self.

Listening to Prince's guitar solo at the end of his epic song *Purple Rain* on Hugh's impressive Hi-Fi system, while getting drunk on a few bottles of Barossa Valley red wine, was the perfect way to end the day... and begin a new chapter in my life.

When Jerry and I got back to Sydney, there was a letter waiting for me from the Australian Film Commission, asking if I would give a talk to the Australian Film Industry about in-camera special effects and they also had a small budget to cover the costs of flying someone from

342     *Give Me Love, Give Me Life*

overseas to Sydney to be the main guest speaker. I knew I couldn't do it on my own, so rang Jim Frazier to ask if he would also give a lecture, as I knew everyone would be fascinated by what he was doing with his deep focus lenses. He was thrilled to be asked and told me he had just completed a prototype of his optical system and couldn't wait to show me the results, so I went to see him later in the week. It was very impressive but could only be used with a 16mm camera, so I suggested he consider upgrading his system to 35mm so it could be used on TV commercials and feature films.

'It's funny you should say that,' Jim said, 'as I have a mate in England who suggested exactly the same thing!' When I asked him who it was, he told me about his friend Peter Parks, who was a marine biologist, engineer and cinematographer, as well as being considered one of the best micro-photographers in the world. I thought Peter sounded fascinating, so I asked Jim if he thought his friend might be willing to come to Australia to give a lecture to our film industry. Jim thought he would leap at the chance so would contact him on my behalf and sound him out. The answer was a resounding yes.

Peter Parks was one of the founding members of Oxford Scientific Films (OSF), an English company which produced award-winning natural history documentaries using innovative filming techniques. He had also provided some visual effects shots on several feature films, so he couldn't have been a better choice. After his talk, which went down very well with the audience, which mainly consisted of Australian cameramen and camera assistants, I took Jim and Peter out for dinner and this was when he told us about his plans to build a new studio within the grounds of Oxford Scientific Films, so he could focus on providing in-camera visual effects shots for feature films.

In the morning, I gave Peter a lift up to Dural, so he could see Jim's prototype lens system and the two geniuses could discuss their innovative theories together. Jim's lens system would, once refined and upgraded, give the appearance of a massive depth of field which would allow the foreground and background to be in focus at the same time. It was a brilliant invention in theory but there was still much work to be done and I am sure Peter's advice was a big help to Jim at the time.

While driving back to the CBD, Peter asked me if I would be interested in coming back to England for a couple of years and work for him as his producer and general sidekick. It was an incredible opportunity and I was very flattered he thought I could be of any help to him. By the time we pulled into the hotel car park we had agreed a deal, which he promised he would follow up in writing.

When I told Jerry about the offer, he thought it was one I couldn't and shouldn't refuse and then told me he was planning to go back to England soon, as his family were missing him and although he loved Australia, he never planned to make it his home forever.

Although I was sad to leave Australia, spending a couple of years in the UK to further my career was a sensible move and having a temporary resident visa meant I could always come back. The only real problem left was to decide which new album to buy to listen to on the plane. In the end I decided on *Swing* by INXS as I wanted to have some Aussie Rock with me on my next adventure. I had already heard the single *Original Sin,* which Chic's Nile Rodgers had produced and persuaded Daryl Hall to do the backing vocals for, so was interested to hear the rest of the album once I was airborne.

On the 6th of September 1984, having now got a two-year contract from Peter, I set off for the UK stopping off in Singapore for two nights to stay at the Raffles Hotel and slept in a King-size bed and not the fold-up-Z-bed I'd endured the last time I was there. The room wasn't cheap but I felt I deserved a bit of luxury before flying on to Sri Lanka where I had arranged to take a short holiday before starting my new job.

After nearly 150 years of British rule, Ceylon became an independent country in 1948 but the colonial influence could still be seen everywhere, including those of the Portuguese and Dutch, who had both ruled there before the days of the British East India Company. In 1972 Ceylon became the Republic of Sri Lanka but maintained its link with the British Commonwealth. However, by the 1980s there was political unrest and the country was having major problems with the Tamil Tiger Rebels. On the 23rd of July 1983, a deadly ambush occurred causing the death of 13 Sri Lankan soldiers. The following night, anti-Tamil rioting began and over the next week thousands of Tamil civilians were killed in revenge attacks.

It was because of the recent violence I had been advised to hire my own driver rather than use public transport. After a short search I found a driver called Nuwan who had his own Peugeot 104. He was very affable and his fees surprisingly affordable, so after making a deal which suited us both we set off for Hikkaduwa.

When we arrived at the seaside resort the ocean looked a bit too choppy for a swim, so I went for a long walk on the beach while Nuwan studied his map and worked out the best routes for the rest of the week. My accommodation at the old trading port of Galle on the first night was a bit basic but clean. I only had to pay for my room, as drivers are given free food and accommodation for bringing tourists to whichever hotel they choose for them.

I got up at the crack of dawn and walked down to the sea where I saw a group of fishermen balanced precariously on cross-shaped beams called stilts waiting for the fish to bite. It was fascinating to watch the men fish in this traditional Sri Lankan way and I was glad I had brought my camera with me. When I got back to the hotel, Nuwan had organised breakfast for me, which consisted of a potato curry with dahl and some roti made from coconut and flour. Afterwards, we went for a walk around Galle and I took some photos of the 16th-century Fort and its impressive clock tower. In the afternoon we drove a short distance to another beach called Unawatuna, which was crescent-shaped and had crystal clear water, so I liked it a lot more than the one at Hikkaduwa. The sea was much calmer here, so I finally got to swim in the Indian Ocean. In the evening, I was disappointed to discover the only thing on the menu for dinner was potato curry with dahl and roti, but I was too tired to make a fuss and just ate what I was given before heading for bed.

In the morning, I went for a walk listening to music through my headphones as I did on most days but when I got to the beach, the sound of the gentle waves lapping on the shore was so soothing I decided to give myself a break from music for the rest of my time in Sri Lanka and just enjoy all the natural sounds this beautiful country had to offer.

The first sound was of an elephant trumpeting. As soon as I saw a group of them bathing in the Maha Oya River, I could understand why the Pinnawala elephant orphanage had become one of the top tourist attractions on the island. Motherless calves are raised here by human foster parents who ply them with bottled milk five times a day in an effort to help preserve the dwindling wild elephant population. One of the calves I saw was so young it still had hair all over its body and looked more like a baby Woolly mammoth.

When we got to the outskirts of Colombo, Nuwan asked me if I would mind stopping at his home for a while before we drove any further north, as there was a special family gathering, he needed to attend. I happily agreed and when we arrived at his house, his young daughter was standing by the doorway waiting for him. She was wearing some red shoes, which were at least five sizes too big for her. The driver told me they belonged to his grandmother and added respectfully, 'Big shoes to fill Mr Jamie.'

As we went into his house, I slipped off my shoes and left them by the door and also took off my prescription dark glasses, which meant I was now legally blind and could only see things clearly which were close to me. My normal glasses were still in my bag in the car. When Nuwan guided me into a rather dimly lit room, there was a large group of people inside talking in hushed tones in what I assumed must be Sinhala, one of the official languages in Sri Lanka. As I looked around for somewhere to sit, I could just make out the shape of a chair next to a small bed in the furthest corner of the room, so headed towards it. I was about to sit down when I noticed someone was lying in the bed. I presumed it must be Nuwan's grandmother whom he had mentioned as we went in, so I stood up to be polite and said, 'Ayubowan', which means hello, but as I got no reply, I wondered whether she was a bit deaf, so I said it again but this time a bit louder. When I still got no response, I tried one more time almost shouting. 'Aayu-bo-wan!' Nuwan must have heard me, as he rushed across the room and asked me what I was doing, so I told him I was trying to introduce myself to his grandmother. His reply is something I will never forget, 'Oh Mr Jamie, you will have to speak much louder than that. She has been dead for three days. This is the wake!'

The drive to Sigiriya was excruciating, as I was mortified at what I had done, but Nuwan thought it was terribly funny and was still giggling to himself when we arrived. It took me nearly an hour to climb to the top of the huge ancient rock fortress, but the view was well worth the effort but the sound of the wind was deafening. Lion Rock was built in the 5th Century by King Kashyapa, who overthrew his father, pushed his brother, the rightful heir, to one side and pronounced himself the new leader in a Palace coup. Any doubt as to whether he was a complete and utter bastard or not was dispelled when I discovered he had his father buried alive in a wall.

The next day, we visited Polonnaruwa to see the Brahmanic monuments built by the Cholas and the ruins of a garden city created in the 12th century. I was surprised to see quite a few grey langurs and toque macaques there, two of the three different species known to have made their home there. Purple-faced leaf eaters are the third. We then drove to the ancient village of Tanthirimale to see a Sedentary Buddha statue carved into the rock and a reclining Buddha, which Nuwan reliably informed me was 45-foot-long. The stone steps to the cave temple at Dambulla were very steep so when I eventually got to the top I was completely knackered and decided to head straight to Cave Number 2, as I had been reliably informed it contained 50 of the 150 Buddha statues on display, which was more than enough for a lifetime let alone a single day.

On the way to Kandy, we passed a man using a hand-held plough being drawn by two water buffalo in a muddy paddy field, so I asked Nuwan if we could stop, as I was interested to see how it was done. He told me ploughing had been done this way for thousands of years, and it was 'damn hard work sir', so I took a photo to remind me to be more grateful the next time I ate some rice.

When we got to Kandy we took a walk around part of the artificial lake in the middle of the town, which was quite attractive and full of terrapins. We then visited Buddhism's most religious shrine, the Sri Dalada Maligawa better known as the Temple of the Tooth... home to one of Buddha's decaying teeth... allegedly... and the most popular tourist attraction in Sri Lanka...apparently. I was surprised to see so many people queuing up to pay homage to the sacred relic but Nuwan told me nearly everybody in the country did this at least once in their lives. Afterwards, Nuwan told me the street food in Kandy was the best he had ever eaten, so we went in search of something tasty for lunch. As we walked the streets I could smell cinnamon, cardamom, cloves and curry leaves, which were all quite pleasant but then I smelt something rather pungent. It was dried fish. I wasn't keen to try it but Nuwan assured me it was delicious and ordered some for both of us. It was very spicy and twenty minutes later I desperately needed to find a loo. Luckily for me, Nuwan knew where I could find the best one in town. The Queen's Hotel is a former Governor's residence and one of the oldest British Colonial-style hotels in the country. It is at the end of Main Street if you are ever in a similar position... so to speak.

On the way to the hill country, Nuwan told me the exciting hanging rope bridge scene in Steven Spielberg's movie *Indiana Jones and the Temple of Doom* was filmed just north of Kandy, and 'Mayapore village' was constructed on the grounds of the Hantana tea plantation. I asked if we could go there but he said there was a better one where I could watch the whole process, so this is where we went next.

When the British ruled the country, they quickly worked out the fertile land in the nearby hills was perfect to grow tea and set about producing it in vast quantities to export around the world. As I watched the tea pickers, who were all women, pluck the leaves amongst the rows of tea plants, one of them let out a terrified scream. After a few yelled exchanges, two of the other pickers ran towards her and started hitting something on the ground with their leaf-picking sticks. Nuwan explained it was most probably a poisonous snake and this this was a common occurrence. There was no sign of a health and safety officer, so I presume they must have been away on this particular day. After I had taken a few photos, it was time for my first ever tea tasting, but it wasn't as easy as I'd expected, as it involved identifying all the key flavour notes, the different aromas and the various textures and all I could taste and smell was... tea.

The old colonial-style Hill Club is a gentleman's club, in Nuwara Eliya. It was first established in 1876 as a retreat for colonial tea and coffee planters and the well-to-do in high society. When I saw the ancient-looking billiard table, I wondered if my father might have played a game or two on it when he was billeted nearby in WW2 while he was training British and Australian pilots to fight against the Japanese. The idea of playing on the same table was very appealing, so I challenged Nuwan to a game but he was far too good for me despite trying his hardest to let me win.

Our last stop was at a wildlife sanctuary called Yala. We left the Peugeot in the car park and got into a Land Rover owned by one of the rangers who offered to show us around, as there weren't any official tours organised at the time. We didn't see much to start with but our guide had more experience than us and pointed whenever he spotted something in the trees. We saw jungle fowl, a grey hornbill, a couple of wood pigeons and numerous peacocks but no mammals even though we knew leopards were lurking there somewhere. When we came upon a group of elephants, we turned off the engine and watched them for at least an hour. Asian elephants are smaller than the African ones but when a bull elephant decided he didn't like us he made it patently clear and charged towards us aggressively. Thankfully our guide was a confident driver, at least while driving in reverse and at speed, and we were able to get away without being trampled.

I am not sure about the elephants, but it was a dramatic moment I will never forget.

It had been a good idea to have a break from loud music for a while but I was now ready to get back into 'the swing'. Literally in this case as on the flight home, the first tape I wanted to hear was INXS's *The Swing* again.

If you pay attention to the lyrics first when listening to music you might be a more analytical person than me, as I don't listen closely to the lyrics on the first run-through and tend to *feel* the melodies first, or get distracted by the beat. A friend once told me this meant I was intuitive...or was it inane? Definitely one of those words anyway.

When I arrived back in England, my parents invited me to stay with them until I got myself sorted. After I unpacked and freshened up a bit, I rang Peter Parks to let him know I had arrived safely and was ready to start at OSF at the beginning of November as agreed but to my surprise and more than a little disappointment he told me he didn't need me until the new year now, as there wasn't enough work for me to do until then. Although it was frustrating there wasn't much I could do about it and at least it would give me a chance to catch up with my family and friends.

As I was interested to find out what new rock music was currently popular in the UK, I was keen to watch the first of a new TV series of *The Old Grey Whistle Test*, which was now being presented by Mark Ellen, David Hepworth and Andy Kershaw. It was immediately obvious to me they were all passionate about music, so I knew the iconic show was in good hands. The Violent Femmes performed *Prove My Love* and *Country Death Song*, a light-hearted ditty written by Gordon Gano about an unhinged farmer who kills his daughter by throwing her down a well and then hangs himself, which in hindsight perhaps wasn't the best song to listen to just before going to bed.

On the 31st of October I watched the news with my parents and was horrified to discover Indian Prime Minister Indira Gandhi had been assassinated by her two Sikh bodyguards on her way to be interviewed by the British actor Peter Ustinov in New Delhi. She was cremated on the 3rd of November, which also happened to be the day I turned 30.

To celebrate... my birthday not her death, I caught up with some of my old mates for lunch at The Chequers in Lymington. It was great to

350 *Give Me Love, Give Me Life*

see them again especially Nicol, who was now working for the British Racing and Sports Car Club (BRSCC) as Clerk of the Course based at Brand's Hatch and driving a rather fancy Ford Sierra Cosworth, which also acted as the pace car. I have to admit I was more than a bit jealous.

A few days later, I decided it was time I owned a new car too, so I bought a Renault Fuego Turbo with 12.8 PSI of boost to generate 107 horsepower and 120 pound-feet of torque. I had no idea what this meant of course but as it did 0-60mph in about 10 seconds it was good enough for me and I would never be able to out-race Nicol anyway.

The next day I drove up to Long Hanborough to have a meeting with Peter Parks at Oxford Scientific Films, and stopped off in Woodstock to ask the local real estate company if they had anything for me to rent in the new year. There was absolutely nothing available, so when the agent suggested I consider buying instead, I took his advice seriously.

When I met up with Peter, he told me he was very grateful I had agreed to delay my starting date and after he guided me around the OSF offices and their current studio, he showed me the plans for his new studio and took me to the exact spot where he was planning to build it. It felt good to be a part of something new and exciting and I couldn't wait for the new year to begin.

My next priority was to see some live music so I drove up to London to meet up with Honor, who I travelled from Nepal to England with in 1977, and after dinner we went to see Helen Folasade Adu at Hammersmith Odeon. The Nigerian-British singer, better known as Sade, started her set with *Why Can't We Live Together* and ended with *Smooth Operator,* or so we thought and were just about to leave when the band went straight into an instrumental called *Snake Bite*, which was a great way to end the gig.

Being offered regular employment for 24 months was such a rare event in the film industry, my parents advised me to make the most of the opportunity and buy a house rather than rent one, as it would be more cost-effective, although part of their reasoning was in the hope I would finally settle down. A few days later I caught up for a drink with

Sara, my old girlfriend from my days at Bournemouth, and she told me her brother Charles was the bank manager in Woodstock, which was a bit of serendipity so she would ask him if he would help me get a mortgage with his bank.

Two weeks later I bought my first ever house in a tiny village called Yarnton just off the A44, which meant it would only take me 10 minutes to drive to work each day. The three-bedroom house was on a new estate and I was its first occupier. My Australian belongings, which included a few bits of furniture arrived a week after purchasing the property and for the first time in my life I now owned my own home and had a full-time job to pay for it.

'Sorted!' as Jerry would have said....and two weeks later my old Sydney flatmate came to visit me having just flown back from Australia to spend Christmas with his family. It didn't take long for us to find out the best pub in the area was The Royal Sun, so we decided to go there to celebrate my good fortune.

'I'll have a bottle of your very best red wine please.' I said to the landlord looking forward to catching up with my mate over a glass or two.

'Sounds like a good idea. I'll have one too please landlord!' Jerry said in all seriousness.

I have never forgotten the stunned look of the other customers in the pub when two wine bottles and two wine glasses were placed on our table, one in front of each of us.

It was priceless, unlike the wine.

Number 1 in the UK charts at Christmas was *Do They Know It's Christmas?*, a song written by Bob Geldof and Midge Ure and sung by supergroup Band Aid to raise money for Ethiopian famine relief. *Like a Virgin* by Madonna had the top spot in the USA.

With the money my mother gave me for Christmas, knowing I preferred to buy my own presents, I bought a new diary and *In the Eye of the Storm*, Roger Hodgson's first solo album since leaving Supertramp. I was impressed with the opening track *Had a Dream (Sleeping with the Enemy)* but it was *Give Me Love, Give Me Life* which really resonated with me as the opening lyrics echoed what I was feeling at the time. 'It's feeling like it's time to ring the changes. It's feeling like it's time to be reborn.' There is a moment halfway through the song where Roger sings 'Give me reason to hope' followed by the sound of a live crowd cheering, which gets me every time and makes me want to join in. The last track *Only Because of You* is an epic which gave me goosebumps, although in hindsight this might have been caused by the draft coming from under the door in my bedroom.

On New Year's Eve, we did the Mummer's Play again but this year Bruce changed the script to keep it fresh and cast me as the Noble Captain. My costume consisted of a double-breasted blazer, a staff cocked hat like Wellington wore at Waterloo and a fake white beard, which any self-respecting Santa would have rejected in a heartbeat. I looked completely ridiculous of course but as everybody else was similarly attired, I blended in seamlessly, which is more than can be said for my performance, which was full of flaws and errors.

We performed the play at five different pubs in the New Forest before arriving at our final destination, The Gun, my old watering hole in Keyhaven, by which time we were all 'a bit squiffy' due to all the free beers we had been given at each drinking establishment we had been to during the evening. It was at this moment I caught the eye of a rather stunning looking woman sitting in the corner of the pub on her own.

'She looks like trouble!' I thought... so naturally spent the rest of the evening trying to chat her up. Amanda was a chiropractor and had a unique sense of humour, which became apparent when she told me she had a cat called Rover and a dog called Mistletoe. At midnight we celebrated the new year with everyone else in the pub and then decided it might be more fun to 'see in' 1985 on our own...so we did.

*Music gives a soul to the universe, wings to the mind,*
*flight to the imagination, and life to everything.*

Plato

## CHAPTER 6: LET'S GO CRAZY

The first week of 1985 was extremely cold, so choosing Stevie Ray Vaughan's *Couldn't Stand the Weather* to listen to on my drive up to Oxford seemed very apt. I loved his unique style of playing the blues and by the time I reached my destination I was in high spirits.

The first shoot I helped Peter Parks with at Oxford Scientific Films was on an IMAX format film called *On the Wing* for the Smithsonian National Air and Space Museum. The brief was to create a scene showing a prehistoric dragonfly flying through a primeval jungle, as seen from its point of view looking over its head and wings. After a few tests, Peter came up with a clever plan and worked out how to achieve it all in-camera. I thought it was ingenious but as all these types of shoots are, it also proved to be quite complicated.

Peter's assistant Philip Sharpe and another modelmaker called Uta Trix designed and made a very impressive and realistic-looking dragonfly, which was about 8-inches long with a 10-inch wingspan, and the prehistoric jungle was created by a team of local modelmakers led by Francis Coates and Jez Harris, using a combination of various plants and the tops of dead Christmas trees, which some of the OSF staff brought in for us to use.

The goal was to film the dragonfly flying at speed through the jungle in one camera pass. This involved using a two-ton overhead servo-controlled snorkel camera rig which had to be manually pushed 45 feet across the studio to film the background of the jungle, and at the same time film the model dragonfly, also servo-controlled, using an aerial image screen which allowed us to see the insect in the foreground against the background, which was also sharp, while tracking and doing body, head and wing moves as it ducked and weaved over and through our mock jungle.

OSF had become famous for making high-quality Natural History films using specialised equipment and camera techniques. Their team of young cameramen were all becoming experts in macro, micro, slow-motion and time-lapse photography, mainly because they were being taught by one of the best, a man called Sean Morris who, along with Peter, was one of the founding members of OSF. The company were also getting a reputation for producing innovative and award-winning TV Commercials and their young cameraman Steve Downer, not only knew how to do all the same specialist photography as the others but also knew how to light products beautifully, which was essential in the advertising industry, so I hoped I would get the chance to work with him one day.

When Peter asked me to drive him to Twickenham Studios for a meeting with the famous film director John Boorman, I was more than happy to do it. As we drove there, Peter explained how he had managed to create some very specific and intricate moves of an eagle descending and glancing side to side for his latest movie *The Emerald Forest*, by using a radio-controlled puppet which Philip had made from the carcasses of two buzzards and suspending it on a wire rig in the studio. Meeting Boorman, albeit briefly, was a real thrill as I had loved his earlier films *Point Blank*, *Deliverance* and *Zardoz*.

Although I was loving working with Peter, I was missing going to concerts so when Meatloaf was on tour promoting his *Bad Attitude* album in February, I drove down to Hammersmith to see him perform at the Odeon with my friend Vicki. I hadn't heard the album before so it was good to hear a few of the tracks played live. He finished with a very loud version of *Bat Out of Hell* and my ears were still ringing by the time I got home.

Amanda drove up to Yarnton to visit me every other weekend and I drove down to see her in Poole on the alternate ones, popping in to see my folks in the New Forest either on the way there or the way back, which meant I was doing a lot of driving but I loved my new Fuego and it gave me the chance to play music at full volume.

On the 11th of March, Eric Clapton released *Behind the Sun*, so I added it to my collection. Phil Collins was one of the co-producers on the album and played additional percussion. Toto's Steve Lukather played rhythm guitar on a couple of tracks and Fleetwood Mac's Lindsey Buckingham did the same on another. Donald 'Duck' Dunn played bass on most of the tracks and Nathan Easton on the others. I could really 'feel' the bass through my car speakers and my favourite tracks to drive to were *She's Waiting, Same Old Blues, Forever Man* and *Just Like a Prisoner.*

When Amanda next came to visit me, we had just had some snow and the local rivers were frozen. While we were walking by a brook, Mistletoe decided to run across the ice, which suddenly and dramatically broke under her weight and she plunged into the freezing water. I know it was sheer madness but I had to save this dog, as I really loved her. Amanda was screaming at me but I ignored her pleas for my safety and inched myself forward on the ice as quickly as I could using one elbow at a time like a commando towards the hole where I had last seen her. The water was so dark I couldn't see anything under the surface, so there was only one thing I could do. As I put my arm into the brook, I let out a scream as it was so damn cold but the pain was worth it, as less than 30 seconds later I could feel Mistletoe's body and somehow managed to grab her collar and yank her to the surface. She then got her front paws onto the edge of the hole and heaved herself up and over my prostrate body before running back to Amanda. I was now shivering like mad but able to crawl back to the edge without going under the ice myself. From this day on Mistletoe followed me around like a shadow.

Needing another fix of live music, I went to London to see Art Blakey and the Jazz Messengers at Ronnie Scott's with Nicol. We were both mesmerised by Art's crisp drumming style and Terence Blanchard's skill on the trumpet. When we met the club's manager Pete King after the show for a drink, he told us he thought Art's band were some of the best jazz musicians who had ever graced the stage there, so we were very lucky.

While the studio was being built, Peter was working on his own idea, which featured a rather cute character called Umbrij, who I would get to know and love quite well over the next few months because we talked about the project every day. I thought if Peter's incredibly detailed illustrations were anything to go by then he was onto a winner.

One day, Peter's wife Suzi kindly invited me to have dinner with them, so I got to meet their two children Toff and Heidi, who had just as imaginative minds as their father. I was treated to Suzi's wonderful cooking quite a few times while I was at OSF and felt very honoured to be treated as part of their family on those occasions.

I then met a member of my own family who I'd previously had no idea existed before. When my cousin Jamie from California and her husband Mark came to the UK to see me, they told me they had been doing some research on our family tree and had discovered we had a Great Aunt in common. I was intrigued, so rang my mother to ask her about it. She knew all about Great Aunt Irie and told me they still kept in touch but only once a year with Christmas cards, so the next time I was visiting my parents, I gave my Irie a call to ask if I could come and visit her and bring my American cousins with me. She was thrilled to hear from me and invited us for tea the following week.

When we arrived in Skirmett, a hamlet in the parish of Hambledon, Irie's beautiful old house blew us away. It was like walking onto the set of a film set for an Agatha Christie TV series and when I saw my Great Aunt for the first time, I couldn't help but think I had just met Miss Marple. Irie's was sharp as a tack, very well-read, well-travelled and had exquisite taste. She told us about what it was like to fly to Australia in 1935 on one of the first passenger planes operated by Imperial Airways and Qantas Empire Airways. It took her just under two weeks and would later be called the Kangaroo Route because of all the long-distance hops. We loved meeting Irie and after my cousins had returned to the States, I took Amanda to meet her and they got on like a house on fire.

A few days after the new studio was completed at Long Hanborough, we had a very special visitor. Terry Jones of Monty Python fame. I had been a huge fan of the comedy sketch show when I was younger, so I was a little in awe of him but he soon put me at ease with his natural charm and good humour. The reason he was at OSF was because he had written the first draft of a movie called *Labyrinth* for Jim Henson, the creator of the Muppets, who had suggested he discuss some of the special effects sequences in the script with Peter, just as he had done a few years earlier for his movie *The Dark Crystal*. Terry told us there were only going to be two actors in the movie, Jennifer Connelly as Sarah and David Bowie as the Goblin King, Jareth, so this meant he could focus his attention on the creatures, so he wanted to get Peter's opinion on what he thought was and wasn't possible within their budget. Being a fly on the wall and witnessing the discussion between Terry and Peter was more than a little surreal but a very special memory for me.

As we had a gap between jobs, Peter asked me to edit a showreel for him to help us attract more feature film work but as there was so much good material to choose from, it was hard to know what to keep in and what to cut out, so once I had made a rough assembly, I showed it to Peter and suggested we should consider making a one-hour documentary as well as the 5-minute showreel. He liked the idea and told me the story should be about how OSF had started as a natural history film company but was now working on TV commercials and feature films as well. He then told me he had the perfect title in mind.

*From Fishpond to Fantasy.*

As I would need an assistant editor, Peter put an Advert in the local paper but we only got one reply and when the young fresh-faced girl turned up for the interview and told me she had never had a job before let alone one in the film industry, I thought this was the last we would see of her, but Peter thought she was smart enough to learn 'on the job' and he would ask OSF's in-house editor, Ramon, if he was willing to teach her, so she could then spend time working on wildlife films with him as well as helping us on our film whenever we needed her. And this was how I met Nikki Oldroyd, who after being my assistant and then Ramon's would go on to become a well-respected editor herself.

In June, I went to see Ian Dury and The Blockheads at the Hammersmith Odeon on their *Hold On To Your Structure* tour with my friend Nicol. Wilko Johnson was on guitar duty, which was an added bonus. The first song was *Billericay Dickie* followed closely by *Wake Up And Make Love With Me* and the last song was *Sex and Drugs And Rock And Roll*, so 'we woz well 'appy' an' went 'ome with plenty of reasons to be cheerful'.

On one of my many visits to see my Great Aunt Irie, she told me her neighbour was a film editor, so after lunch I went next door to meet him. To my surprise, her neighbour was none other than Gerry Hambling, the man who had edited Alan Parker's movies and kindly taught me how to use a Moviola editing machine in 1980. He invited me in for a chat and told me what it was like working on some of the films he had edited since we first met, including *Pink Floyd: The Wall, Absolute Beginners* and *Mississippi Burning.*

On the 12$^{th}$ of July I went to see Dire Straits at Wembley. It was a memorable gig as *Brothers in Arms* had been released in May, so hearing the band play a few tracks from the album live, including *Money For Nothing* and the title track, was worth the ticket alone. We then had a lovely surprise when Hank Marvin from The Shadows came on stage to perform the encore with the band. *Going Home*, the theme from the movie *Local Hero*.

The 13$^{th}$ of July was one of the biggest musical events in history. Live Aid, which was organised by Bob Geldof from the Boomtown Rats and Midge Ure from Ultravox. There were many great performances but my favourites were Status Quo who opened the event, Bryan Ferry with David Gilmour on guitar, Dire Straits, who must have been exhausted after playing the night before, Queen who rocked us as promised in one of their songs and stole the show being the Champions they were, followed by David Bowie and The Who. At the end everyone came on stage together to sing *Do They Know It's Christmas?* We watched it from beginning to end on TV along with 1.9 billion of our closest friends. It raised £150 million to help famine in Ethiopia. The live event was broadcast by the BBC with a large team of presenters including Mark Ellen and David Hepworth, who I had seen before on *The Old Grey Whistle Test.*

Before heading back to Oxford, I popped into Tower Records, which had recently opened a store in Piccadilly Circus. It was like stepping into an Alladin's Cave. I spent hours browsing through all the albums and cassettes on display but there wasn't enough time on this trip to see everything. However, I knew I would return... and often.

Our next project was to provide some special effects for the Disney movie *Return to Oz* directed by Walter Murch. Our job was to create a visually exciting sequence for the scene where Dorothy tumbles through a cavern of emeralds. This was achieved by building a 40-foot trough with translucent latex walls and a profusion of acrylic crystals. Once it had been constructed Peter backlit it and filmed the shots with a tracking snorkel system capable of holding everything in sharp focus. The background plates looked amazing but unfortunately the live-action footage of Dorothy falling, which was shot by another company against a blue screen, didn't look very convincing so when the two shots were combined afterwards, the result wasn't nearly as good as any of us would have liked. I was a bit disappointed but sometimes you just have to do your best and move on.

A week later, Jim Frazier and his assistant Glen flew to the UK to visit us. Jim stayed with Peter and I put Glen up at my house. It was great to see them again and while they were there, I got them to help me do a few extra shots which we could use in the documentary *From Fishpond to Fantasy*, including a series of slow-motion shots of Jim firing an arrow through three smoke filled balloons which popped one after the other as his arrow went through them. It looked spectacular.

While Jim and Glen were still with us, we had another visitor but this time from America. Hoyt Yeatman was a visual effects supervisor and one of the co-founders of Dream Quest Images. He was very clever, full of fresh ideas and we all liked him a lot.

While he and Peter had a chat, Jim played me a cassette with a music demo on it by a young man called Mars Lasar, who apart from having a very cool name was a brilliant composer. Jim had only met him in Sydney recently and as he loved his music, he wanted me to hear it as well. Mars had composed everything on a digital synthesizer and sampler called the Fairlight CMI, short for Computer Musical Instrument, which had been created by Kim Ryrie and Peter Vogel in Australia. After giving Mars a call to get his permission, I used one of his tracks to edit the images for our showreel, and when Peter heard it, I could tell he was impressed but when we discussed who we should get to compose the music for *From Fishpond to Fantasy,* we decided to try Mike Oldfield's older brother Terry, because we had both heard his original music for *In Search of the Trojan War*. Which had recently been on TV. Terry was a wonderful flautist and his music was perfect for our project. He was also a lovely man and we soon became friends.

After Jim Frazier and Glen had returned to Australia, Peter got a call from producer Duncan Kenworthy, asking if he could visit Jim Henson on the set of *Labyrinth* at Elstree Studios. When we arrived, Jim was busy shooting a scene with Sarah, played by Jennifer Connelly and The Fireys, a group of creatures which she encounters in the film. The unique and slightly scary-looking puppets were dancing around her to a song which David Bowie had written for the film called *Chilly Down*. It was a privilege to be allowed to watch the rehearsal. Afterwards, Peter had a quick chat with Jim but didn't introduce me as there wasn't enough time. However, when Jim drove up to OSF to see Peter a week later, he walked into our studio, came straight up to me and said, 'Hello, I'm Jim Henson. I'm sorry I didn't have time to meet you last week. You are coming to lunch with us aren't you?'

This single act of kindness meant a great deal to me and said a lot about the great man.

Lunch was at The Bear in Woodstock and apart from Jim, Peter and I there was also his daughter Lisa and his producer Duncan Kenworthy. As Jim looked at the menu, his face was hidden behind it for a moment and then I heard the unmistakable voice of Kermit the Frog say, 'I hope they don't have frog's legs on here!'

On a day trip to Bristol, Peter and I meet up with two young stop-motion animators called Peter Lord and David Sproxton to discuss an upcoming project which might need their services. When we entered their studio, they were busy making a TV commercial for Scotch VHS tapes. Peter Lord was moving various parts of a model skeleton, known as Archie, and David Sproxton was standing behind the camera making sure the set was lit properly. As I had directed a few stop-motion commercials at Gillie Potters, I was fascinated to watch them working. It only took a couple of minutes for me to realise their animation was far superior to anything I had ever been involved with. This was the first time I met the owners of Aardman Animations but it wouldn't be the last.

When I eventually finished editing *From Fishpond to Fantasy* and got Peter's approval of the fine cut, I went down to London to do the online edit and colour grade. As there were so many different shots in the film it was going to be a long day, so when I was asked if I would mind taking a break for an hour to allow another client to use the edit suite, I was more than happy to oblige.

Imagine my surprise when the artist then known as Prince walked into the room with his editor, who introduced himself as Ray, and told us he had been flown in from LA just to cut a new music video of the song *Let's Go Crazy,* which they had shot using eight cameras the night before at his performance at the Theatre de Verdure in Nice. When I asked if they would prefer me to leave the room while they did the edit, Ray said, 'No stay and watch. I think you might enjoy this!'

Eight small TV monitors were brought into the edit suite and lined up in row on a fold-up bench at the front of the room, so Prince could see all the images he had shot on the eight cameras at the same time. As they had been placed underneath the post-house's large permanent screen, this meant he could also see the image from whichever camera they had just cut from. Ray told me all the footage had already been synced to the same playback of the track, so all he had to do was cut from one camera to another depending on what order Prince decided intuitively worked best on the day.

When everything was set up, Prince nodded at Ray who then pressed the play button and all eight monitors came to life. The next thing I heard was Prince's opening words to the song. 'Dearly beloved.

We are gathered here today to get through this thing called life.'

Prince then shouted over the top of himself, '4... 5...7...2...4...3...8...1...' and so on until the song was over. As he called out the random numbers, Ray cut from one camera to the other just as he would have done if it had been a live edit on the night of the performance. They played it back twice, made five minor changes and after screening it another two times, Prince nodded and patted Ray on the back, turned around and smiled at me, got up to shake my hand, said a quick 'Thank you' for allowing him some time in the edit suite and then he was gone.

It was quite something to witness the musical genius at work and I felt incredibly inspired. We then continued our own online edit and colour grade until it was completed, but it was hard to concentrate after such an unexpected but welcome interruption.

The following month, I got a call from John Gaydon, a well-respected artist manager and the CEO of Media Lab Music, inviting me to meet ex-10cc musicians Kevin Godley and Lol Crème, who were now having great success directing music videos, as they were interested in me joining them as an in-house director. It sounded very exciting and would have been right up my alley but during the interview Kevin explained what they actually wanted was for me to just act as the technical director for a photographer called Koo Stark, who was currently dating Prince Andrew. It was a privilege to meet them both but I decided to turn the opportunity down as I was really happy working with Peter Parks and as I still had a year left on my contract with him, I wanted to do the right thing.

On the 19th of November, I went to Ronnie Scott's again with Nicol to see Charlie Watts, the drummer with The Rolling Stones. He had created his own big band which included some of Britain's best jazz musicians as well as his friend ex-Cream bassist Jack Bruce who also played cello during the evening. After the concert, Nicol and I had drinks with Pete King, the club's manager and he introduced us to the legendary Ronnie Scott himself who was still grinning ear to ear, as he had loved the gig so much.

The next day I bought Molly Hatchet's double live album *Double Trouble* on cassette to play in the car as Nicol had told me it was the best live album he had ever heard. It was hard to disagree with him as every track was excellent. My favourites were *Gator Country, Boogie No More* and *Fall of the Peacemakers* but they also did a cracking cover of Skynyrd's *Freebird*. Dave Hlubek and Duane Roland traded some of the best guitar licks you will ever hear.

At the end of the month, I mixed the soundtrack for *From Fishpond to Fantasy* at a sound studio near Taunton which Terry Oldfield had recommended. The mix went well and after we had played it back to our satisfaction, the sound engineer sold me his Cherry Red Fender Telecaster Custom 1978 Telecaster for £400. It was more than I could afford but I felt it was time I owned a 'grown-up' guitar and as soon as I started to play it, I knew I had made the right decision.

After being on such a high, it all came crashing down a couple of weeks later when Peter told me he couldn't afford to keep me on for another year, as he was going to detach himself from OSF and form his own company called Image-Quest, which meant there was no guarantee of any income for either of us for a while. It was a total shock and I was completely thrown by this unexpected turn of events, as the only reason I had bought a house was because I thought I had financial security for at least the next two years. I completely understood Peter's difficult position and couldn't expect him to employ me without any paid work on the horizon but as there was little chance of getting any other film work in the area, I would have to look for work elsewhere. London was the most obvious choice and I considered ringing John Gaydon to see if his previous offer was still open, but would mean me either having to commute every day or rent a room in somebody else's house in town during the week while still paying for my mortgage. Neither option was very appealing and as there was no guarantee of any film work in the immediate future, I didn't know what to do. The stress was overwhelming and trying to work out how to continue paying my mortgage without any income on the horizon was all-consuming. The most obvious answer was to unburden myself of the financial problem and focus on finding a suitable solution which would allow me to regain control of my finances.

Ten days later, I put my house up for sale and as I got a very reasonable offer almost immediately, I sold it and decided to go back to Australia. I thought I was more likely to get work as a director there than in England.

When I told Amanda my plans she said although she had always fancied the idea of living there, her chiropractic business was doing well at the moment, so she didn't want to come with me right now but promised she'd visit me one day. Maybe.

The house sale went through quite quickly and I ended up making enough profit to cover the hefty loss of the sale of my Turbo Fuego. As I had clocked up over 26,000 miles since I'd bought it, I couldn't really complain but being British, of course I did.

I had a quiet but happy Christmas with my parents, did one more Mummer's play with my friends Bruce, Bob and Nicol, this time playing the part of The Fool, and then on the 4th of January 1986 after saying au revoir to Amanda, I made my way to Heathrow.

As I boarded the plane, I wondered whether I had made the right decision. Although I had made my mind up to go back to Australia, part of me didn't want to leave my family behind yet again but the call to adventure, as usual, was too strong.

Once I was in my seat and had made myself comfortable, or at least as much as is possible in Economy, I put my headphones on to listen to some music and chose Dire Straits' *Brothers in Arms* for company. The opening track *So Far Away* is a song about a man whose itinerant lifestyle keeps him away from the one he loves.

'Tell me about it!' I thought to myself.

A moment later Mark Knopfler kindly obliged.

*The old skin has to be shed before the new one can come.*

Joseph Campbell

## CHAPTER 7: NOW WE'RE GETTING SOMEWHERE

January isn't the best time to go to Bali, as it's the wettest month but between the intermittent tropical downpours there were occasional patches of sunshine. The mixed weather conditions suited how I felt at the time, as I was suffering from occasional bouts of depression one minute with moments of unfounded optimism the next. Depression affects different people in different ways. I have recurrent depressive disorder, which can come on without warning at any given moment but is usually not too severe and only the people closest to me would be aware that something isn't 'quite right'. It's not something I can just snap out of but listening to music on my headphones while out for a walk helps me manage my condition by giving me 'time out' from the real world and 'time to' acknowledge whatever situation I have got myself in, try to learn from the mistake and then move on. The yellow brick road to success is paved with an obstacle course of failures and you can't truly become resilient unless you are willing to fall down a few cracks from time to time.

Music has always been my safe place and certain songs put me in a more positive frame of mind almost immediately. My top five are *Light My Fire* by The Doors, *Gimme Shelter* by The Rolling Stones, *Sweet Home Alabama* by Lynyrd Skynyrd, *Won't Get Fooled Again* by The Who and *Whole Lotta Rosie* by AC/DC. The reason these particular tracks affect me in such a positive way is because they all have memorable melodies and upbeat tempos, which release feel-good hormones called dopamine directly to my brain's reward system. This is also why I reward myself with a new album after each successful job as by doing this I strengthen the connection between music, success and my well-being.

They say it's good to have a daily routine to help combat emotions, so I took a walk along Kuta beach and had a swim in the sea every morning, had a relaxing massage in the afternoon and drank half a dozen cold beers at a bar in the evening while listening to live music.

This regular regime worked surprisingly well and by the end of my short stop-over on the Island of the Gods, I was in a much better frame of mind and ready to return to Australia.

While I was in the air, I came to a sudden realisation. Travelling had become almost important to me as my passion for music because spending time in a different culture and interacting with the locals always makes me appreciate what I already have. Enough.

Travel also gives me the opportunity to use my greatest gift, which is being able to see the world through the eyes of a child. My curious nature has rewarded me on numerous occasions by rejoicing in the smallest things, which is why I take photos of the shapes cast by shadows, colourful reflections, ripples and rainbows, which many other people walking along on the same path often never 'see', or at least not in the same way.

On the 13th of January 1986 I arrived in Sydney and found a room to rent in a flat in Cremorne near one of my favourite watering holes, The Oaks. Now all I needed was to find some work.

After making over a dozen phone calls to people I knew in the film industry, I got lucky and was offered an interesting job by a company called Golden Dolphin Productions, which was a huge relief and meant my *Return to Oz* had been a good decision.

The co-owners, Bob Loader and Tristram Miall, wanted me to co-direct a 50-minute documentary called *The Mystery of the Full Moon,* which told the story of how the moon influenced life on Earth. Tris had already shot the interviews, including one with the Apollo 12 commander, astronaut Charles 'Pete' Conrad Jnr, the third man to walk on the moon, and another with American author Joseph Campbell, who wrote *The Hero with a Thousand Faces*, a book I had read when I was at Film School. Joseph had many interesting theories about the mythology of the moon and in one of his pieces to camera he said, 'The Sun is a killer and the Moon refreshes. Dew is thought to come from the Moon. The drink of immortality, ambrosia, is supposed to come from the Moon, and there are legends of the Moon as a vessel. You can see it filling up with the ambrosia as it gets full and then dispensing it to the world as it dies, so out of the Moon's death comes life to us all.' I have never looked at the Moon in quite the same way since. The reason they hired me was to add some humour to the film, as they both felt it was a bit too serious and needed to be more accessible to a general audience, so I suggested to counter the serious tone of the interviews, we could create some dramatic live-action sequences or do some animation in the style of Monty Python. In the end, we did both and it worked well.

The day after completing my job for Golden Dolphin, I got a letter from Peter Parks to tell me *From Fishpond to Fantasy* had won a Gold Award at the Chicago Film Festival as well as the Best of Festival award, which did my self-confidence a power of good.

To celebrate the prestigious awards, I went to see Dire Straits at the Sydney Entertainment Centre. Their set was almost identical to the one at Wembley apart from the addition of *Industrial Disease* and *Latest Trick*. After a particularly energetic version of *Solid Rock* to end the show, *Countdown* host Molly Meldrum got up on stage and persuaded the audience to sing *Waltzing Matilda* as a thank you to the band. The encore was *Going Home*, which made me stop and think about where I now felt most at home. The UK or Australia?

My family and oldest friends were all in the UK but Australia had given me opportunities I would never have had if I had stayed put in London and not taken the risk to travel to the other side of the world when I was twenty-one. The UK offered me emotional security and unconditional love in the form of my parents but Australia gave me a joy factor I still hadn't found anywhere else, so the next day I made a decision and applied for Australian Citizenship.

One of the best things about Australians is their easy-going attitude and their dry sense of humour, which has always appealed to me, the more irreverent the better as far as I'm concerned, as it matches my own. I was a big fan of Australia's longest-running TV comedy show *Hey Hey It's Saturday* because of the constant ad-libbing between the host Daryl Somers and voice-over artist John Blackman. There was also a musical element to the show, which I enjoyed, usually involving ex-Skyhooks guitarist Red Symons, Ol' 55 saxophonist Wilbur Wilde or *Countdown* host 'Molly' Meldrum, who were all household names in Australia in the 80s along with Vegemite, Tim Tams and Golden Gaytimes, a toffee and vanilla flavoured ice-cream coated in chocolate and covered in minuscule biscuit crumbs.

If I was serious about becoming a true-blue Aussie then it was important to know about these Aussie icons along with the fact Australia invented the Hills Hoist, a height adjustable rotary clothesline, and the Ute, a two-door vehicle with an open tray at the back to carry 'whatever' cargo was required. I also needed to know a little Aussie slang, which was great fun to learn. For instance, if someone tells you the manager is 'flat out like a lizard drinking' it means he is extremely busy so can't possibly see you at the moment. If you then ask to speak to the assistant manager, you might be told there is not much point as they are 'as useful as a one-legged man in an arse kicking contest', sometimes followed with a second reference like, 'He isn't the sharpest tool in the shed anyway' which simply confirms their first observation.

I love Australians because of their positive attitude to life and their self-deprecating humour, both of which were starting to rub off on me.

When Amanda flew to Sydney to visit me in March, we rekindled our romance and had two lovely weeks together. The day before she left, we talked about the possibility of living together in Australia but as her business was still thriving in the UK it wasn't dwelled on for long and we decided to just stay in touch and see what happened. A week after she had gone back to the UK, I flew down to Adelaide to direct a couple of commercials and with the proceeds I was now able to afford a new car.

The only downside of buying a soft-top Suzuki Sierra was having to buy a steering-wheel lock and a portable stereo system, which I had to pull out of the console and take with me every time I parked the car, but it was a small price to pay, as you can't drive a soft-top without having some decent music blaring out of the speakers at full volume.

The first cassette I played was *Master of Puppets* by Metallica. The recently released album was hailed as a masterpiece by the critics and British rock magazine Kerrang! claimed it 'finally put Metallica into the big leagues where they belong'. Hell Yeah!

Although rock music is often connected to aggressive behaviour, for me, listening to loud music allows me to release my inner anger in a non-harmful way and reduces my stress levels considerably. I have a number of good friends who enjoy heavy metal as much as I do and they are all kind gentle souls who wouldn't harm a fly or say boo to a goose, despite wearing leather jackets, studded belts, black combat boots, black jeans and black T-shirts with Judas Priest, Saxon, Megadeth and Motörhead printed on the front of them. My mother always taught me to never judge a person by the way they look and to be curious about them instead, as you might miss out on a great friendship. She was quite right...as mothers usually are.

To keep in touch with what was currently 'popular' in Australia, I listened to 2MMM, also known as Triple M. It was my favourite Sydney FM radio station at the time because the breakfast time slot was hosted by a very funny man called Doug Mulray, aka The Reverend Doctor Doug who had an array of fictional characters with silly voices who would phone-in to talk to him, including Madam Zenda who made ridiculous horoscope predictions, and Jack Africa who was convinced the chooks were out to get him.

One morning, I heard a unique song on Uncle Doug's show called *Sounds of Then (This Australia)* by a band called GANGgajang. It was written by Mark 'Cal' Callaghan and co-produced by their drummer Graham 'Buzz' Bidstrup. The lyrics were brilliant and captured what tropical Queensland is like when it's hot and steamy, which I experienced when filming the CSR sugar mills with my friend Edwin.

'Out on the patio we'd sit. And the humidity we'd breathe. We'd watch the lightning crack over cane fields. Laugh and think, this is Australia.'

This great song sparked the germ of an idea, which then turned into a documentary called *Sounds Like Australia*. The concept was to use the sights of nature to inspire music and the sounds of nature to create it. It was an ambitious concept but Film Australia liked it and offered to fund it. This was partly due to the fact Tris had recently become their Executive Producer and put in a good word for me.

The first thing I did when the funding was approved was to ask Mars Lasar if he was willing to co-compose the music with Kevin Peek, the guitarist from SKY, who I hoped would be willing to collaborate with him. I wanted Mars on board to sample all the nature sound effects we were able to record on location into a Fairlight, which I knew he could do better than anyone else as he had worked as a demonstrator for Fairlight Computers on their first multi-track sequencer, so knew the computer musical instrument inside out. When I rang Kevin, he loved the idea and couldn't wait to get started as he was a big fan of the Fairlight.

Another fan of the Australian invention was Peter Gabriel. He had bought the very first one in the UK and used it on his 4th album. The marimba at the beginning of *San Jacinto*...isn't a marimba but a sound produced by a Fairlight CMI. In May, he released his 5th album, *So*, and although he continued to use the Fairlight, these songs were a bit more commercial than on his previous records, especially *Sledgehammer*, which became a huge hit and Peter's duet with Kate Bush on *Don't Give Up* must be one of the most powerful songs ever written. It was so uplifting and filled with so much emotion it made me have compassion for my younger self, the boy I had once been but was no longer, simply because I didn't give up, even though I'd felt like doing so on more than one occasion. Even today, whenever I am feeling a bit depressed, I still listen to this song before making a decision about what to do next.

The 1st of June 1986 was a special day because the 'Master of the Telecaster' was in town. Albert Collins & The Icebreakers played at the Hordern Pavilion and the gig was sensational. Albert had the longest guitar cable I had ever seen and when he walked through the audience while playing a solo, it took three roadies to stop it from being trod on or pulled out of the amp. *Cold Feeling* and *Frosty* were the standout tracks but as I was just about to go on location the song which meant the most to me was *I've Got a Mind to Travel.*

Four days later Steve Windon, the cameraman and Max Hennser, the soundman, and I drove north to Dorrigo National Park to begin filming *Sounds Like Australia.* Our first location was Dangar Falls where I wanted Steve to get shots of the stunning waterfall from as many different angles as possible. We then continued driving to the New England National Park to look for Tom's Cabin where we wanted to spend our first night so we could be in place to film sunrise coming up over the Northern Tablelands.

The accommodation was fairly basic but suited our needs perfectly. When we woke up, the valley below was covered in mist and the hills were numerous shades of blue. It was a beautiful scene and the dawn chorus was just as mesmerising. Max was recording it all on his new Nagra tape recorder and as he listened to it back through his headphones, he gave me the thumbs up.

As soon as we got back to Sydney, we dropped the car and went straight to the airport. Next destination Darwin. We had a lot of luggage to check in, as apart from our suitcases we also had our film equipment to put in the hold except for Steve's camera, which he preferred having on his lap for the duration of the flight to lessen the risk of damage in the hold. But when we stopped off at Alice Springs to refuel and got off the plane to have a pee, he decided it would be safe to leave the camera on his seat while we were in the terminal. After relieving ourselves, we thought we would have time to have a quick cup of tea. We were wrong! When we walked back onto the tarmac, we saw our plane take off right in front of us... with all our gear still on board. As there hadn't been any announcements in the terminal to re-board, we had assumed we still had plenty of time before re-boarding but instead we were now stranded in Alice without our luggage and equipment.

'No worries, she'll be right!' one of the local airport staff told us confidently after we had explained our unfortunate situation to him, and then added, 'You're not the first dickheads to miss their flight and leave their stuff on the plane,' which I thought was rather unnecessary even if factually correct. He then told us to wait while he made a call and to our relief returned ten minutes later with some good news. 'The crew are going to take everything off the plane for you in Darwin and it will be waiting for you in lost property when you get there. You are lucky as there's only one more flight there today but it's not due for another 4 hours, so you'd better make yourselves comfortable!'

When we finally got to Darwin and were reunited with our belongings, we all let out a collective sigh of relief and then went straight to our motel. While drinking a few beers together to unwind we watched *Countdown* on the TV in my room. When they screened the music video of Sydney DJ 'Uncle Doug' Mulray & The Rude Band's latest irreverent song *You Are Soul* we couldn't resist joining in the chorus 'You Arsehole', which made us laugh and forget our stupid mistake earlier in the day. There were a number of other music videos on the popular Aussie TV show but the most memorable was the one for Peter Gabriel's *Sledgehammer*. It was directed by Stephen R. Johnson with some innovative Claymation and Stop-motion animation provided by Aardman Animations and Brothers Quay. Having met the owners of Aardman the previous year it came as no surprise the video was so imaginative and I hoped I would get the chance to work with them one day.

We had to get up at the crack of dawn the next morning as it was a four-hour drive to get to Katherine Gorge. As soon as we arrived Steve shot some beautiful images looking down into the impressive sandstone gorge and then found our way down to the river where I hired a boat to take us through the gorge to get footage of freshwater crocodiles basking at the edge. The next morning, we got up even earlier so we could get to Yellow Water Billabong in Kakadu National Park, just as the sun was rising. The sky was an ominous blood red when we arrived but had turned three shades of yellow by the time, we were on our flat-bottomed boat cruising down the South Alligator River. We spotted our first 'Saltie' within fifteen minutes and this was when the Park Ranger who was acting as our guide, suggested to Max, who had been testing the temperature of the river with his fingers, he might like to take them out of the water, 'Presuming you want to keep them of course!'

When we got to a secluded spot where it was safe to get out of the boat, we started looking for other wildlife to film. Seeing a Jabiru fishing for the first time is quite something. The black-necked stork was much larger than I had imagined and had an extremely long beak which it was attempting to catch either a fish or a frog with, quite successfully by the look of it. We then saw an enormous saltwater crocodile sunning itself at the edge of the river with its mouth wide open, so I told Steve to set up the camera and try to capture the moment when it closed its mouth and slid back into the water, as it would make a terrific shot. Jim Frazier had taught me crocodiles did this behaviour to release heat from their body after eating and it was called mouth gaping, which coincidentally was exactly what my mistrusting crew were doing when I told them I was heading off for a couple of minutes to find the next shot and leaving them on their own. It was evident both my crew were more than a little scared of the huge crocodile, so I tried to assure them I *thought* it had *most probably* just eaten something and this was why it was now resting with its mouth open and was trying to cool off, so it was highly unlikely to attack them...well *fairly* unlikely anyway. As they were standing a good 5 metres away from the croc and filming it on a zoom lens, I thought they were pretty safe but they didn't know this of course and when I returned, they were in exactly the same position.

'Haven't you got the shot yet? Do I have to do everything around here?' I asked, pretending to be a bit cross. I then noticed the crocodile was closing its mouth, a sign which made me think it might be about the move, so I said, 'Oh well, come on then... turnover... camera... sound.... and ... action!' Two seconds after I shouted the magic word, the crocodile slowly slid majestically down the bank into the water and completely submerged itself leaving only the faintest of ripples. Afterwards, Steve and Max looked at me in such awe I had to turn away to hide my smile, as the timing had been pure luck but I wasn't about to share this fact.

On the way back to our motel, we saw an enormous bushfire, so stopped by the roadside to film it. Five minutes later a large car pulled up right beside us and when the driver got out I realised it was Jim Frazier, who had seen the smoke and hurried to the scene to film it. I had flown Jim to Cairns and on to Darwin a week earlier to get some specific wildlife shots for the film, so it wasn't a surprise he was already in the same area as we were. While Steve filmed the fire, Jim filmed the black kites which were hovering near the edge of the fire watching for potential prey like lizards and insects fleeing from the extreme heat.

When we had enough shots in the can, we dropped our gear at the motel and then looked for somewhere to have dinner. While we were eating, Jim told us he had once seen a kite create a fire by dropping a small burning branch onto an open area so it would catch fire on purpose so it could then locate its next meal trying to escape the flames.

After the others had gone to their rooms to check their gear, Jim told me he had managed to get some fabulous footage of a Victoria's Riflebird performing its courtship dance while he had been in the Atherton Tableland near Cairns. This had only happened because his great friend John Young had built a special hide high up in the treetops, which allowed Jim to get the sequence we needed. He had also managed to get a shot of a Palm Cockatoo tapping a twig on the top of a branch, which I thought might be able to use at the start of a piece of music like a conductor tapping his baton on a podium.

While we were in the Northern Territory, we got some great shots and sounds of frogs croaking, emus gulping, corellas squawking and a couple of pied-butcher birds singing a duet, which sounded remarkably like the theme tune to *Close Encounters of the Third Kind*. We also filmed some egrets fighting each other over a fish and a comb-crested jacana walking across some floating vegetation. Jim called them JC birds, as it looks like they are walking on water.

On our last evening, we saw a large flock of birds silhouetted against the sunset, so we quickly pulled over to the side of the road. Jim and Steve filmed them while Max recorded the extraordinarily loud sound they were making. Jim told us what we were witnessing was ten thousand whistling ducks all taking off at the same time and the incredible sound was made by their wings. It was pure magic and something which will live with me forever.

In the morning, Jim flew south to Melbourne where he was going to try and get some footage of a superb lyrebird in Sherbrooke Forest and we flew west to Kununurra to meet up with Kevin Peek, a superb guitarist, and take him to the Bungle Bungles. We took two helicopters to get there. One for the crew and one for Kevin so we could film him in one of them from the other.

On the way to our destination, we flew over Lake Argyle, which seemed to go on forever. The pilot told us it was Australia's second-largest freshwater man-made lake reservoir by volume, which explained why it was taking so long to fly over it.

When we finally saw the Bungle Bungles I was lost for words. I had never seen anything like them before. The orange and black striated sandstone domes, high ridges and deep gorges were truly spectacular and it felt like flying over a range of giant glowing beehives.

After we landed, we then walked for about 15-minutes until we reached a natural amphitheatre, known as Cathedral Gorge and this is when Kevin got his guitar out and started to play. The acoustics were amazing and we managed to get a lovely shot of a master musician doing what he did best. It might have been the smallest audience he had ever had but I am sure it was also the most memorable.

Just before sunset we took off in our helicopters to get some aerial images of the rock formations changing colour as the sun went down, making sure we got back with enough time to set up camp in a dry river bed in one of the narrower gorges before it went completely dark.

Sleeping in a swag under the stars with a small fire burning nearby was magical and when we woke up in the morning there was a full moon and sunrise at the same time. The Bungle Bungles had only been discovered three years earlier when another film crew had flown over it, so it was a real privilege to be allowed to spend some time on such ancient and sacred land. I remember thinking at the time this would be the closest I would ever get to the feeling of being on another planet. It was...other-worldly.

After arriving at Kevin's studio in Perth, we filmed him composing a short piece of music using the gulps of the emus to provide the beat and the duet of the pied-butcher birds as the melody. He then added some guitar on top and it sounded incredible. The next day we all flew back to Sydney together to film the scenes we needed with him and Mars Lasar composing music together at Film Australia.

'That's a scrub wren, crimson rosella, whip bird and that... well that sounds like a helicopter!'

Jim told us with a big smile as watched his mind-blowing footage of a super lyrebird imitating whatever it had heard in its area in Sherbrooke Forest. It then performed a spectacular dance which left us speechless. Jim told us he had heard of some lyrebirds which had imitated a trail bike and even a chainsaw but our helicopter impression trumped them all.

During a quick break outside to get some fresh air, we noticed six Kookaburras sitting on a branch so Jim and Steve quickly grabbed their cameras to get some shots of them. While they set up, I asked Kevin if he would play his guitar under the tree to see if the birds reacted to his music. One of the Kookaburras shook its head from side to side, which sounded just like a pair of castanets, so Kevin, now inspired by the natural sound, proceeded to play some Flamenco. The Kookaburras turned their heads to watch his performance beneath them but one of them clearly wasn't as impressed as we were and released a poo which landed right on Kevin's shoulder. Jim and Steve got the whole thing on camera and Max had managed to capture both the music and the Kookas 'laughing' at Kevin, so we now had a comedic scene to add to the film. It worked well musically and also showed how self-deprecating Kevin was, which endeared us all to him even more.

As Mars Lasar had brought his Fairlight to Film Australia, we asked him to improvise something with Kevin on guitar using all the natural sounds which we had managed to record on location, which had now been sampled and were inside the Fairlight. The result was beautiful to hear and this impromptu jam allowed both musicians to convey all their thoughts and ideas, which were floating around in their head, without the need for words. It was a privilege to be a fly on the wall and witness the process of their shared creativity.

We kept the Fairlight at Film Australia overnight, as in the morning I had arranged for an animal wrangler to bring in an echidna and a blue-tongued lizard, which I placed on the musical instrument to create some interesting looking shots we could use for publicity and then I got Steve to film similar setups which we could use in the title sequence of the film.

As I wanted to be the first person to use Jim Frazier's special new lens system and also include Densey Clyne in my film, the three of us drove out to Broken Hill a few days later and found a location where we could film a grasshopper in the foreground in focus with Densey in the background recording the sound it made, also in focus. It worked so well we did another shot with some ants and another with a frog. While we were there, we also filmed some galahs and recorded their high-pitched screeches.

To make the opening title sequence even more spectacular I asked Jim if we could film some of his crystal art as timelapse shots so we could see the shapes magically forming. He was very happy to do it and when I told him I planned to intercut these images with some of the best scenic shots we had got on location, he said he would use coloured gels to light them, so I could then dissolve from a shot of green crystals to a green rainforest or from orange crystals to an orange bushfire and so on. I then spent the next few weeks doing the editing at Film Australia with my assistant editor Claire and we loved every minute of it.

When I finally had an edit, I was happy with, I showed it to Tris and Jim, and then made a few changes which they suggested to make it tell the story better. We then did a sound mix and this was when it all came together. Kevin and Mars wonderful soundtrack using the sounds of nature was totally unique and Steve and Jim's images were outstanding. On the night we completed the film, I went to see Johnny Winter perform at the Hordern Pavilion. Although his best song was *Johnny B. Goode* the most appropriate was *It's All Over Now*.

The following month, I put down a deposit for a one-bedroom apartment on the 15$^{th}$ floor of a high-rise in Waverton, a short walk to North Sydney. Although it was very small, it came with a lock-up garage and the use of a communal swimming pool, and at least I was on the property ladder again. A couple of weeks after moving into my flat, I went to see Elvin Bishop at The Basement. The former member of the Butterfield Blues Band was a phenomenal guitarist and had a unique style all of his own. When he sang *Fooled Around in Fell in Love* it made me miss Amanda, who I had just received a letter from to tell me she would be coming back to Sydney at Christmas and was thinking about applying for Australian residency.

As a housewarming present to myself, I bought a brand-new Sunbeam 'Express' kettle, which meant my old 'jug' could now be retired and I would never have to use a bare element again. These stylish kitchen appliances had only been available in Australia since 1984 and were allegedly able to boil two cups of water in 60 seconds. 'Whatever will they think of next!', I thought, as I waited patiently for my latest purchase to prove its mighty claim.

Stevie Nicks was the next international artist I went to see at the Sydney Entertainment Centre. I particularly liked her cover of Tom Petty's *I Need to Know* and loved her song about the old Welsh witch *Rhiannon,* which she usually performed with Fleetwood Mac. Simple Minds played at the same venue in October. *Waterfront* and *Don't You (Forget About Me)* were exceptionally good and the Scottish band ended their set with a medley of *Love Song/Sun City/Dance to the Music.*

The following month American singer Jennifer Warnes released an album called *Famous Blue Raincoat: The Songs of Leonard Cohen* as a tribute to the Canadian singer-songwriter. My favourite track was *First We Take Manhattan* but I have to admit my positive opinion was biased as it was based on the slick guitar licks provided by Stevie Ray Vaughan.

On the 7th of December, Elton John performed one of the most memorable concerts ever staged at the Sydney Entertainment Centre. In the first set, he played with a 14-piece band. The song *Benny and the Jets* went on and on forever, which made the audience go crazy. When he came back on stage to start the second set, he was dressed as Wolfgang Amadeus Mozart and had an 88-piece orchestra with him, conducted by James Newton Howard, so every song had a completely new feel to it, which the audience loved.

A week later Genesis played on the same stage on their *Invisible Touch* tour and this was the first time I saw Phil Collins do the infamous drum duet with Chester Thompson as an intro to *Los Endos*. Watching two of the best drummers in the world interact with each other with such intensity was something to behold and I felt privileged to witness their musical chemistry live.

Amanda arrived a week before Christmas and within days she was driving me crazy, rearranging everything in my apartment in a way which upset my slightly compulsive sense of order. I was used to my personal belongings being neatly arranged in a way which made sense to me but now my flat looked like a bomb had hit it. I wasn't a total 'neat freak', I could cope with wet towels left on the bathroom floor, leaving the toothpaste cap off, undies left to dry on the back of the chairs and even dirty cups and plates left in the sink, but hiding my precious vinyl collection behind the sofa so my LPs were no longer either accessible or in alphabetical order was a step too far! Although my OCD symptoms might be considered minor compared to others, my need for things to be in their 'correct' places was going to be an issue. Sharing such a small space was always going to be difficult but as we had not encountered this problem in the UK, I didn't understand why it was becoming one now. However, when Amanda had stayed at my house, we spent most of the time either at the pub or in bed and at her house, it didn't matter to me whether it was a mess or not as I didn't have to live there fulltime but now it was a real issue and we started having rows, which we usually regretted immediately and it didn't take long before we were back to being like any other compromising couple, and let's be honest, there is a lot to be said for make-up sex.

On Christmas Day we were invited to a Waifs and Strays party hosted by my good mate Baggers on the roof of his apartment block with all the other residents of the building who hadn't got families to go to. It was a lovely evening and we had a happy day together but the armistice only lasted until the end of the week and then we agreed to go our own ways.

I spent New Year's Eve listening to my favourite records while putting the LPs back in order from Aerosmith to ZZ Top.

My first live gig of 1987 was on Valentine's Day when I saw The Eurythmics at the Sydney Entertainment Centre on their *Revenge* tour. By the time they sang *Here comes the Rain Again,* Annie Lennox had the crowd in her hand and everyone was singing along with her and dancing. My favourite moment was Dave Stewart's extended guitar solo, which was worth the price of the ticket alone. Backing singer Joniece Jamison almost stole the show when she sang a duet with Annie on *Sisters Are Doin' It for Themselves* but the best was kept for last with a heartfelt version of *The Miracle of Love* still ringing in my ears as I went home.

A few days later I was hired to direct an In-Flight video for Qantas, which featured TV presenter Margaret Throsby interviewing Graeme Murphy, the talented Sydney Dance Company choreographer and Juan Ignacio Rafaelo Lorenzo Trápaga y Esteban, a highly entertaining singer better known by his stage name Ignatius Jones. Once the studio interviews were approved, Qantas flew me and a two-man film crew down to Melbourne to interview Australian Tennis star Pat Cash at his home. Pat was very friendly, answered all my questions openly and told me how much music helped him focus on his game, so when I got home I made Pat a mixed tape with all my favourite rock songs on it starting with *La Grange* by ZZ TOP and ending with *Freebird* by Lynyrd Skynyrd.

Pat Cash defeated Ivan Lendl in the Men's singles at Wimbledon later in the year. I'll let you decide whether you think, like me, it must have been my tape, which spurred him on to victory!

The last part of the job for Qantas was to film Ken Done, a very popular Australian artist and designer at the time, at his home in Chinaman's Beach. In the 1980s, hundreds of households had something in their house designed by Ken Done. I had a doona cover and a set of pillowcases…and I wasn't afraid to use them.

Despite his commercial success the Art establishment refused to consider him a 'proper artist', which must have been frustrating for him if not demeaning. When we arrived at Ken's lovely home, I could immediately see where his inspiration came from. The views were spectacular, so we filmed him walking along the beach and then did the interview in his studio. Ken was fascinating to talk to as we discussed what 'proper art' meant I realised my knowledge of Australian artists was non-existent, so at the weekend I took myself to the Art Gallery of New South Wales to look at paintings by three artists Ken thought I would appreciate.

The first was Russell Drysdale (1912-1981) whose emotive paintings made me stop and think what it must have been like to live in Australia when times were tough during drought and the Depression. The second was Tom Roberts (1856-1931) whose work I liked a lot as his impressionistic style really captured the beauty of the bush, or at least how I imagined it looked. However, my favourite was Indigenous artist Albert Namatjira (1902-1959) as his intricate watercolours of the Australian outback were breathtaking and his deep spiritual connection to the land was there for all to see.

I had originally only intended to teach myself a bit more about the 'history of art in Australia' but ended up learning a little about 'Australia's history through art', which intrigued me so much, I vowed to come back to the gallery as soon as I had more time.

On the first day of March, Tris Miall rang to tell me *Sounds Like*

*Australia* had just been bought by ABC and National Geographic. I felt like celebrating so as ZZ Top were playing at the Sydney Entertainment Centre two days later, I bought myself a ticket. It was a terrific gig and they played all my favourite songs, including *Got Me Under Pressure, Legs, Sharp Dressed Man* and of course *La Grange.* It always amused me how the drummer Frank Beard, was the only member of the band who didn't actually have a beard.

It had been a great year so far with some interesting and well-paid film work and plenty of live music, so I was feeling pretty happy with life and decided to stay at home for a few days to relax by the pool and listen to the radio. On the 9th of March U2 released *The Joshua Tree.* After hearing Doug Mulray play the entire album on his show, I bought a copy the very next day. The tracks I liked the most were *With or Without You, Where the Streets Have No Name* and *I Still Haven't Found What I'm Looking For* as they sounded timeless but I thought the whole album was truly outstanding.

On the 14th April 1987 I became an Australian Citizen. It was one of the proudest days of my life and from a practical point of view, having dual nationality meant I could now travel in and out of the country whenever I wanted without having to reapply for a new visa every time. It also gave me the one thing which had been missing in my life…a real sense of belonging.

To celebrate this landmark achievement, I bought Crowded House's debut self-titled album, which as my Aussie mates pointed out was a bit daft as they were a New Zealand band, so I must be 'a few stubbies short of a six pack', but the reason I wanted to have it so badly was because there was a song on the album called *Now We're Getting Somewhere*, which resonated with me as it looked as though I finally was… at last.

*Travel is never a matter of money, but of courage.*

Paulo Coelho

## CHAPTER 8: WELCOME TO THE JUNGLE

Having just bought a record by a Kiwi band, it was a happy coincidence to get a call from my friend Peter Avery in New Zealand, whom I had first met when I was working with Alastair Macdonald. Peter had been an art director back then but was now a successful TV commercials director himself and had his own production company in Wellington called First Light. He told me he was currently looking for another director so wondered if I would be interested in working with them for the next six months.

As I now had Aussie citizenship, this meant I could now work in New Zealand without having to get a work visa, so the next day I flew to the 'Windy City' to talk to Peter about the job in more detail and met his producers Peter 'Huey' Hewitt and Jeff Williams who I liked immediately, so it was an easy decision to make and after we had agreed terms, I signed on the dotted line, promising to return to Wellington a month later.

I only just arrived home when I received a call from another director, asking for my help on a TVC for James Hardie. I was very flattered as Peter Wall had worked with the likes of Orson Welles, Candice Bergen and the two Ronnies, Barker and Corbett. His business partner, Peter Hopwood was an ex-racing car driver who had now retired from the sport and had become a cameraman. Their office was on a yacht, which they moored at d'Albora Marinas on The Spit at Middle Harbour. It felt slightly surreal to be having a production meeting on a yacht but this is what we did and after chatting about the job over a few cold beers I agreed to help them with their special effects.

The shoot went well and we wrapped in time for me to see The Pretenders at the Sydney Entertainment Centre. They did a great cover of Jimi Hendrix's *Room Full of Mirrors* as well as their best-known songs *Back in the Chain Gang* and *Brass in Pocket.*

As my mate Baggers had just sold his flat and needed somewhere to live while he searched for a new one, the timing couldn't have been better for both of us, so while I was flying back to Wellington, he moved into my flat in Sydney and would pay me enough rent to cover my mortgage until I got back.

I landed on the 'Land of the Long Grey Cloud' on the 11th of May and stayed at Peter's large wooden house in Kilbirnie, which he shared with his partner Trudy. As they were going on holiday for the next five weeks, Peter said I could stay in their house for free as long as I fed the cats but would have to find my own pad by the time they came back. The two cats were neurotic and paranoid, not their real names but they might as well have been as it described them perfectly.

Over the next two weeks the First Light producers, Huey and Jeff, took turns taking me to the local advertising agencies to show them my commercials reel in the hope they would be impressed enough to ask me to direct one for them. A week later one of the agencies rang Jeff to say they had a great job for me to direct for AWA Computers but as the Rugby World Cup was about to start, we would have to wait until it was over because the client was a 'rugby tragic' and didn't want to miss a match. The All Blacks were the favourites to win, as their team included David Kirk, Sean Fitzpatrick, John Kirwan and Grant Fox who were considered some of the greatest players in the world at the time. In the end, the Kiwis did win the cup after defeating France 29-9 in the final on the 20$^{th}$ of June.

We started shooting the commercial for AWA Computers three days later, hiring a local cameraman called Warrick 'Waka' Attewell to shoot the live-action sequences, which we would intercut with some highly imaginative animation created by a very talented artist called Fane Flaws, who we agreed should share the director credit with me as his visual contribution was so exceptional. The editor was my old friend Paul Maxwell who had worked at Alastair Macdonald Productions with me in Sydney and it was a real bonus to be able to work with him again after so long. Once we had shot all the footage we needed, Jeff told me I had to fly to Auckland to do the online edit, as there weren't any professional post facilities in Wellington at the time.

After getting into a taxi at Auckland airport, the driver said, 'Welcome to the Jungle!' which I thought was a rather odd thing to say, considering there was no rainforest to be seen in the immediate vicinity, but then I realised he was just telling me the name of the song currently playing on his car radio was *Welcome to the Jungle.*

Taxi drivers are often a great source of musical knowledge as they listen to the radio for many hours each day. My cabbie today was a mine of information and told me about the American hard rock band Guns N' Roses who had recently released their debut album *Appetite for Destruction* and he thought the song presently doing damage to my eardrums was one of the best tracks on the record. The other two standout songs in his opinion were *Paradise City* and *Sweet Child O' Mine.* Their singer, Axl Rose, which is an anagram for 'oral sex', had a very distinctive and powerful voice but it was their sensational guitarist, Saul 'Slash' Hudson, who caught my attention as his solos were soulful and seductive. Apparently, Slash had been given the memorable nickname by his father's best friend, the actor Seymour Cassel, because as a kid he was always in a hurry, zipping in and out of the house going from one thing to another and never taking time to sit down and relax.

When Peter got back from his holiday, I moved into a shared flat with two middle-aged women called Jane and Patricia, who both had pianos and took snipes at each other all the time, so it was a bit like living with the popular British musical drag act Hinge & Bracket. I loved them both, as they taught me how to cook, which I hadn't realised was so much fun until then. The only downside was the effect it had on my appetite, as being surrounded by all the wonderful smells, tantalising tastes and sensational sights made me feel less hungry when it was my own cooking. The plus side was how preparing and cooking a meal helped me feel relaxed and allowed me to unwind after a busy day. It was truly therapeutic.

As I poured myself another glass of red from the rather impressive Stonyridge Vineyard on Waiheke Island, one of 600 dotted around

New Zealand's coastline, I decided it was time to see a bit more of this beautiful country, so as we had no filming the following week, I hired a car and drove myself to Tūrangi, a small town on the west bank of the Tongariro River and not far from Lake Taupo, known as the inland sea of New Zealand.

The reason I chose this particular spot was because it was where Justine, the widow of one of my godfathers, lived and after I had spoken to her on the phone, she invited me to come and stay. My godfather Pat Toynbee had been in the Fleet Air Arm in WW2, which is when he became a friend of my father and he had also been part of the expedition team for Sir Vivian Fuchs who led an overland crossing of Antarctica in 1957-8.

Pat had sent me a couple of books about his adventures when I was at school but sadly, I never got the chance to meet him before he died, which was a pity as apart from being interested to hear about his expeditions to the South Pole first hand, I would have liked to know more about my father.

Justine's second husband Ron was keen for me to go fishing with him, so we got up early the following morning and headed to the nearest river to catch our breakfast. I was thrilled when I caught a couple of decent size trout and having now got a taste for a new sport, I booked myself into Tongariro Lodge to have a professional fly-fishing lesson. The exclusive lodge supplied the waders, rods and tackle and took me to a part of the river where they thought I would get the best chance of a catch. It took ages to get the hang of casting correctly but once I had got the knack there was no stopping me and I caught three reasonably sized trout. We released the smallest two back into the river but kept the largest to have for dinner It weighed 5.5 lbs, which the Lodge chef told me was quite a *bug fush*. After cooking the trout and serving it with a side portion of *chups,* I ate it on their *dick*.

It had been an excellent day in The Land of the Long Flat Vowel.

When Waka asked me if I would edit a music video which he had just filmed in a school hall for a band called The Warratahs, I said I'd be happy to do so, as the band were a bit different to the norm, which appealed to me. They were made up of rock and jazz musicians who wanted to play country music, and although not my cup of tea, they were very good at it and the song *Hands of my Heart* was very catchy, so much so I couldn't get it out of my head for weeks afterwards. I then got a series of five commercials to direct for Toyota, which kept us busy and also topped up my bank account. We flew Australian DOP Vince Monton over from Sydney to light the spots and he did an excellent job as did the Kiwi DOP Jim Bartle on my next commercial for Holden Camira.

As a reward for my efforts, I bought *Crest of a Knave* by Jethro Tull, which I thought was their best album in years, perhaps because it was more guitar-based than usual. Martin Barre sounded more like Mark Knopfler than ever before on *She Said She Was a Dancer*, and Ian Anderson was in fine flute form on *Farm on the Freeway,* a song which tells the story of a farmer who has to sell his land to make way for a new road. But my favourite track was *Budapest,* a song about a young man who goes exploring to escape his monotonous life but discovers he has the same problems wherever he goes.

In mid-September I met an aspiring young actress called Julie and asked her to come with me to see renowned guitar picker Brownie McGhee who was performing at Wellington's Town Hall. I have always loved the blues but this was the first time I felt transported right back to where it all began. One of his songs was called *Blues All Round My Bed* so I took this as a positive omen of things to come. I'm glad to say it was and the following night, Julie and I started going out with each other.

I couldn't wait to start the next commercial as it was for New Zealand Post and I really liked the script. The quirky idea was to show a variety of weird objects like a metronome wrapped in brown paper tied with string and a fluffy toy Kiwi with a name tag on one of its feet, being weighed on a set of scales and then sent to its destination with the guarantee they would all arrive safely. We hired Alan Locke to be my DOP and a professional modelmaker from Sydney to create all the weird and whacky packages and Richard Briers from *The Good*

388                  *Welcome To The Jungle*

*Life* did the voice-over in the style of his character Tom Good, which added extra humour to the spot

Two days after doing the online edit at Images in Auckland, Julie and I were back at the Wellington Town Hall to see Chris Rea on his *Dancing With Strangers* tour. *Windy Town* got the biggest cheer of the night because of Wellington being regarded as one of the windiest cities in the world and when he sang *Let's Dance*, everyone danced in the aisles.

The last show I went to in New Zealand was Billy Connelly. It was his first world tour and I wanted to see if Julie enjoyed his humour as much as I did, which of course she did. We went with Paul Maxwell and his wife and although we all laughed our socks off, the evening was a little bittersweet for me, as my six months were almost up, which meant it was time for me to go back to Australia.

Saying goodbye to Peter, Huey and Jeff was pretty hard as they had done so much for me, but the hardest part was still to come. Although Julie had known right from the start I would be returning to Sydney when my contract expired, her career was just taking off, so it wasn't the right time for her to consider coming with me. After a tearful farewell at the airport, she gave me an envelope and told me not to open it until I was in the air. She then walked away without turning back. I kept my promise but as soon as the seatbelt sign was turned off, I opened the envelope and read her card, which contained this heartfelt poem.

'If every drop of rain meant I love you, and if you asked me how much I loved you, it would rain all day.' When I looked out of the plane's window it was covered in tiny drops of rain, which to me represented the tears I was holding back.

Before going home, I stopped off in the Cook Islands for a few days, as I had never been to the South Pacific before and wanted to see what an unspoilt paradise really looked like. I wasn't disappointed as the white sandy beaches on Aitutaki Island were spectacular, and swimming in the crystal-clear lagoon was sheer bliss.

One morning, I took a small boat to One Foot Island where many years ago, a chief had forbidden his people to go fishing there, so when a man and his son were spotted there one day, they were immediately sentenced to death but the father saved the life of his child by concealing his footprints with his own and this is how the island got its name.

Although some new resorts were being built on Rarotonga, the largest of the Cook Islands, I was glad to discover none were allowed to be higher than a coconut tree. When I went to the bar at my hotel to order a sundowner, there was nobody there to serve me so I sat down to wait. Suddenly I heard a voice from above say, 'I'll be with you in a minute.' The man was clearly British and a couple of minutes later he descended a wooden ladder from the thatched roof and introduced himself as the manager. While Chris poured me a cold beer, we had a chat and discovered we were both brought up in the New Forest, which was quite a coincidence in itself but after talking a bit further we then worked out it was his mother who had taught me how to ride when I was a boy. It's a small world indeed. He then produced two guitars and we had a short jam, which went so well Chris invited me to perform with him at another hotel in the evening. It wasn't a paid gig but we were given food and free drinks all night. We played a number of songs together including J.J Cale's *Call Me the Breeze* and *After Midnight,* which couldn't have been a more perfect way to end my adventure in the South Pacific.

I got back to Sydney on the 23$^{rd}$ of October 1987 and as Baggers had moved out the week before, I was able to move straight back into my one-bedroom flat. My friend had left it spotless and also made sure my Suzuki had a full tank of petrol, so I was able to resume my old life instantly.

After a quick shower and change of clothes, I was in a taxi and on my way to the Sydney Entertainment Centre to see Eric Clapton. 'God', as he was called by some of his fans, started his set with *Crossroads* and ended it with *Further on up the Road*, which described my last six months perfectly. My time in New Zealand had been a blast.

Robbie Robertson singer-songwriter with The Band had jammed with Clapton on the same track on the 1976 Martin Scorsese movie *The Last Waltz,* so when his self-titled solo album was released a few days later I was eager to hear it. The opening track *Fallen Angel* took me by surprise as it featured a duet with Peter Gabriel. The other track which I loved on first hearing was *Somewhere Down the Crazy River,* which features a chord sequence played on a Suzuki Omnichord, an electrical instrument producer Daniel Lanois had been introduced to by ex-Roxy Music musical magician Brain Eno.

The next overseas artist to perform at the Entertainment Centre was Billy Joel. The 'Piano Man' included some great covers in his set, including *You Are So Beautiful* (Billy Preston), *Hotel California* (The Eagles), *The Power of Love* (Huey Lewis and the News) and *Let It Be* (The Beatles), as well as 27 of his own songs, so it was night to remember, for Billy especially, as there were a lot of lyrics to memorise.

At the beginning of November, *Sounds Like Australia* won two ACS Golden Tripod Awards for the Best Wildlife Film and Best Documentary at the Chicago Film Festival, as well as the Gold Award at the Hawaii Film Festival and the People's Award at the Italian Film Festival. I immediately let everyone who had worked on the film know about its success, which wouldn't have received any of the prestigious awards if it hadn't been for their hard work. As a small reward for my part in the film's success, I bought myself a cassette of *Kick* by INXS to play in my car. The album included *New Sensation, Devil Inside* and *Need You* Tonight, all of which I thought were tremendous but the track I liked the most was the ballad *Never Tear Us Apart* because Michael Hutchence's lyrics about what it is like to have an instant connection with someone were so full of emotion. When I received a call the next day from Peter Avery to let me know the AWA Computers commercial I had directed for him had just won the Gold Award at the International Advertising Awards in New York, I couldn't help but laugh, as it felt a bit like the old joke of waiting ages for your bus and then an hour later three all come along at once.

It was an honour to receive all these awards, as it meant I must be doing something right, but for some reason the success didn't improve my feeling of self-worth at all. It is thought low self-esteem often begins in childhood, so perhaps there was something in my past which was holding me back and affecting both my career and my relationships. I had no idea what it could be but decided it might be time to find out why, so after getting over the stigma of seeing a 'shrink', I made an appointment with my doctor to ask him to refer me to one before I changed my mind.

The first time I saw a clinical therapist was a bit intimidating as he asked me so many questions, many of which seemed irrelevant, but after I had spilled my guts, I was surprised at how liberating it was to talk to a complete stranger. My fears had been unfounded.

After 'taking me back' to my childhood, I told him about the bullying I had suffered at the hands of the other boys at my boarding school, the mental and physical abuse by one of the teachers, and how my natural curiosity had often been mistaken for questioning authority, which I was then unjustly punished for.

In those days, the word *anxiety* was used to describe what we would now be called depression. I'm not even sure whether it was considered a genuine illness at the time but more of a psycho-sematic nervous disorder associated with being stressed by the pressures of life. The doctor had another name for it. Melancholia. He told me he thought I chose to be moody at will and intentionally remained in this state because I took pleasure in its 'darker aspects', although I never found out what this meant.

After three lengthy but cathartic sessions, my therapist told me how he thought my difficulty in maintaining relationships might partly be due to being sent away from home to live with strangers where I was exposed to separation from everything which was familiar to me and represented security. The repeated experience of coming home for the holidays and then being forced to leave again to go back to school just as I was feeling settled had created a psychological pattern and this subconscious habit along with the death of my father at such a young age combined with the constant bullying at school would all have had an impact on my mental wellbeing.

When I asked him why I felt so little joy after winning my awards, he thought I might have something called imposter syndrome, which is when someone thinks they don't deserve the accolades bestowed on them and fear they will be 'found out' at any moment for being a fraud. Despite the evidence being to the contrary. Phew! It was a lot to take in.

To overcome my feelings of worthlessness he advised me to try to have more compassion for my younger self, as it wasn't 'his' fault, and to try to let go of my need for perfectionism.

'Many perfectionist tendencies are rooted in the fear of being judged when you get things wrong,' my therapist said in his last session with me, 'I suspect this personality trait began after your experiences at boarding school, we don't have to get things right every time, errors are acceptable, so try not to be too harsh on yourself and when you do have a win for God's sake celebrate it!'

I took his advice and 'celebrated' my recent awards by going to see David Bowie on his *Glass Spider* tour at the Sydney Entertainment Centre. Bowie's set was an eclectic mix which included a few songs I wasn't familiar with like *Up the Hill Backwards*, a cover of *Bang Bang* by Iggy Pop, *Chant of the Ever-Circling Skeletal Family* and *Beat of Your Drum*, but I was glad he did perform these less well-known tracks as it made me appreciate what a brilliant storyteller he was as well as being a fabulous singer, gifted artist and cracked actor. The songs I enjoyed the most were *Loving the Alien, China Girl, The Jean Genie, Let's Dance* and *Modern Love.* Bowie's back-up band featured Peter Frampton on guitar and his expressive solos inspired me to practice on my own guitar more often. The hard work paid off, as the next time I saw Mars Lasar he asked me to play a solo on one of the tracks on his new album and even gave me a credit, which was a big thrill, especially for such a small contribution.

When a production company called Ashenhurst-Hughes offered to represent me, I was very flattered because John Ashenhurst was a legend in the Advertising Industry, having created the look for the iconic 'Singapore Girl-Singapore Airlines' commercials, which were all beautifully shot by the maestro himself. His experienced producer Annie Hughes, told me John liked the fact I worked intuitively, as he did too, which was a massive compliment but I knew I would never reach the heights of such a master craftsman, so I just tried to listen and learn as much as I could from him while I had the opportunity.

The most important event to happen to me in 1987 took place on the 3$^{rd}$ of December, as this was the day, I got my first Australian Passport. When I proudly showed it to my friends at the pub, they all shook my hand and then said typically Aussie things like, 'Fair go mate!', 'Good on ya!' and 'Drink up buddy, it's your round!'

While we were drinking, *Run to Paradise* by The Choirboys suddenly blared over the pub speakers and everyone stopped talking and began singing along to the recent hit song about misspent youth on Sydney's northern beaches. I had never experienced anything quite like it and shook my head in disbelief.

'Come on mate! If you want to be a true-blue Aussie you have to sing along to our national rock anthem!'

After the song was over, everyone resumed chatting to their friends normally as though nothing had happened.

But it had. I had just been accepted. I belonged.

As becoming an Aussie was worth celebrating in style, I went to see Jimmy Barnes at the Sydney Entertainment Centre with the same group of friends five days later. The support acts Johnny Diesel & The Injectors and Noiseworks got the crowd in the right mood but it wasn't until Jimmy came on stage that the party truly started. *Too Much Ain't Enough Love* and *Driving Wheels* from his *Freight Train Heart* album went down well but when he sang Cold Chisel's *Goodbye (Astrid Goodbye)* and followed it with *Khe Sanh* the roof came off and we all started screaming almost as loud as 'Barnesy', which as anyone who has heard him scream in front of a live audience will tell you is impossible.

After the show, we took ourselves down to Woolloomooloo to have a late-night snack at Harry's Café de Wheels. The moveable food van had become famous over the years for serving 'Tiger Pie', which contained plenty of meat and was topped with mashed potato, mushy peas and gravy after one of their gigs. The pie got its name from the original owner Harry 'Tiger' Edwards who had been given the nickname due to his boxing skills. Sadly, the van was forced to move in 1981 because the Navy wanted to redevelop the dockyard but the good news is there is now a permanent site near Fingers Wharf, so you can still get your mitts on a 'Tiger'. If you are ever thinking of going to Australia, it's important to know the 'Tiger Pie' has nothing to do with the more commonly known 'Pie Floater', which originated in South Australia and where the pie is placed upside down in a bowl of thick pea soup and then drowned in enough tomato sauce to make the aftermath of the Valentine's Day Massacre look trivial by comparison.

I agreed to see my therapist for one more session as he was interested to know if 'becoming an Australian' had helped give me a sense of belonging, so I told him it had and how the commitment had also given me a national identity to be proud of, which I had never felt in the UK, perhaps because I was born in Scotland and felt allegiance to the country of my birth rather than of my education. As I was about to leave the therapist said, 'Good luck with your career and in the nicest possible way, I hope I don't see you again!'

Just before Christmas, my neighbour's water pipes burst and flooded my flat in Waverton. The living room carpet was ruined and had to be pulled up and thrown away. Thankfully their insurance would cover the cost of buying a new one but in the meantime, I would be without a carpet until the new year, as nobody was available to replace it until then.

When I went to Baggers new apartment for a Waifs and Strays party on Christmas Day, I met a rather attractive woman who said she was a teacher and after I told her about my recent carpet catastrophe, she put a hand on my shoulder and said with a dead-pan face, 'Oh, I'm sorry to hear that. How about a shag?' I must have looked shocked because she roared with laughter and said with a wicked grin, 'I can't believe you fell for it. Shag. Carpet. Get it?' I did, but must admit to having been slightly disappointed as if it had been a serious offer, I doubt I would have refused.

When my new carpet was finally fitted, I invited her to dinner so she could inspect my new acquisition. This time when she asked me the same question she added, 'No pun intended!' so I knew where I stood...so to speak.

1988 started in spectacular fashion when the first Tall Ships arrived in Sydney on the 19th of January, having sailed from Hobart as part of the International Tall Ships Race. Richard, one of my old friends from kindergarten, and his wife Judi who had been at 6th form college with me, arrived a day later with their son Rory and my friend Vicki, who I had travelled around America and Canada with, so I now had a flat full of Poms to share the upcoming festivities with.

On the 26th of January, we all went to a Bicentenary party hosted by our mutual English friends David and Tricia, whose house in McMahons Point was right on the harbour, so we had a splendid view of the First Fleet re-enactment of their arrival in Botany Bay in 1788. The aptly named 'Parade of Sail', which featured a flotilla of classic riggers, skiffs, motor boats and yachts was a truly spectacular sight, especially having the Sydney Opera House and Harbour Bridge in the background.

I was having so much fun at the party, the question of whether we should have been celebrating 200 years of white occupation of Australia, was something I didn't think about until the next day when I watched the news and learnt had been protestors holding signs with the slogan 'White Australia has a Black History.' I felt deeply ashamed I hadn't bothered to try and understand the bicentenary celebrations from the Indigenous point of view. It was a wake-up call and as I listened to *Blackfella, Whitefella* by the Warumpi Band, the only indigenous song I had in my collection at the time, I vowed to learn more about their history and culture. The lyrics in this powerful song say it all.

'Blackfella, whitefella, it doesn't matter what your colour, as long as you a real fella, as long as you a true fella.'

My passion for live music was about to be well and truly catered for over the next few months. On the 30$^{th}$ of January, I went to see Pink Floyd perform at the Sydney Entertainment Centre. *A Momentary Lapse of Reason* was the first tour without Roger Waters. Guy Pratt, who had spent some time with Icehouse, was now on bass duties. It was a great gig and I enjoyed hearing songs from their new album, especially *Yet Another Movie* and *Sorrow* but it wasn't until I heard the crowd clapping along to Guy's bass riff at the start of *One of These Days* off *Meddle,* I knew he had won over the fans.

In February, I was lucky enough to see Leroy 'Roy' Buchanan when he played at the Tivoli. The American Blues guitar legend had a very distinctive guitar style and I particularly liked the way he bent his strings to make his guitar wail and used his tone knob to either mute or swell a note at any given time. He would also occasionally strike one of the strings with his plectrum and his thumb at the same time, which created harmonics called 'whistlers'. His frantic cover of Henry Mancini's *Peter Gunn* was crazy but the best was still to come when he played *The Messiah Will Come Again,* which almost brought me to tears as his guitar sounded like someone crying. Perhaps this was because it was written while he was struggling with drug and alcohol abuse. On the way home, I stopped off for a nightcap at a bar in Crows Nest and as I sipped my second Scotch, I wondered about my dependence on alcohol but was pretty sure I had it under control…at least for now,

Although, I'd had a wonderful summer with plenty of live music and fun with my friends, I'd had no paid work at all but I wasn't overly concerned, as I had managed to save most of what I had earned in New Zealand so had enough to keep me going for a while. When I next went into the office, John Ashenhurst told me not to worry too much as the film industry often had quiet periods and suggested I go overseas for a while until things picked up again. Although we hadn't had the chance to work together on any commercials yet, what I did gain from the experience of spending time with such a generous man was more belief in my abilities.

This was an important turning point in my life as I no longer felt quite as undeserving of my success as I had in the past and was able to move on with renewed confidence. I knew there would be other setbacks in the future but I now felt better equipped to cope with them. And now I had an Australian passport it not only allowed me to stay in the country indefinitely but also meant I could work overseas for as long as I wanted to or as in this case, needed to until the film industry was back on its feet again, so after renting my apartment through a local estate agent, I took a taxi to Sydney airport and as I boarded my flight, I remembered a quote attributed to Yankees hero Yogi Berra, 'It feels like Déjà vu... all over again!'

*Fools rush in where angels fear to tread.*

Alexander Pope

## CHAPTER 9: ROCK AND A HARD PLACE

I arrived in England on April Fool's Day 1988 but as I was in no rush to go where angels fear to tread, I took the tube from Heathrow to Parsons Green rather than a taxi. While I looked for some work in London, I stayed with my godmother's daughter Mops who had a lovely house off Munster Road. Although her real name was Liz, she was given the nickname 'Mops' as a child because of her mass of curly hair and it had stuck. As she also worked in the film industry, she understood how there were often long gaps between jobs, so it was a big help to me to have her support and understanding.

One of the first things I did once I was over the jetlag was to buy a couple of music magazines. The front cover of NME had a photo of REM on it with the caption 'The Band Who Fell to Earth' underneath it and Q magazine featured a photo of Tina Turner with 'AWL-RAHT' written over the top of her. I had been buying New Musical Express since the 1970s but Q had only been around since 1986. It was founded by Mark Ellen and David Hepworth who had previously presented *The Old Grey Whistle Test*, so I knew it would be worth reading and always bought a copy whenever I got the opportunity.

Although Gillie Potter had retired some time ago, Ken and Mary were still working together out of the same office in Holborn but were now called The Film Company. When I popped in to see them one morning, they welcomed me with open arms and told me my timing couldn't have been better as they had just been hired to produce a series of comedy sketches and were looking for a director. I couldn't believe my luck and started work the next day. The show featured Scottish comedian Tony Roper, who had starred in the TV shows *Naked Video* and *Rab C. Nesbitt*. Filming in the same studio where Ken had taught me how to direct my first TV commercials and title sequences made me feel quite nostalgic and it also gave me the perfect opportunity to thank him for being my mentor.

After the job was approved by the client, I drove down to the New

Forest to see my parents for the weekend in my new second-hand Renault 5, which I bought with my director's fees. It was great to catch up with my folks and hear about the rest of my family. They loved having the grandchildren to stay but found it a bit exhausting as they were so full of energy. While I was in the area, I caught up for a drink with my friends Richard and Judi whom I had last seen in Sydney Harbour earlier in the year when we were watching the tall ships together. Judi's sister Pauline, who was a doctor, was also at the pub, which was a lovely surprise, as she was a highly intelligent young woman and good company.

In May, I took Pauline to see Fleetwood Mac at Wembley on their *Shake the Cage* tour. Their charismatic singer-guitarist Lindsey Buckingham had gone his own way and been replaced by singer Billy Burnette and session guitarist Rick Vito, which suited me fine, as I knew Rick could really play the blues. They performed their hits *The Chain, Dreams, Go Your Own Way* and *Don't Stop* but also played *Oh Well* and *Stop Messin' Around* from their previous incarnation when Peter Green was in the band, so we were treated to the best of both Macs. *Gold Dust Woman* gave Stevie Nicks a chance to shine and *Little Lies* allowed Christine McVie to remind us what a great singer she is as well as a talented songwriter Mick Fleetwood's unique drumming style was as instinctive as ever and John McVie's crafted bass lines kept the band tight all night.

It felt good to be back in London for a while as the music scene was always vibrant and I was often spoilt for choice. On the 6th of June, I went to see Midnight Oil on their *Beds Are Burning* tour at the Town and Country Club in Kentish Town. The band were tight thanks to Rob Hirst's impressive performance behind the drumkit, the two guitarists' impeccable timing and Peter Garrett's unique voice and exaggerated dance moves. The set included *The Dead Heart,* a song about the mistreatment of Indigenous Australians and *Beds Are Burning,* which criticised how many of them were forced off their land. When they sang 'it belongs to them, let's give it back', everyone in joined in and meant it.

On the 24th of June I was fortunate enough to see Blues legend Stevie Ray Vaughan at the Hammersmith Odeon. Stevie's backing band Double Trouble consisted of Chris Layton on drums, Tommy Shannon on bass and Reese Wynans on keyboards. *Scuttle Buttin'*, *Say What!*, *Texas Flood* and a cover of Stevie Wonder's *Superstition* were the highlights for me but then he came back on stage and did two encores. *Love Struck Baby* and a cover of Jimi Hendrix's *Voodoo Child (Slight Return)*, which blew the whole audience away, including Eric Clapton who was sitting four seats away from me in the same row.

The following week, I went to Wembley Stadium to see Bruce Springsteen and The E Street Band on *The Tunnel of Love Express* tour with some friends from Australia who were in the UK visiting family. The band included The Horns of Love led by trombonist Richie 'La Bamba' Rosenberg. 'The Boss' opened with *Tunnel of Love* and after performing another 30 songs, including *Born in the U.S.A*, *Dancing in the Dark*, and *Glory Days,* he finally ended his mammoth set with *Twist and Shout,* but by then we all had sore feet from dancing and hoarse throats from singing, so were unable to do either.

Being able to attend so many live music gigs was a real treat but I now needed to get some work to pay for them, so when The Film Company asked me if I would like to direct a commercial for Milka Chocolate, I was happy to oblige. The brief was to show how the chocolate was made using only three ingredients, coco beans, sugar and a special milk powder which had come from the Alpine. Ken and I devised ways of making it look better than it actually was by filming the beans in slow motion tumbling into a silver bowl, pouring sugar over the edge of a black piece of card using multiple exposures so it looked like a waterfall and pouring chocolate coloured milk in slow motion into a glass bowl from underneath to make it look more appetising. The special powder was never seen but we did film plenty of pack shots of the chocolate bars. The logo for the Swiss company was a purple cow called Lila with a bell around her neck. Thankfully the client supplied a mock-up photo of a purple cow, which was a relief, as for one awful moment we thought we might have to paint a real one.

At the beginning of July, I caught up with Linda, who had once been a flatmate of mine in Sydney, and she agreed to come with me to see Jethro Tull at Wembley Arena. As it was their *20th Anniversary* tour their set list covered songs from all their albums since they had first formed, including *Nothing is Easy, My God* and *Thick as a Brick*. Original drummer Clive Bunker came on stage to play congas on a fine rendition of *Fat Man* and violinist Ric Saunders from Fairport Convention, who had been the support act, joined the band for a fabulous version of *Budapest*. Ten days later, my friend Nicol and I went to Ronnie Scott's to see the Cuban-American jazz trumpeter and pianist Arturo Sandoval. His jazz was a bit different to anyone else's, as he managed to fuse Afro-Cuban rhythms with his compositions. As soon as he started playing *El Misterioso* we were 'gone man, solid gone!' Since I had last seen my old friend, he had secured a position working at Brands Hatch, which was the ideal job for him because of his love of motorsports. I was happy for Nicol and felt lucky to have such a good friendship with someone I might not see for ages but then when we did catch up, we could carry on as if we'd only been apart for a day.

As Pauline had been working so hard, she hadn't come to any of my recent concerts but was determined not to miss Maina Gielgud's production of *Sleeping Beauty* at the Royal Opera House in Covent Garden. Lisa Pavane, the principal artist with the Australian Ballet, was the Lilac Fairy and her performance was spectacular. Afterwards we met up with Graeme Murphy, the Australian choreographer who I had filmed for Qantas the previous year, and I was happy to hear he had recently been awarded the Order of Australia for his services to ballet.

On the 14th of August, Roy Buchanan, whose gig I had been to in February, hanged himself in his prison cell in Virginia, America. He was being held in jail overnight after a domestic dispute. It was quite a shock as although his drinking habits had been a concern in the past it was thought he had got his act together and was now sober. In an interview he did before he died he was quoted as saying. 'Probably the reason I never made it big is because I never cared whether I made it big or not. All I wanted to do was learn to play the guitar for myself. You set your own goals for success. And when you succeed it don't necessarily mean you will be a big star, make a lot of money, or anything. You'll feel it in your heart, whether you've succeeded or not.'

I have never forgotten those words and they still resonate today as I have never cared whether I made it big and became rich and famous either. At the end of August, I flew to Paris for the bank holiday weekend. I had hoped to take Pauline with me but her busy work schedule put an end to my romantic intentions, so as I had been neglecting my passion for photography recently, I took my camera instead. Having managed to save a few quid from my last job, I decided to splash out and put myself up at the Hôtel Sydney Opéra for a couple of nights, ate at the best restaurants and went to see the impressionist paintings at the Musée d'Orsay and the Musée de l'Orangerie. While standing in front of the *Water Lilies* by Claude Monet I met a young woman who introduced herself as 'Eleezaberth' who told me she was a freelance writer. When she offered to show me Paris from a local's perspective, I readily agreed as this was the inspiration I needed. Our first stop was Montmartre, which I had only ever been to at night before so I was excited to be there during the day and see where artists like Renoir, Van Gogh, Matisse and Picasso had once lived and breathed. As we walked, we discussed our respective careers and it felt good to talk to another freelancer who understood the pressure of what it was like to have long gaps between jobs. While we were drinking our coffees at a typical Parisian café, I heard the now famous cappella song *Don't Worry, Be Happy* by Bobby McFerrin being played on the radio for the first time. I still smile every time I hear the song and it takes me right back to Montmartre and its cobblestoned streets full of history.

On the 13<sup>th</sup> of September Jeff Healey released his album *See the Light*. As soon as I heard the opening track *Confidence Man*, a cover of the John Hiatt song, I was hooked. Jeff was blind, having lost his eyesight at the age of one due to a rare form of cancer. He played his guitar sitting down with his guitar on his lap because it felt more natural to him and then played chords with his left hand and used his right to pick and strum. His unique sound was instantly recognizable and I became a huge fan of his music.

I received a call in October from a producer called Simon Mallinson who was interested in representing me in Scotland, so I flew to Glasgow to meet him. We got on well so the next day he drove us both to Edinburgh to see a couple of agencies and after getting a positive reaction to my showreel, I felt optimistic I might get some work with his company.

When I got back to Mops' flat in Parsons Green there was a message for me saying Jackie was in London, so I called her back and arranged to have dinner. Within five minutes of being in each other's company it was clear our feelings for each other hadn't diminished. Before she flew back to Hong Kong, I took her to see The Robert Cray Band at the Hammersmith Odeon and afterwards we said goodbye and went our own ways...again.

At the end of the month, Pauline took me to see *Still Life at the Penguin Café* at the Royal Opera House. The ballet began with the voice of Jeremy Irons telling us how the Great Auk had recently become extinct and the first scene was set in a café where humans and penguins danced together. The choreography by David Bintley was extraordinary and the original music by Simon Jeffes was perfect. Each scene then featured an endangered species or culture until the climax where all the creatures and characters got together on an ark-like vessel in the pouring rain. The conservation theme appealed to me and the music was so inspirational I bought the album of the soundtrack.

The next morning, I started work on a video for Ladybird Books at the Film Company, which featured Gemma Craven who had made a name for herself in the BBC drama *Pennies from Heaven*. Her role was to read *Little Red Riding Hood* dressed as a Granny and *The Golden Goose* dressed as a Princess to a group of children in a studio set made to look like the attic of an old Tudor House.

In the evening, one of the crew played us the first album by The Travelling Wilburys. The 'Supergroup' comprised of Nelson Wilbury aka George Harrison, Otis Wilbury aka Jeff Lyne, Lucky Wilbury aka Bob Dylan, Charlie T. Jnr. aka Tom Petty and Lefty Wilbury aka Roy Orbison. The album was truly joyous. My favourite songs were *Handle With Care* and *Last Night* simply because the whimsical lyrics made me smile.

George Harrison got Monty Python's Michael Palin to write the liner notes, which read: 'The original Wilburys were a stationary people who, realising that their civilization could not stand still for ever, began to go for short walks – not the 'traveling' as we now know it, but certainly as far as the corner and back.'

Over the next few weeks, I had to fly up and down to Glasgow numerous times as Simon had found us a cinema commercial to produce for a lingerie company called *Entice*. As it wasn't a big budget, we had to think about how we could get the best production values for as little money as possible. Simon did a recce and found the answer by suggesting we film our spot at a beautiful Edwardian stately home called Manderston in the Scottish Borders, which was home to the 4th Baron Palmer. It had the world's only silver-plated staircase, a grand marble bathroom, long corridors and a sundial, so was ideal for our needs.

We hired a very attractive Dutch-Indonesian model called Astrid to wear the different pieces of lingerie the client wanted us to film. Despite being freezing cold, she was a trooper and in between takes rather than just trying to keep warm in the thick dressing gown and fluffy slippers we had provided for her, she went to the chilly kitchen and made us all cups of tea, which endeared her to all of us. Baron Palmer was a generous host and provided us with endless biscuits. (Huntley & Palmers obviously!)

Derek Suter, whose nickname was Sooty, had previously been a 'gaffer' (lighting technician) and was looking to get a break as a cameraman, so we gave it to him. It was his first gig as a DOP and he lit all our setups beautifully. As Astrid was so beautiful it was hard to get a bad shot of her and every piece of lingerie fitted her perfectly...with the addition of a few pins, needles and gaffer tape when required. To add a bit of drama to the commercial, we filmed a trained dove flying in slow motion over the sundial and along one of the long narrow corridors, which added a certain *je ne sais quoi*. Instead of just adding a logo on the end in post-production, we got a 35mm transparency slide with the word 'Entice' on it and by placing a projector on the fluid head of a second tripod we were then able to pan the word across a marble column, across Astrid's face and on the marble floor. This simple in-camera technique gave the commercial a classy look and the client was absolutely delighted.

A week later, Pauline and I went to see George Benson at Wembley Arena. I had never heard anyone sing so many songs with the word Love in the title. *Love is Here Tonight, Love X Love, Moody's Mood for Love, Love Ballad, The Greatest Love of All* and *Turn Your Love Around*. I was all loved out towards the end and quite relieved when he sang a cover version of Leon Russell's *The Masquerade* and on his final song *On Broadway,* he did a brilliant skat and guitar duet, which topped off a very entertaining night.

The following week I got a call from a friend in Sydney asking me if I could housesit for them from mid-December for a month, so I treated it as a sign it was time to go back to Australia. After spending a few days with my parents, I got on a plane and headed back to Sydney just in time for the annual Christmas party at Spectrum. It was great to catch up with a few of my old colleagues and to discover the Australian film industry had picked up a bit while I was in the UK. When one of the film editors told me he had been to see a therapist to cope with the stress of having such a long gap between paid jobs, I confided to having also seen one the previous year. Another editor who must have overheard us, interrupted our conversation and said, 'I have a much simpler way of dealing with stress.' We were both intrigued, so asked him to tell us what it was.

'I just stand up and yell fuckity-fuck-fuck-fuck three times at the top of my voice and then start again!'

I have tried doing this a few times since and must admit it works admirably well.

After having a rather boozy Christmas Day with my Pommy mates, I thought I would have a quiet night in alone on New Year's Eve at the house I was looking after, but when my rather attractive neighbour popped around to ask if I would like to have a drink with her, it was an offer I couldn't refuse, so I followed her back to her house. Two minutes later, I was confronted by the sight of four slightly inebriated women sitting in a Jacuzzi, all drinking champagne from plastic flutes and giggling like schoolgirls. When one of them suggested I join them in the hot tub, I did. Well, it would have been rude not to.

On New Year's Day 1989, I got a call from a young woman called Laura, who was the sister of a friend of mine in the UK who was currently on holiday in Australia. As the house I was staying in had a huge pool I invited her to come and have a swim. We got on so well we ended up having a short holiday romance, which put a big smile on both our faces.

On the 3$^{rd}$ of February, I took Laura to see B.B. King at the Sydney Entertainment Centre. The 'King of the Blues' included a cover of Aaron Pinetop Sparks' *Every Day I Have the Blues* in his set and also played Roy Hawkins' *The Thrill is Gone*. I loved the way B.B could bend a single string up and down and create such a distinctive and expressive vibrato effect. He was mesmerising to watch and a huge influence on the way I attempt to play.

When my house-sitting duties were over, I wasn't sure where I was going to stay next but by a stroke of good fortune a friend of a friend needed someone to look after their house for the next month, so I now had another temporary home for a while. While I was living there, I was offered a one-off job with a company called ZAP, owned by a big bear of a man called Zoran Janic, who I greatly admired as he was a wonderful animator.

The commercial was for Pelican Beach Resort. I asked Steve Windon, who had shot *Sounds Like Australia* to be my DOP and he agreed to do it for mates-rates. The resort was in Coffs Harbour but as the budget was so small the client couldn't afford to fly us up there, so we had to improvise and filmed the spot in a car park at one of Sydney's many beaches on the North Shore. We created a mock infinity swimming pool by placing a large metal tray painted turquoise, filled with water about an inch deep in the foreground and asked three swimsuit models to stand on a bench about 100 yards away, so when everything was lined up correctly it looked like the girls were standing on the far edge of a crystal-clear swimming pool with the Pacific Ocean glistening behind them. The only problem we had was every so often a car would go in or out of the car park and spoil the shot, so we had to time everything perfectly. Malinda who was one of the models, as well as our production manager, was a proud Bundjalung, Gidhabal and Galibal woman, which was wonderful for me as not only had I made a new friend on the shoot but now I also had someone to teach me about Indigenous Australian culture firsthand. When she told me her ambition was to be the youngest Indigenous director in Australia, I had no doubt she would achieve her dream and go on to become a brilliant storyteller.

After the owners whose house I had been looking after returned home, Laura and I decided to drive up to Coffs Harbour together and stayed at the real Pelican Beach Resort. As I had just shot for a commercial for them, we were treated like VIPs and even had our own pool right outside our villa. After two nights of being treated like rock stars, we continued north to Brisbane to see my mentor Edwin Scragg and his family who had recently left South Australia and were now living in Queensland. It was lovely to see his daughters Emma and Sarah again and we had great fun kayaking on the river by their house.

We got back to Sydney in March just in time to see Joe Camilleri and The Black Sorrows at Harbourside in Darling Harbour. They played songs from their album *Hold On To Me*, including the title track, *Chained to the Wheel* and *The Crack Up*. It was the first time I had seen the Tongan-Australian backup singers Vika and Linda Bull but I knew it wouldn't be the last. The talented sisters were truly amazing and stole the show.

Two days later I got a call from Simon in Scotland to tell me he had a commercial for me to direct for the Strathclyde Regional Council and as the budget was quite reasonable, it would cover a return airfare to the UK. I hadn't planned to go back again quite so soon but with no commercial work in Australia, it was an opportunity to update my showreel, so after saying goodbye to Laura, I flew back to London and then on to Glasgow. Simon picked me up from the airport and then we went on a recce to find the best locations, which included the enchanting Isle of Bute, a short ferry ride across the Firth of Clyde.

Scottish rock band Simple Minds had recently released a great black and white music video for the song *Belfast Child*, so we thought it would be a good idea to try something similar. Adrian Wild was getting a good reputation for his stylish camerawork, so we hired him as our DOP and he did a great job. We thought shooting it in black and white would look terrific but the client wanted us to shoot it in colour, so we compromised and shot it in colour but did two grades, one in black and white and the other in colour. In post-production we superimposed 'anything' which and 'anyone' who represented the council in colour onto the black and white backgrounds. When the client saw it, he was tickled pink.

As a reward to myself I bought Tom Petty's *Full Moon Fever*. His solo album was produced by Jeff Lynne who also co-wrote many of the songs including *Free Fallin'*, *I Won't Back Down* and *Runnin' Down a Dream*, which featured some stunning guitar licks by Mike Campbell. As for my own dream, I decided to put it on hold for a while. With no work to go back to in Australia, I thought I might as well postpone my return and spend the summer in the UK.

When I told Mops my plan, she kindly said I could have her spare room for as long as I needed it, which was a real godsend.

On the 1st of July 1989 I attended a very special concert at a charity event at Wintershall Estate in Bramley, Surrey. The magnificent grounds made the perfect setting for a picnic by the lakes. Mops and I and my friends Emma and Karen sat on a rug, eating canapes and drinking champagne until the music started. We then wandered up to the open-air stage to see Band Du Lac, who had a rather impressive line-up. Eric Clapton on guitar and vocals, Steve Winwood on guitar, keyboard and vocals, Gary Brooker on keyboard and vocals, Mike Rutherford on guitar and vocals, Andy Fairweather Low on guitar and vocals, Dave Bronze on bass, Henry Spinetti and Phil Collins on drums with Danny Hammond adding extra percussion, Mel Collins and Frank Mead on saxophones and supplying some sweet backing vocals were Sam Brown, her Mum Vicki and friends Carol Kenyon and Margo Buchanan. The show was sensational with each talented musician being allowed to shine and play two of their own songs with the rest of the band backing them up.

The crowd was small enough for me to be standing only a few feet from the stage, so I had the perfect spot to see so many of my musical heroes. It was a pity no cameras were allowed on the day, as I would have got some memorable photos. Steve Winwood sang *Freedom Overspill*, Eric Clapton played *Old Love* and Sam Brown performed an incredible version of her hit *Stop* with E.C providing a sensitive if somewhat extensive solo. Standing right next to me was Sam's father Joe Brown. Thankfully, I managed to stop myself from singing *Mr(s) Brown You've Got a Lovely Daughter* and the special moment wasn't ruined for him. They played *The Living Years*, *Cocaine* and *A Whiter Shade of Pale* and ended with The Spencer Davis Group's *Gimme Some Lovin'*.

Afterwards there was a rather impressive fireworks display over the main lake and then everyone took off their green wellies and went home in their helicopters or range rovers…as you do at such celebrity-filled charity events.

At the end of the month, I saw Simple Minds at Wembley Stadium on their *Street Fighting Years* tour. *Waterfront* was powerful, *Belfast Child* was emotional and *Biko*, a cover of Peter Gabriel's song, was unexpected. The energetic gig ended with *Alive and Kicking*.

A few days after the concert I got a call from a producer called Ron Bareham to tell me he had just done a deal with the Turkish branch of the advertising agency Saatchi & Saatchi, to supply a director and a DOP to work on ten commercials, but there was a catch…they had no scripts and they all had to be shot in ten days. This was the perfect job for me as I loved being put on the spot and having to improvise and use my imagination.

On the 30th of July, I flew to Istanbul with an elderly cameraman called Ray Parslow and I couldn't have had a better DOP, as he was an intuitive person like me and was really up for the challenge. Ray had been the cinematographer on Antonioni's 1966 movie *Blow-Up*, starring David Hemmings and Vanessa Redgrave but I remembered the film more for the soundtrack by Herbie Hancock.

When we arrived, we were taken straight to the Hilton Hotel where we would be staying for the duration of the shoot. The agency producer and creative team were charming and grateful we had come, which was a good start. They told us the client was the Turkish Sports For All Federation, although the correct name might have been lost in translation. They then explained how they were a non-profit organisation but wouldn't become official until the following year. Their goal was to encourage everyday people to do more physical activity, so they asked ten Turkish sports personalities to give up a day of their time to make a commercial which promoted their particular sport. We looked at the list of athletes, discussed a few ideas with the agency and eventually agreed we should come up with a few comedic scenarios, which exaggerated how bad they were at their chosen sport when they first started doing it but eventually became the best in their field.

The schedule was agreed purely on who was available on each day, so improvisation was the order of the day… every day. Our first commercial was the equestrian event, so we put Turkey's most successful horse rider on the smallest Shetland pony we could find and asked the animal trainer to make it come to a halt every time it came up to a jump. It looked quite ridiculous of course but when the film crew all laughed, we knew were onto a winner. I was pleasantly surprised at how the famous equestrian not only agreed to make fun of himself but also hammed it up perfectly. The second commercial featured a well-known basketball player talking to his agent on the phone while bouncing a ball with his other hand at the same time. The continuous bouncing eventually made part of the floor collapse and his ball disappeared down the hole. When the athlete looked down, he was surprised to see the owner of the flat below climb out of the hole and hand his ball back to him. The ideas were getting quirkier with each athlete. The best one was kept for last, as it needed to be filmed at night. The idea was to see Turkey's best hope of winning a Gold Medal for breaststroke having to swim a length of the pool while being chased by sharks. The illusion of killer sharks on the hunt was created using plastic triangles, painted matt black and then superglued to polystyrene bases which had fishing sinkers and weights attached to them so the mock-fins would stay upright when pulled through the water. These mock-shark fins were then attached to fishing lines each thread through hooks at both ends of the pool, and four crew members pulled the fins across the water at speed, so that when the weighted floats were submerged at the correct level, it gave the impression the swimmer was being stalked by the sharks was quite convincing. To help the trick work and look more dramatic, Ray lit the scene from behind and from just one side of the pool so the fins were in silhouette. It was cheap and amateur but very effective.

Before we left Istanbul, Ray and I had time to see a few tourist attractions together. It was wonderful to see the Hagia Sophia Grand Mosque and the Blue Mosque again and walk through the old streets just like I had done in 1977. When we saw a young boy wearing a Fez trying to sell other fezzes at his street stall, Ray put one on his head and did a great Tommy Cooper impersonation, my friend Baggers would have been proud of. He then proceeded to teach the local lad how to say 'Just like that!' while showing him how to do the same hand gestures the English comedian did when saying his famous catchphrase. It was a sight to behold and the photo I took of the two of them remains one of my favourites.

It was just as well I had decided to save all the money I earned from my lucrative Turkish gig for a rainy day, as after only being back in the UK for a week, work, unlike the British weather, suddenly dried up completely. Having stayed in England far longer than originally intended I took this as a sign telling me to go 'home' to Australia.

Whether it was fate or coincidence, I will never know, but 24 hours after my so-called 'sign', I received a call out of the blue from The Film Business, one of Australia's leading film production companies, asking me if I would like to join them as a TV commercials director based out of their Melbourne office. I wasn't too keen to live in 'Melbs' again, as I preferred Sydney and had been hoping to move back into my flat, but this unexpected opportunity felt like fate was trying to give me a helping hand. In the end, I decided the risk of going back to Oz was no worse than the risk of staying put, so agreed to their terms.

On the $11^{th}$ of September, The Rolling Stones released *Steel Wheels*. My favourite song on the album was *Rock and a Hard Place,* as thankfully I was no longer between either.

Before heading down under yet again, I had a farewell party in a restaurant on Munster Road with about 30 of my friends and at the end of the night, I was presented with a wooden boomerang and a T-shirt with Jamie *'Boomerang'* Robertson printed on the front of it.

The nickname has stuck ever since and the rest is…geography.

*A good traveller is one who does not know where he is going to,*
*and a perfect traveller does not know where he came from.*

Lin Yutang

## CHAPTER 10: HOLD ON TO ME

Before I left, Mops had given me a cassette of Chris Rea's new album *The Road to Hell* to listen to on my flight back to Australia. Apparently, the raspy-voiced singer had been stuck on the M4 motorway when he got the idea for the song. Thankfully I didn't suffer a similar fate on my way to Heathrow and managed to catch my flight on time.

I landed in Melbourne at dawn on the 28th of September 1989. Having done the long-haul flight so many times before, you would have thought I was used to the arduous journey by now but this wasn't the case. I was completely knackered, so it was just as well I had been given 24 hours to recover before having to report for duty.

The Film Business had a lovely office in South Melbourne and on my first day, I was introduced to the team who were all very friendly and made me feel welcome. There were two other film directors at the company who had their own distinctive styles and seemed to be very busy, which was a good sign of things to come. When I looked at their impressive showreels, I realised my work looked almost amateur by comparison, so I would have to work a lot harder from now on if I wanted to become anywhere near as good as them in the future. It was time to take my career much more seriously.

Over the next two weeks Michael Cook, the owner and producer, took me to see all the top advertising agencies so their creative teams could see my latest showreel, which now included both the commercials I had shot in Scotland. Michael and his partner Gary invited me to dinner on more than one occasion, which was exceptionally kind of them and now I was back in Melbourne I was also able to reconnect with my first boss in Australia Mike Reed, and my Aussie family the Fitzgeralds. The next step was to find somewhere to live and after a short search, I was lucky enough to find a charming little Victorian house to rent in Albert Park, one of the trendier inner suburbs near Middle Park Beach. The building was made of wood and painted light blue with yellow frames around the door and windows. There was one small bedroom at the front of the house, a sitting room with polished floorboards, a small kitchenette in the middle and a bathroom right at the back. Once I had furnished it with some second-hand furniture it felt more like a home and I could finally invite my friends around for a barbie.

Melbourne Cup is always a huge event in November but this year was a bit special for me, as I had been invited by the Fitzgerald's, to go to the races with them. When Bernadette, a friend of mine from Sydney, rang to ask if she could come and stay with me for the weekend, she was added to the list without a problem. 'Bernie' was a fabulous dress designer, so looked a million dollars in the outfit she had made for herself and somehow managed to persuade me to wear a suit and tie as well as my fedora hat. Personally, I thought I looked like a complete dickhead but she was adamant I looked very stylish and 'quite' handsome. However, my brief ego boost was soon crushed when we got in the taxi and she quipped. 'Everyone will be looking at me and not you anyway darling, so it doesn't matter what you're wearing!'

When it was time to put a bet on the Melbourne Cup race, I chose a horse called Super Impose but it was a New Zealand bred horse called Tawriffic which won on the day.

I didn't get my first commercial until the beginning of December but when I read the script, I felt confident I could do it justice. The TVC was for a margarine spread called Less and the brief was to see the hero pack of the product surrounded by loaves of homemade bread in the middle of an ancient forest with shafts of light coming through the trees to illuminate the scene. Our visual reference was a frame from Ridley Scott's movie *Legend* and to achieve this rather grandiose look we hired Keith Wagstaff as the DOP. As I had worked with him before, I knew he would do a good job with the lighting. It took two days to turn the studio into a magical forest and in an attempt to make it look natural, Keith used a dozen mirrors to bounce the light through the model trees and a smoke machine to create the magical mist. It looked very impressive if a little over the top for such a small budget commercial. However, the client loved what we had done and my career in Australia was back on track.

As Jackie was in Melbourne to have Christmas with her parents, we all went to see The Black Sorrows at the Greek Theatre together. When they sang their big hit *Hold on to Me,* Jackie took hold of my hand. In hindsight it would have been the perfect moment to ask her to leave Hong Kong and to come and live with me in Australia, but I didn't have the guts. Although I didn't realise it at the time, this would be my last chance.

I spent Christmas with the Fitzgeralds and after a huge feast we all listened to Fabian sing and play the piano for us, which was a special moment, as 'Fabes' had a lovely voice and was also an exceptional musician. I felt blessed to be considered part of this special family and their love and support really helped me feel settled in Melbourne.

The first concert I went to in 1990 was Lonnie Brooks at the Corner Hotel in Richmond. Fabes and his sister Emma came with me. The Chicago Bluesman had a very distinctive style, which was a concoction of country, swamp and electric blues known as Voodoo Blues. Lonnie's 'otherworldly' guitar work had us in a trance all evening.

On the 2$^{nd}$ of February anti-apartheid activist Nelson Mandela was finally freed after 27 long years in prison. Two weeks later I saw Split Enz and Crowded House at the Sidney Myer Music Bowl. When Tim Finn sang *I Hope I Never (see you again)* I imagined this is what Nelson would be thinking about his prison guards on Robben Island. The Kiwi band also sang *Hard Act to Follow* and *History Never Repeats* but the only song I remember Crowded House singing was *Don't Dream It's Over.* The reason it stuck in my mind was because I received a letter from Jackie the following day telling me she had met someone in Hong Kong and was about to move in with him. I was more upset than I thought I would be, as I had rather hoped once I had got more settled, I might be able to persuade her to move to Australia.

He who hesitates...as the proverb warns.

Although I'd had a great start to the year music-wise, getting some paid work was a different matter and I was just starting to get a wee bit concerned when The Film Business got two commercials for me to direct in a row. The first one for ANZ Bank, which John 'Oggy' Ogden shot for me, was very straightforward but the second for Stanley Tools shot by David Eggby, who had been the DOP on the movie Mad Max, was anything but.

The script called for three young men to drive a bright yellow Volkswagen Beetle to the edge of a huge lake and then after turning the car upside down, use the tools to convert it into a raft and then row themselves across to the other side of the lake. To achieve this rather ambitious amphibious idea, we bought two old beetles, one from a second-hand car dealer, which was driveable, and the other from a scrapyard, which was no longer roadworthy but was good enough body-wise to create the raft. We shot the commercial at Lake Eildon, about a four-hour drive from Melbourne, which proved to be the perfect location for our needs. When we did the shots of the raft, David donned his fishing waders so he could film the action at water level without getting wet. The three actors were then taxied via a small motorboat out to the raft before carefully climbing on board one at a time. I made the tallest actor stand up at the front of the raft and asked him to row the amphibious beetle across the water using an oar in the same way as if he was in a gondola. I then asked the other two actors to sit at the back of the raft to act as a counterbalance while pretending to look comfortable, which was almost impossible as the raft was so wobbly. It took a few takes to look convincing but we got there in the end without any mishaps and everyone went home happy.

In March, I took Fabes' sister Emma to see Melissa Etheridge on her *Brave and Crazy* tour at the Palais Theatre. The American singer was both. I loved her voice but it got so raspy by the time she sang *Bring Me Some Water* I hoped somebody in the audience might be kind enough to do as she asked. A week later, I was hired to direct a TVC for Black Magic chocolates. The tongue-in-cheek script required the ad to look a bit like a 1960s Hammer Horror movie. The brief was to follow a beautiful young woman wearing a long red dress, as she walked barefoot through a misty forest at night during a full moon like one of Dracula's brides. We would then see a driverless horse-drawn carriage galloping towards her and after pulling up right beside her, she would notice the elegant box of chocolates strategically placed on the leather seat, and, unable to resist the temptation, she would climb into the carriage and be whisked away into the night. We found a stunning model with long dark hair who was perfect for the part and I asked my friend Bernadette to design a long red dress, which would emphasize the girl's slender neck and bare shoulders and also allow her to walk without tripping up. We chose a talented DOP called Jeff Darling to shoot this live-action commercial, as he was known for his dramatic lighting. As we were filming such a large area at night, we had to use a bank of huge lights on tall stands to illuminate the action. We also had to block off Fitzroy Gardens in the middle of the city for two consecutive nights, so there were quite a few volunteers on crowd control as well as a large crew and a couple of Police officers to ensure everyone's safety. It was great fun to shoot and thankfully it all went smoothly. My old mentor Mike Reed edited the commercial and then took me to a Thai restaurant after work to celebrate a 'job well done'.

At the weekend, I flew up to Sydney to see some of my mates and while I was up there, I bumped into David Denneen, who was considered the top commercials director in Australia at the time, so when he stopped me in the street to tell me he thought I had done a decent job on the Black Magic commercial it was high praise indeed, especially as his company, Film Graphics, had also quoted on the job. David's generous compliment was just what I needed to hear and it filled me with confidence. I will always be grateful to him for taking the time to talk to me and for the way he treated me as an equal.

When I got back to Melbourne, I edited a new showreel so it now included all the commercials I had done for the Film Business on it, and then Michael and I spent the next few days doing more 'go sees' to try and get more work.

On St Patrick's Day I was invited to a friend's fancy dress party. While I was talking to the host, I suddenly felt someone pinch my bottom. When I turned around to see who the pincher was, I was surprised to see a rather gorgeous woman with a mane of long blonde hair smiling at me. She then whispered in my ear, 'I just wanted to get your attention!' Well, it worked. She now had my complete and undivided attention for the rest of the evening...the whole night and most of the following day.

Virginia was a senior nurse and a midwife and worked at the Royal Women's Hospital in Melbourne. She had a great sense of humour and enjoyed teasing me about the fact I was beginning to go bald. As she thought I looked a bit like the ex-Genesis drummer Phil Collins, I took her to see the real Mr. Collins at the National Tennis Centre on his *Seriously, Live!* tour. It was the perfect gig for a romantic evening as he started his set with *Hand in Hand* and ended with *A Groovy Kind of Love, Easy Lover, Always* and *Take Me Home.* It was not my kind of music but when you are falling in love you pretend to enjoy whatever songs your new lover likes in an attempt to bond with them. It works both ways of course, as I found out a week later when I took Virginia back to the same venue to see Fleetwood Mac on their *Behind the Mask* tour. She put on a brave face but I don't think she enjoyed the gig as much as I did. Having different musical tastes isn't the end of the world but having a similar sense of humour is vital if you want a relationship to last, so I was interested to see what Virginia thought of Billy Connelly when I took her to his latest show. I need not have worried as she giggled helplessly all the way through the gig. The Scottish comedian's observations of human behaviour were spot on as usual. We both commented on having sore jaws the next day from laughing so much.

For our first romantic weekend away together, we decided to drive along the Great Ocean Road to look at The Twelve Apostles, a group of wind-eroded limestone rock formations which rise out of the Southern Ocean. I got some dramatic photos of them at sunset and then we stayed in Lorne for the night. In the morning we drove on to Port

Fairy, which had lots of old-fashioned looking cottages Virginia took a fancy too but what I really wanted to see was the old lighthouse on Griffiths Island, as it was built by Scottish stonemasons way back in 1859. The last lighthouse keeper who had lived in it was there from 1929 until 1954, the year I was born. Over the weekend, we got much closer and my girlfriend told me she thought I was 'a keeper,' which made us both laugh.

In April, I went to see Vincent Damon Furnier aka Alice Cooper on his *Trashes the World* tour at the National Tennis Centre with an old friend called Catherine, as Virginia wasn't a fan and didn't want to come but didn't mind me going with another woman, as she trusted me. The long set was a mixture of old songs like *I'm Eighteen* and *Welcome to My Nightmare* and new ones off his latest album *Trash*. The most entertaining moments were when Alice got decapitated by the Guillotine and when the audience sang along to *Schools Out*, *Department of Youth* and *Under My Wheels*.

The next commercial I got was for Australian car manufacturer Holden. The brief was to film an old farmer helping untangle a young calf trapped in barbed wire and carefully place it in the back of his Ute before driving the vehicle back to his farm. A simple idea but a really emotive one if shot correctly, so we decided it would help the story if we shot it at dawn to capture the early morning light. Unfortunately, on the shoot day the sky was overcast yet again, so our DOP Malcolm McCulloch suggested we try again the following week. Thankfully we had much better weather this time and got what we needed. As we hadn't recorded any sound on the day to save the cost of taking a soundman with us, we added the sound effects and the one line of dialogue the farmer said when he picked up the calf, in post-production. Pretending to be the old farmer, I mumbled 'C'mon little fella' into a microphone and when we played it back the timing was a perfect match to the farmer's mouth movements but my voice sounded too young, so we recorded my voice again but at half speed, which made it sound lower, as well as slower. This was much more convincing and when the client saw the fine cut he had no idea it was me who had said the line and loved it.

As Virginia wasn't into the blues, I asked Fabes if he would like to come with me to see Johnny Copeland at the Corner Hotel in June. The guitarist's genre of music was called Modern Electric Texas Blues and we loved every darn tootin' note, especially on *Cut Off My Right Arm, Wella Baby* and *Learned My Lesson.*

A few days later Virginia and I went on a short holiday to Far North Queensland. We spent the first night at a hotel in Cairns and the following morning drove up to Port Douglas. I hardly recognised Four Mile Beach as it looked so different from when I had first seen it back in 1977. Since then, a businessman called Christopher Skase had opened the luxurious Sheraton, Grand Mirage Resort, right on the beachfront. When we looked at the price of a drink, we nearly fainted so had a quick swim in their pool just so we could say we had been there and then we went in search of a cheaper watering hole in Port Douglas. Over the next two days, we took a boat to Low Isles, a tiny coral cay about 15 km off the coast to do some snorkelling and did a day tour to Cape Tribulation. We were taken by a knowledgeable tour guide called Strikie, who took us on a crocodile spotting cruise on the Daintree River and then to Mossman Gorge where it was croc-free so safe to have a dip in the clear mountain river. On our last day we took a coach to the wonderful Milla Falls and I was glad to see the wonderful waterfall hadn't changed too much since I had first seen them thirteen years earlier.

On the 27th of August Stevie Ray Vaughan was killed in a helicopter crash after a gig in Wisconsin where he and his band Double Trouble had been the support for Eric Clapton. The tragic accident brought back memories of losing my friend and mentor Alastair. It was hard to believe it was already eight years since the crash. I still missed him a lot and hoped he would be proud of what his protégé had achieved since his untimely death.

In September, we went to see Peter Ustinov at the Comedy Theatre. He was a wonderful raconteur and told some hilarious anecdotes in his brilliant one-man show. In the same month, we also saw classical guitarist John Williams and Flamenco guitarist Paco Pena perform with an amazing Andean troupe called Inti Illimani who played a variety of flutes and small stringed instruments called charangos and cuatros. I enjoyed taking Virginia to these events and sharing the experience definitely helped us bond as a couple but I was also aware I was living beyond my means and couldn't afford my current lifestyle unless The Film Business found me some more commercials to direct soon but the advertising industry had gone terribly quiet lately and all I could see in my insecure little mind were dark clouds on the horizon.

When I heard the rousing opening riff to *Thunderstruck* for the first time, I was completely blown away. The first track on AC/DC's new album *The Razors Edge* was sensational. However, *Money Talks* also hit home because I was now down to my last few dollars and with no paid work on the horizon, I was beginning to doubt myself again.

When I got a call from the estate agent who rented my flat in Sydney to let me know my tenants were moving out and therefore it would soon become vacant, I took it as a sign to move back to Sydney. There was no guarantee I would have any more luck finding work there than in Melbourne but I felt I needed to do something proactive and as The Film Business had an office in the heart of Sydney's CBD, they said it made no difference to them where I based myself.

When I told Virginia I was leaving Melbourne, she was understandably upset but after telling her I wanted her to join me as soon as I had some regular income again, she wished me well and we said goodbye. As I packed my car for the long drive ahead, I remembered a quote by the American actor Lionel Stander, often wrongly attributed to Oscar Wilde, which made me smile, 'Anyone who lives within their means suffers from a lack of imagination.'

An hour after leaving Melbourne, I replayed the tearful farewell I'd just had with Virginia in my head and it made me feel so distressed I had to pull over and stop for a few minutes to get my act together.

What if I had made the wrong decision? Maybe I should turn around and go back? I suddenly felt completely directionless and started questioning my motives for moving. I wished my father was still around so I could ask his advice but as this was not an option, I would just have to work it out for myself.

Once I had sufficiently recovered, I put a cassette of *The Good Son* by Nick Cave and the Bad Seeds into my tape deck and continued on my way. *The Weeping Song* was the perfect song to match my miserable mood and when Blixa Bargeld sang The Father's lines to Nick, they made me think about what my own father and what he would have thought of me at this precise moment. Not much I suspected, so I pulled over once more, swapped the tape for the latest AC/DC album, pressed play and then with Brian Johnson asking *Are You Ready*, got back onto the highway hoping to hell I had made the right decision.

Moving back into my apartment in Sydney proved to be a smart decision, as it was somewhere I was familiar with and close to my old friends who all offered their support.

It was at The Film Business office in Sydney where I met a producer called Maury who was American and passionate about music, so we soon became friends. Her favourite band was Aerosmith, who just happened to be in town so we decided to go to the gig together. Maury managed to get us front row seats but there was no chance to use them, as the whole audience stood up the moment the concert began so we did the same and then danced in front of the stage all night like hyperactive teenagers. *Janie's Got a Gun, Sweet Emotion, Dude (Looks Like a Lady)* and *Love in an Elevator* all went down well with the crowd who knew all the words to every song but the best reaction of the night was during *Walk This Way* when everyone in the audience went totally bonkers.

When I next went to see Jim Frazier and Densey Clyne, I discovered they had a couple of rather distinguished guests staying with them. TV Presenter David Attenborough and Mike Gunston from the BBC's Natural History Unit. They had all worked on the series *Life on Earth* and when I arrived, were exchanging some amusing anecdotes about working together. After a quick cuppa, I offered to give David and Mike a lift back to their hotel in Sydney. I longed to ask them a few questions about filming animals in the wild, but they were so busy discussing an upcoming meeting with the ABC Natural History Unit I had no choice but to keep quiet the whole way there. After I had dropped them off, I wondered whether I might be the only 'taxi driver' in the world, albeit a temporary one, to have ever remained silent for the duration of a journey.

In November, I went to see Eric Clapton at the Sydney Entertainment Centre. He started with *Pretending,* a track from his *Journeyman* album, which hit home as 'pretending' was exactly what I had been doing whenever Virginia called to ask if I had found any work yet. I wasn't doing well at all and had had no income for months but I didn't want to sound like a loser, so told her everything was 'fine'. Eric included three of my favourite songs in his set, *I Shot the Sheriff, White Room* and *Can't Find My Way Home* and amongst the rest there was still time for a hattrick of loves, *Bad Love, Old Love* and *Sunshine of Your Love.*

Virginia flew up to Sydney for Christmas and after picking her up from the airport, I told her how things were looking far more positive now workwise and I was hoping to get some TV commercials to direct fairly soon. Quite why I kept up this pretence is hard to say but I think part of me felt ashamed for being unemployed despite there being a recession, which according to our treasurer Paul Keating was 'the recession we had to have'. It was Australia's worst since the Great Depression.

To make sure the weekend was as romantic as possible, I decided not to mention my fears and financial insecurities to Virginia while she was staying with me. On Christmas Day we had a barbie on the roof of Baggers flat with a few of our mutual mates and on Boxing Day my dear friend Robbie invited us for a drink at her fabulous house overlooking Balmoral Beach. We watched the New Year's Eve fireworks from Rich and Marcia's flat directly opposite the Sydney Opera House and on the first day of 1991, Virginia flew back to Melbourne.

I had no paid work in January at all. Being unable to find work in my chosen profession was doing my head in and my intake of alcohol increased significantly during this time, which resulted in me becoming very depressed. My self-worth was at an all-time low equalled only by my lack of energy and feelings of helplessness so I did what I always do when I can't cope with what is going on around me. I went to my safe place. Music.

On the 4th of February, Queen released *Innuendo,* which I thought was their best album in years. I was impressed with the classical guitar contribution on the long title track by Steve Howe of Yes, loved the melancholic *These Are the Days of Our Lives* and was amused by the lyrics on *I'm Going Slightly Mad*: 'This kettle is boiling over. I think I'm a banana tree.' The silly song appealed to me simply because I was going slightly loopy at the time too and it helped me to laugh at myself. However, it was *The Show Must Go On,* which got me off my arse and encouraged me to keep going and face life's challenges head-on.

A little ray of hope came in the last week of February, when The Film Business got me a well-paid commercial to direct for a well-known breakfast cereal in Malaysia, but there was a catch…It couldn't be shot until the end of March as the packaging with the new logo wouldn't be available until then. As the job would mean me having to fly to Kuala Lumpur for the pre-production meeting, I asked my producer Michael if he would mind me flying to the UK first and then attend the meeting in Kuala Lumpur on my way back to Sydney. He assured me it wouldn't be a problem and as the budget would cover my return flights to Malaysia, all I had to do was cover my airfare from KL to and from London. When I rang Virginia to let her know I had finally scored a lucrative job and would be overseas for a few weeks, she wished me good luck and then made me promise to stay in touch by mail.

After staying with my parents for a week, I took a train up to London to see my mate Nicol, as he had scored us a couple of tickets to see the legendary blues guitarist Albert Collins at the Town and Country Club in Kentish Town. 'The Master of the Telecaster' was on in the form of his life especially on *Travellin' South,* a track off his excellent album *Iceman.* I loved Albert's ice-cool sound especially the high sustained notes, which he achieved by playing his guitar through a Quad Reverb Amplifier.

My short and sober holiday in England was over in a heartbeat but it was just what I had needed to get me out of the doldrums and back into a positive frame of mind. By the time I had got to Kuala Lumpur and was being taken to my room at the Hilton Hotel, I was my old self again and ready for work. Now I'm more than happy to slum it when I have to but when a bit of luxury is offered on a plate, courtesy of the client, I will make the most of it, so after taking a hot shower and slipping on a white towelling bathrobe, the only decision I had to make was whether to have beer, wine or spirits from my mini-bar or to abstain until the job was over. I compromised and only had one of each.

In the morning, the pre-production meeting with the advertising agency all went according to plan and in the afternoon the casting session was straightforward as we only needed to cast a couple of Malaysian teenagers who looked healthy and could dance to a pre-recorded music track in front of a blue screen backdrop. Before heading back to the airport, I checked out the studio where we would be filming in April and thankfully it was just what we had hoped it would look like, so I couldn't foresee any problems.

I was only back in Sydney for eight days but this was more than enough time to brief the animators about what had been agreed with the agency at the meeting in KL and then I flew back to Malaysia to do the actual shoot. Sitting next to me in Business Class, was Steve Newman who we had hired to be my DOP, as he was something of an expert filming with blue screens. Unfortunately, when we arrived at the studio, we discovered their manager hadn't bought the chromakey blue paint we had asked him to and required for our filming purposes but had bought two cans of normal household paint instead and although they were both blue, one was Sky blue and the other Navy blue. To our surprise and slight concern, the man had painted the wall with the two different shades side by side so there was a very obvious and distinctive line between the two shades of blue. Instead of having a tantrum, Steve being the professional he is, calmly suggested we film the boy against the Sky blue and the girl against the Navy blue, as we could always 'Fix it in Post', which was an expression creeping more and more common into our industry language when things didn't work out quite as well as they should have done on the shoot. It wasn't an ideal solution but Steve quipped, 'When you only have one option you have yourself a plan!'

To our immense relief, the shoot went reasonably smoothly, so when it was over Steve and I took a drive down the coast to Malacca, or Melaka as it is pronounced and spelt in Malaysia. We meandered through the narrow streets of the old trading port admiring the architecture, which was a mixture of British, Portuguese and Dutch styles from the various times those countries occupied the Peninsula. I particularly liked the brick-red 18th Century Anglican Christ church that was built by the Dutch and the fountain next to it dedicated to Queen Victoria. Steve's favourite place was Jonker Street, the main street in Chinatown where we found a good place to eat as well as presents for our other halves.

When we arrived back in Sydney, Virginia was waiting for me at the airport and her beautiful smile made my heart skip a beat, so I either had arrhythmia or I was in love.

*Wherever you have friends that's your country,*
*and wherever you receive love, that's your home.*

Dalai Lama

## CHAPTER 11: NEVER TEAR US APART

After the Malaysian job was completed, I took Virginia to see INXS at the Sydney Entertainment Centre. The band kicked off proceedings with *Suicide Blonde* and by the time they performed *What You Need* they had the crowd eating out of the palm of their hands. The stand-out track was *Never Tear Us Apart,* which Michael Hutchence sang with such emotion it brought tears to both our eyes and still feeling a bit emotional after the gig, I asked Virginia if she would like to move up to Sydney and live with me. There was an awkward pause and then thankfully she said yes … but only if we rented somewhere bigger, as she felt it would be too claustrophobic living together in my pokey bachelor pad, so the next day I put my flat on the rental list at the local estate agent and started looking for somewhere more suitable.

On the 4th of May 1991, we moved into a two-bedroom apartment in Mosman and a few days later we flew down to Melbourne together to pack Virginia's ancient car to the hilt with all her 'stuff', and then drove back to Sydney the pretty way taking the coastal route via Lakes Entrance, Malacoota, Eden, Merimbula, Batemans Bay, Ulladulla and Kiama.

Our new life together was really good for a while and if there hadn't been a recession at the time, I think it would have got even better but as I hadn't had any paid work for ages, my bank balance started to shrink at the same rate as my self-esteem, which put a lot of stress on our relationship. It wasn't just us feeling the pinch of course. The ongoing recession was making life hard for everyone and unemployment was at an all-time high.

Before we moved in, we had agreed to go halves on the household costs but as I had no regular income, Virginia agreed to pay the lion's share for the first couple of months, and this financial inequality made me feel inadequate and unworthy of her love, so much so I started drinking heavily as well as taking antidepressants.

Although listening to music usually helped me when I was feeling low, nothing seemed to work this time and I spent hours sitting on my own staring into space, which wasn't a good sign but then in mid-June, Lynyrd Skynyrd came to my rescue when they released *Lynyrd Skynyrd 1991*, their first album since the tragic plane crash back in 1977. Five of the surviving members, Gary Rossington and Ed King on guitars, Leon Wilkeson on bass, Billy Powell on piano and Artimus Pyle on drums decided to reform the band and recruited Ronnie Van Zant's younger brother Johnny as their new vocalist. They also brought in Randall Hall on guitar to take over from Allen Collins who had been paralysed in a car crash in 1986 and Kurt Custer on additional drums and percussion. After listening to the album all the way through, I felt the band were really missing Ronnie's unique storytelling skills but there were some good tracks on it nonetheless. The opening track *Smokestack Lightning* was full of energy and when I heard the last track, *End of the Road*, I sincerely hoped it wasn't…for them or me.

The re-incarnation of one of my favourite bands gave me a much-needed boost and although I was drinking more than was healthy for my liver, I began to feel a lot better mentally. The new music helped me connect with something greater than myself and lifted my spirits.

A month later Tom Petty and the Heartbreakers released *Into the Great Wide Open*. Jeff Lynne co-produced the album and wrote eight of the songs including *Learning to Fly* and the brilliant title track. I had just finished listening to the last track on side one, *All or Nothin'*, when I got a call from a recruitment agent in New York who had seen my showreel and thought he could find me some work in America. When I told Virginia my news, she got quite excited and told me the idea of moving to the States rather appealed to her, which was good to know.

The agent rang again the following day to let me know he had spoken to a producer in San Francisco who was interested in talking to me about directing TV commercials for their company. When I asked if he knew who they were he said, 'Have you heard of George Lucas? Well, it's his company. Industrial Light and Magic! You know, the guys who do all the special effects for all the big-budget movies!'

Of course, I knew exactly who ILM were, as they were the company who had been responsible for the visual effects on all the *Star Wars* films as well as many other mega-movies I had seen. Getting a job with them would solve all my financial problems in one go and would get me much closer to my end goal of working in Hollywood, so there was a lot riding on my upcoming trip. After another phone call, it was agreed I would fly to San Francisco in August to have an interview with ILM and they would cover all my travel expenses in advance. It felt too good to be true but the next day a large sum of money was transferred into my bank account, so I bought a Round-the-World ticket, which would allow me to go to the UK after my interview and see my family on the way back.

As Metallica had just released their fifth studio album *Metallica*, I decided this would be the perfect music to get me in a better frame of mind for my trip to America. Every time I hear the opening riff to *Enter Sandman,* I still get pumped up today, but it was *Nothing Else Matters*, which spoke to me and made me feel more positive about fulfilling my dream to eventually work in Hollywood, as I took the lyrics of the power ballad to mean having found what I want to do with my life, I should simply get on with it…as nothing else matters.

When I got off the plane in L.A, my cousins took me back to their home for a couple of days to get over the jetlag and then I took a taxi to Encino to see my friend Mars Lasar, who had worked on *Sounds Like Australia.* Mars had rented a big house, which had once belonged to Johnny Weissmuller, the first actor to ever play Tarzan. Although he originated the famous Tarzan yell, the final version was used in the twelve movies he made, was created by a sound engineer called Douglas Shearer who manipulated Weissmuller's voice and then played it backwards. It felt quite surreal having a dip in Tarzan's swimming pool knowing the famous actor and former Olympic swimmer had also swum in it but obviously much faster.

I flew up to San Francisco the next day and stayed the night with Geof and Jana who I hadn't seen since they moved home to America so there was a lot of catching up to do. In the morning they dropped me off in Mill Valley where my friends Mark and Suzanne, whose wedding I had gone to in the Napa Valley, lived. If Virginia and I did ever move to the San Francisco area, it was good to know we would have a ready-made network of friends.

As soon as I arrived at ILM, I was ushered into an office where I met two men who were very polite and tried to make me feel at ease. They came straight to the point and told me they loved my work and could tell I had the sort of experience they were after, but their problem and therefore mine, was that I hadn't worked on any of George Lucas' big movies, so it was going to be hard for them to promote an unknown director to the local advertising agencies. They hoped I understood their position. I did of course, but wondered why they had gone to the expense of flying me all the way there if they had already decided not to hire me.

One of the three men answered my unspoken question by saying, 'If it doesn't work out this time, it doesn't mean we're not interested in hiring you,' he said trying to let me down gently, 'there may well be other opportunities in the future.'

I felt massively disappointed, as getting a job with ILM would have advanced my career in leaps and bounds and I also thought my relationship with Virginia would blossom once I was able to provide financial security for us.

On the way out of the studio complex, I bumped into an old friend from Sydney who was now working at ILM as an engineer. After asking for permission and making me sign a non-disclosure document, he showed me around their workshops, which was fascinating and I got to see some of the intricate models and props they used on *Star Wars, Empire Strikes Back, Raiders of the Lost Ark* and *Back to the Future*. It was a wonderful experience but all it really did was make me feel frustrated I wasn't going to get the chance to work there now.

On the journey back to Mill Valley, my taxi driver asked if I was going to see Lynyrd Skynyrd the following evening. I had no idea they were on tour, so when I got back to Marks' house, he got out a map and showed me where the gig was being held and as it was only an hour's drive, I decided to go in case I never got the opportunity to see them ever again.

On the 31st of August, I finally got to see Lynyrd Skynyrd at the Shoreline Amphitheatre in Mountain View. They opened their set with *Smokestack Lightning* and then played some of their older songs including *I Know A Little* and *Saturday Night Special* before trying out a couple of new songs on the appreciative crowd. When they played *Call Me The Breeze* and *Sweet Home Alabama* I was grinning from ear to ear but the best was yet to come. Seeing *Freebird* performed live for the very first time is still one of my happiest musical memories of all time and made up for the disappointment of not getting the job with ILM.

When I got to the UK, I hired a car and drove down to the New Forest to stay with my parents for a couple of days. I could tell they were both concerned about my well-being and state of mind but gave me their unconditional love and support as always and told me they believed in me and trusted me to sort out my own problems, which is just what I needed to hear at the time. I then drove up to London to meet my mate Nicol who took me to see Status Quo at Wembley on their *Rock 'til You Drop* tour. The band did exactly as they had promised on their poster, playing thirty-eight songs in a row, twenty-four of them in four different medleys... using only three chords. I'm joking of course. This 'fun fictional fact' was music folklore but I still enjoyed teasing my mate about it at every conceivable opportunity.

Quo would always be Nicol's favourite band but the biggest band in the world in 1991 were Guns N' Roses. On the 17th of September the American hard rock band released two new albums on the same day called *Use Your Illusion 1* and *Use Your Illusion 11*. The first contained an epic ballad written by Axl Rose called *November Rain*, which I loved because of Slash's emotive and extensive guitar solo and the second included *Estranged,* which at over nine minutes in duration might understandably be considered at least five minutes too long but instead was the best track on either album. The artwork on both records was almost identical except for the colour scheme. Estonian-American artist Mark Kostabi used yellow and red for the first and blue and purple for the second. The double-release was a defining moment for the band and ensured their place in rock history forever.

When I arrived back in Sydney, Virginia was at the airport to meet me. Absence had made both our hearts grow fonder and it felt wonderful to be back in each other's arms again. When I told her I didn't get the job with ILM she seemed even more disappointed than I was I hadn't got the job with ILM but this may have been because her dream of living in the States had also gone down the gurgler.

Although Australia was slowly starting to come out of recession, the advertising industry was still deathly quiet, so I rang Michael, the owner The Film Business, to thank him for doing everything he could but felt it was time for me to move on. On the 1st of October B.B. King released *There Is Always One More Time*. The opening track was called *I'm Moving On,* which I thought was rather apt under the circumstances.

Hearing I was back in Australia, Jim Frazier rang to tell me Subaru Australia had just hired him to make a short film featuring him driving his brand new 5-door Subaru Forester to Uluru in the heart of the Northern Territory's arid Red Centre and he wanted me to direct it for him.

Virginia wasn't happy when I told her I was going away again so soon after having just got back but appreciated this was a chance of a lifetime for me.

The journey to Uluru, also known as Ayer's Rock, took us four days and on the way, we found some stunning places to camp where we slept under the stars in our swags. Having Jim's company all the way to the Red Centre was wonderful, as he knew all the names of whatever birds we came across from the Australian ringneck parrot to the Zebra finch and could spot the tiniest of creatures a kilometre away while driving at speed.

When we got to Wilcannia, it was like stepping back in time. It had once been a busy river port transporting wheat and wool along the Darling River via paddle-steamer. At Kinchega National Park we saw an historic old wool shed which had been built in 1875 with river red gums and corrugated iron. Legend has it six million sheep were sheared there... back in the day. I took a photo of Jim in front of the rusty wreck of an old Holden. The scene reminded me of Midnight Oil's thought-provoking song *Beds Are Burning*. The opening lyrics are, 'Out where the river broke. The bloodwood and the desert oak. Holden wrecks and boilin' diesels. Steam in forty-five degrees.'

The Australian Outback covers around 70% of the continent. Uluru is right in the middle.

Seeing the massive sandstone monolith for the first time was breathtaking but seeing it again at sunset when the colour of the rock changes was truly spectacular.

Sleeping in a swag so close to the sacred rock was a real privilege as in those days there were very few other tourists and it felt like we had this special place all to ourselves. Forget about a hotel with 5 stars we were now sleeping out in the open with well over 2000 of them overhead and all for free. It was so quiet there I could almost hear my heartbeat.

Early the next morning, Jim carefully placed a grasshopper on a branch near his camera and then asked me to drive his Subaru between the insect and Uluru in the background. By using his special lens system, Jim was able to get the insect, his car and the monolith all in focus at the same time. An hour later, I was taking photos of Jim walking in the sand dunes when he suddenly spotted a snake trail in the sand, so we followed it and found a black and white bandy-bandy, also known as a hoop snake. It was venomous so I didn't want to get too close but Jim thought we should make the most of this unexpected find so we set up a shot with the bandy-bandy in the foreground, his car with me at the wheel driving through the middle of the frame and some red sand dunes in the background. Everything looked sharp at the same time again thanks to Jim's invention, which would one day make him world-famous.

After the filming was done…and dusted…we headed for a motel in Alice Springs so we could wash all the red dirt off our bodies and clean the camera gear in the comfort of an air-conditioned room. After a long hot shower, we walked to a nearby bar and had a couple of ice-cold beers. On the speakers we heard Yothu Yindi's protest song *Treaty*. Mandawauy Yunupingu had co-written the lyrics with singer-songwriter Paul Kelly to highlight the lack of progress on the treaty between Indigenous Australians and the Australian government.

When we eventually got back to Sydney, I could tell Virginia wasn't happy I had left her on her own yet again, so I took her out for dinner to apologise and then we went to the Sydney Entertainment Centre to see Dire Straits. It was the band's *On Every Street* tour, so they played a few songs off their new album including *Calling Elvis, Planet of New Orleans* and *Fade to Black* as well as old favourites *Romeo and Juliet, Private Investigations* and *Brothers in Arms*.

On the 1st of October B.B. King released an album called *There Is Always One More Time*. The opening track was called *I'm Moving On,* which was apt as I had called Michael, the owner of The Film Business, the day before to thank him for doing everything he could for me and then said I felt it was time for me to move on. He wasn't happy about it and felt I should give them more time but I had made up my mind. I then tried calling a few other production companies but none of them were in a position to take me on as they were all in the same boat.

Virginia suggested I look for alternative ways to make some income but the long-lasting effects of the recession meant there wasn't much else around to even consider. However, as I had taken so many photos on both my overseas and outback adventures, I wondered whether I might be able to make some money from them, so I spent the next few days cataloguing my transparencies and putting them in dust-free sleeves, so at a later date I could show them to my publisher friend and possibly also find a photo library willing to represent me.

Now I no longer had anyone representing me for commercials work and therefore had no office to go to during the day meant I was at home a lot more, so we were now on top of each other more than usual and this made both of us feel a bit claustrophobic. On top of this, I also hated having to depend on my girlfriend's meagre income to cover our living costs as it made me feel guilty and resentful, which gradually grew worse as the weeks wore on. Instead of alcohol and anti-depressants giving me a temporary lift as they had done in the past, this time they just made me feel sad, hopeless and lonely and there is nothing worse than being lonely when you are in a relationship. Virginia continued to love and support me as best she could but my mood swings became so unpredictable and I acted so out of character, she must have wondered who the hell she was living with. The result of too many boilermakers (whiskeys followed by beer chasers) mixed with benzodiazepines had some unfortunate side-effects including slurred speech, confusion and memory loss, which made me appear and act like an unhappy drunk. It didn't take long before I started to spiral into a cocktail of self-doubt and self-loathing and when I looked in the mirror, I no longer recognised myself.

I had lost my identity and was 'seeing' myself as a complete failure, someone who was incompetent and unworthy of love. Not knowing who I was anymore made me feel isolated which added to my mental stress and spilled over into our crumbling relationship.

In the end it was my diaries which came to my rescue. As I skimmed through the last three years of my life, I read comments I had written in my past, which explained how every time I had felt like a failure, I had found a way to keep going until I became successful again. It was a cathartic experience and helped me come to a massive realisation.

Failure was only a feeling not my true identity. The unrecognizable face I had seen in the mirror was a false reflection. Now all I had to do was work out who I really was… and more importantly who I wanted to be.

On the 24th of November, Freddie Mercury died from complications with AIDS. The outpouring of grief around the world was overwhelming. To comfort myself I played Queen songs all day.

*Who Wants To Live Forever* made me cry but it was *I Want To Break Free*, which made me stop in my tracks, as the song is about someone who feels trapped in their relationship, which is how I was feeling, not just because of the shame, guilt and frustration of being unemployed and indebted to my girlfriend but also because of the negative relationship I currently had with myself. I wanted to break free of 'him' too. I also feared life would always be like this unless I gave up my dream of working in Hollywood, which I wasn't prepared to do... at any cost. Sadly, everything came to a head one day and the inevitable collision occurred and I made the self-destructive decision to split up.

It wasn't Virginia's fault in any way, as she had been endlessly patient with me, especially as I had been away for most of the time we were supposed to be living together, but in the end, I felt unworthy of her love and pushed her away. Regrettably, I handled the situation very badly and unintentionally hurt this special woman far more than she ever deserved. I could have blamed it on the recession, which was certainly a contributing factor, or the fact I was drinking too much, or on the medication I was taking but this would have been far too easy. The truth was I had been acting like a total dickhead. I had never felt so worthless in my life.

With the Paul Kelly song (*I've Done all the) Dumb Things* swirling around inside my head, I realised I had some tough decisions to make, as having earned so little over the past year I was now in debt up to my eyeballs, so in the end I felt I had no choice but to sell my apartment and anything else which would raise a few extra dollars. I then bought a one-way ticket to London and vowed not to return to Australia until I had sorted myself out once and for all.

*As you proceed through life, following your own path,*
*birds will shit on you. Don't bother to brush it off.*

Joseph Campbell

## CHAPTER 12: BEFORE YOU ACCUSE ME

As Greta Garbo said in the 1932 Oscar-winning film *Grand Hotel*, 'I want to be alone,' but she never said this in her private life. What she did say was, 'I want to be left alone,' which is a different thing altogether. I often like to be on my own. It's a choice. I don't dislike being with other people, I just prefer my own company sometimes. I don't sit at home feeling lonely and depressed. I read quietly or listen to music loudly. For me, solitude increases my happiness and helps me cope better with stress.

Having temporarily lost my sense of identity, it felt good to be able to define myself by what really mattered to me again and seclusion was now back at the top of my list.

To aid my recovery, I went on a diet to improve my energy level and after making a playlist of uplifting songs from the 60s and 70s I started doing my daily walks again. I included *Hey Bulldog* by The Beatles, *Good Vibrations* by The Beach Boys, *Sunny Afternoon* by The Kinks, *Summer in the City* by The Lovin' Spoonful and added *19th Nervous Breakdown* by The Rolling Stones at the end to make me smile and feel grateful I'd only had one.

It took exactly a month of no alcohol or any other form of medication before my brain had recovered sufficiently to regain the ability to suppress the urge for either. Slowly the feelings of worthlessness, anxiety and depression began to fade and I was ready to take control of my life again.

As I slowly descended the stairs one morning, I heard my mother say 'Come on *son*, make an effort,' so I took a deep breath, forced a smile onto my still-sleepy face, and went into the kitchen, which is when I saw Mum looking out of the window and talking to the *sun*, which was hiding coyly behind some clouds. This time my smile was real and the moment I knew everything was going to be fine.

On the 17th of January 1992, I was offered a ticket by a friend to see Phillipe Genty's puppet show *Forget Me Not (Ne M'Oublie Pas)* at the Queen Elisabeth Hall in London. As the person she was originally going with wasn't able to go with her at the last minute, she said I could have the ticket for free if I didn't mind acting as her 'handbag' and promised me there were 'no strings attached!'

The kind gesture from my friend was just what I needed to get me back into the world of the living and I thoroughly enjoyed the performance. In one of the scenes a female dancer swirled a large piece of cloth while four men in René Magritte bowler hats taunted her. In another, a group of women wearing white dresses danced with men in black-suits wearing bowler hats or were they really puppets? It was hard to tell, because it was actually both. No wonder Genty was considered a genius.

At the end of the month, I moved into a shared flat in Fulham with a guy from Wales called Neil. We got on like a house on fire as we were both into the same music.

One of the positives of living in London is the amount of live music on offer.

On the 29th of February, I went to see Lynyrd Skynyrd at the Hammersmith Odeon. Although they played the same set as the one I had seen in America, this time my seat was close to the stage, so I was able to get a much better view of Gary Rossington's incredible guitar skills. By the time the band played *Free Bird*, I was feeling like a new man and ready, willing and able to look for some work.

I was given the opportunity to do so almost immediately after receiving a phone call from one of the producers at Oxford Scientific Films, to ask if I would be interested in directing a commercial for them, which of course I was. When I got to the OSF studio in Long Hanborough, it felt a bit strange to be back there after so long but as soon as I saw my cameraman friend, Steve Downer, I relaxed and we picked up where we'd left off as though no time had passed since we had last seen other.

The commercial was for a Swedish chocolate called Tarragona and our brief was to film the three main ingredients, chocolate, hazelnuts and milk, as though they were being made individually rather than on a production line in a factory plus a pack shot at the end. We filmed the hazelnuts tumbling down a silver metal shoot and being roasted on a small grill using a smoke machine underneath it. We then shot the milk flowing through a twirly glass tube and splashing into a glass fish bowl, which in slow motion looked quite spectacular. The chocolate shots were a bit harder to get right as the product didn't look very appealing when it was melted down, so we made our own chocolate using a mixture of cocoa powder, virgin olive oil, paint and food colouring. As revolting as it sounds the result looked amazing thanks to Steve's clever and subtle lighting and the hard work of his camera crew.

While I was working for OSF, they put me up at The Bear Hotel in Woodstock. Although I was over my last relationship, I wasn't looking for another but I had to admit it would have been fun to have had some female company while I was there, as my room had a huge four-poster bed, so it felt a bit of a waste not to have anyone to share it with.

In March, I received a call from Simon, who I had worked with in Glasgow, to see how I was and when I heard they were going to see Jethro Tull at the Royal Concert Hall, I decided to fly up to Scotland and go with them. As Tull were on their *Catfish Rising* tour, they played quite a few songs off the new album, including *Rocks on the Road*, which I could resonate with having overcome a few obstacles of my own recently.

Going to live gigs always makes me feel good so when my mate Nicol rang to tell me he had bought us tickets to see Tom Petty & The Heartbreakers at Wembley Arena the following week, I was a very happy camper. *Into the Great Wide Open, I Won't Back Down, Free Fallin', Refugee, American Girl* and *Learning to Fly* were my top six of the twenty-four songs he sang during his long, energetic and impressive set.

In May, I went to see Jethro Tull again but this time it was at the Wembley Conference Centre on their *A Little Light Music* tour. It was very different to their last gig as it was a mostly acoustic set. The highlights were *One White Duck, Nursie* and *Life is a Long Song,* which they had never performed live before, so it was a real treat.

A week later, I had a meeting with a well-known photographic stock images library who looked at a selection of my travel images and told me they could sell my slides to publications for a percentage of whatever I made from them, so I agreed and in my first week I made a hundred quid, so I now had an additional way of earning some money. One morning, I got a call asking me if I had any images of Barcelona, so I told them I hadn't at the moment but could have by the following week if they were interested. They were, so I called my friend David Levin, who was a professional photographer based in Barcelona and after he agreed to help me I booked a cheap flight to the Catalonian city.

After David had picked me up from the airport, we drove into the city to see Antoni Gaudi's La Sagrada Familia so I could take some photos of the church, which is considered to be one of the best examples of Gaudi's unique style. We then went to La Pedrera, also known as Casa Milla, a private residential building with an exterior which looked a bit like a rock quarry, and Casa Batllo, which had balconies made of skulls and supporting pillars made of bones, so I was able to get some really interesting photos of both places. Next on our list was La Rambla where I photographed a large mosaic circle by Joan Miró, which many people walk over the top of every day without realising it is a piece of art. As we got back in the car, David read me a quote by Miró which I liked so I wrote it down.

'I try to apply colours like words that shape poems, like notes that shape music.'

As we drove to the Cap de Creus peninsula, David told me he was currently experimenting with using X-ray film, in the same way as conventional film, but to take landscape photos. They looked quite similar to my own black-and-white photos but his clouds were far darker and much more dramatic than mine, which he had achieved by using a red filter. When we arrived in Cadaqués, we climbed onboard a small wooden boat and took a short trip around the bay so I could get some photos of the charming fishing village. After eating some delicious local seabream for lunch, we drove up to the Salvador Dali House Museum in Portlligat. As soon as I saw the giant egg perched on top of the roof, I knew we had come to the right place. Inside the house there were some impressive paintings and a multitude of rather bizarre objects, which the surreal artist, formerly known as Salvador Domingo Felipe Jacinto Dalí i Domènech, Marquess of Dalí of Púbol, had collected over the years, including a stuffed Polar Bear in the lobby, which had been a gift from his friend, the British poet Edward James. In 1936 Salvador Dali gave a lecture at the International Surrealist Exhibition in London wearing a diving suit, which Edward had bought for him at Siebe Gorman & Co. When the shop assistant asked Dali how deep he was planning to dive he had allegedly replied, 'To the depths of the subconscious!'

My Catalonian adventure was far too short but well worth the effort of going as I sold 15 of my images, which paid for the whole trip with enough left over to buy a ticket to see Crowded House at Wembley Arena on their *4 Seasons in 8 Weeks* tour, which featured both Neil and Tim Finn. They played all their hits, including *Four Seasons in One Day*, *Don't Dream it's Over* and *Weather With You* but the songs I enjoyed the most were the covers of *Sunny Afternoon* by The Kinks and *Throw Your Arms Around Me* by Hunters & Collectors because of the intimate interaction between the band and the crowd.

My passion for going to rock concerts had been well and truly catered for recently and it continued when I got given a free ticket to see Eric Clapton and Elton John at Wembley with Bonnie Raitt as the support act. The American singer and blues guitarist returned to the stage during Eric's set to perform *Before You Accuse Me* with him and Queen guitarist Brian May made a guest appearance with Elton on *The Show Must Go On*. Bonnie and Brian then joined everyone else on stage for the final song. *The Bitch is Back*.

Feeling revived by so much great music, it was now time to find some work and start making some money again so when Ken and

Mary asked me if I would like to direct a children's puppet show for them, I couldn't have been happier. Working with my old friends again was very healing for me, as they treated me like part of their family and gave me a safe platform to demonstrate my artistic skills. The show was called *Paper Capers* and featured a goat called Chuck, a fidgety squirrel called Bridget and Rock'n'Roll Mole. The three puppets sat behind a fallen tree trunk, as though delivering the evening news and broke into a different song for each news item, which had been pre-recorded and rehearsed many times before the shoot. The miniature forest set was raised off the ground and we placed a small monitor underneath it, so the puppeteers could see what they were doing. As they had all previously worked at the Jim Henson Company crew, they were very professional, which made my job very easy and also great fun.

The day after we finished the edit, Mary got a call from a Norwegian advertising agency asking if she knew of a freelance director they could hire, as they needed one for an upcoming commercial for TORO pasta sauce, so much to my delight, she recommended me and 24-hours later I was on a plane to Oslo to attend a pre-production meeting.

After being introduced to everyone in the room, the agency producer told me they had just decided to shoot the spot in the South of France rather than Italy because it would be much cheaper to do it there. Going to Provence with all expenses paid was going to be a tough gig... but someone had to do it.

As I was allowed to choose my own cameraman, I asked Nat Crosby, who I first met in 1973 when I was still at Film School, if he would like to be my DOP. Nat had won three BAFTA awards since I had last been in touch with him, so I thought he might not be interested in working on such a small commercial but after telling him what was involved, he said he would love to do it but just had one question, 'What's the joy factor?' After I told him he would be put up in a swish hotel and fed the best France had to offer for dinner every night, he said, 'Okay, I'm in!'

I flew to the South of France in mid-July to do the location recce with a local fixer called Pierre. The client put me up at the fabulous Hotel Beau Rivage, which was one of the oldest hotels in Nice. While waiting for the lift, the concierge proudly informed me Henri Matisse had once stayed there. After I told him the famous artist had died on the day I was born, he quickly assured me he hadn't died at *their* hotel, which I thought was very drôle.

After seeing an old Provencal farmhouse which had been converted into a restaurant called *Le Mas des* Géraniums in *Opio*, I knew we could shoot most of our commercial there, as the front of the building looked more Italian than French and the view from their garden could easily be mistaken for Tuscany. It also had a kitchen which was big enough for our filming purposes but as we needed a different location for the rear of our mock restaurant in the commercial, we kept looking until we found the perfect spot, which was a restaurant called La Seguinière in La Gaude, under an hour's drive east of Opio.

In the evening, our fixer, Pierre, took me to Bar des Oiseaux in Old Nice because he thought it was the best food in town. He was right. It was superb. They also had a marvellous singer and guitarist who played J.J. Cale songs in French and as there was a spare guitar sitting beside him, I asked if I could get up and jam with him.

'Mais bien sur monsieur. This is why I 'av deux guitars!' He replied, so I then asked if he could play *After Midnight*. 'Apres Minuit? But of course!'

I enjoyed playing lead on this great song and when we had finished the customers all clapped, which was a boost to my ego, as I hadn't played in front of anyone for quite some time so had been a bit nervous. We then played *Call Me The Breeze,* which is one of my favourites but I had never performed it with someone singing the words in French before, 'Appelle moi la brise. Je souffle encore sur la route. Bien, maintenant ils m'appellent la brise. Je souffle encore sur la route.'

At the end of the evening, as everyone was leaving, one of the waitresses asked if I would be kind enough to walk her home. And being a gentleman, I could hardly refuse.

As Nora and I strolled arm in arm down the Quai des États-Unis, I noticed a few other couples walking along the beachfront in a similar fashion. I was just beginning to wonder how much further we were going to have to walk when she suddenly put her arms around me and kissed me passionately on the lips. She then whispered in my ear, 'Je veux faire l'amour avec toi.' Unfortunately, as I didn't have my Berlitz French phrase book to hand, I had to make a wild guess at what she had said but her amorous advances gave me a fair indication. And being a gentleman, I could hardly refuse.

The 'Amour d'un soir', as the French call it, was just what I needed to help me move on from my last relationship and I was still smiling when I got to the casting session the following morning where we got everyone we needed except for the main character, a food critic, who I would cast when I got back to England as the role needed a professional actor with perfect comic timing. The wardrobe check went just as smoothly as the theatre had its own costume department so there were plenty of clothes to choose from.

The shoot began in August. All the cast and crew turned up on time and with some simple but effective set-dressing, Le Mas des Géraniums in Opio became *Ristorante Corleone* in Tuscany. The actor I had cast in London to play the food critic was hilarious and made us all laugh before we had even begun to film, which was a good sign.

On the second day we converted the garden at the location in La Gaude to look as though it could be part of the same Italian restaurant as the previous day with tables and chairs placed under the trees. Sitting at each table were our local extras all dressed in costumes to look like Italians. A middle-aged couple at one, a pretty girl with dark hair at another and a very old man with his beautifully dressed granddaughter sitting near the entrance to the kitchen where two waiters were waiting to come out with food on trays when I shouted 'Action!' The actors weren't the only ones in costume. It was such a hot day Nat had borrowed a white linen napkin, doused it in cold water, and placed it on his bald head to keep it cool underneath his Panama hat. I nicknamed him Lawrence of Arrabbiata.

The client was so happy he invited Nat, Pierre and I to dinner at La Garoupe in Cap D'Antibes. The food was *exceptionnel,* the wine list *extensif* but the cost was *très cher,* so I was glad it was all being paid for by our generous benefactor.

In the morning, I flew back to London to search for more work. It took less than 24 hours.

'It's like this,' Ken told me when I went to their office in Holborn, 'We've been asked to make a 30-second commercial for Scandinavian Airlines but there's a twist.'

'It has to be on air in less than a week.' Mary piped in.

'Is there a script?' I asked.

'Not as such,' Ken said slowly taking a puff of his cigar. He then explained the reason for the rush was that the airline had a new route flying direct from Beijing to Stockholm starting at the end of the following week, so they needed the commercial to be on air as soon as possible in both cities. Our brief was to film several Chinese people, young and old, doing everyday things and when they hear an SAS aircraft flying overhead, they stop what they are doing, look up at the sky and then smile and wave at the plane.

As it was a Friday and Bray Studios had been booked for the following Tuesday, we only had three days to come up with a storyboard, get it approved, hire a cast and crew, build whatever sets we needed and hire the costumes and props. Mary had already booked the well-respected actor Bernard Hill to do the voiceover on Monday morning it was going to be a bit tight but as my claim to fame was I didn't like to plan my spontaneity too far ahead, now was the perfect time to prove it.

My storyboard was approved on Saturday morning and then Mary and I went into Chinatown together at lunchtime to look for potential 'actors' who would be willing to work for us on Tuesday. As Mary already knew one of the restaurant owners quite well having eaten at his establishment quite often, she thought it was the best place to start our quest and it proved to be a really good decision.

Mr Tang told us he normally closed his restaurant on Mondays but if we were willing to pay cash, he would swap days and close on Tuesday instead, so he and his staff could all come and be movie stars for a day. As well as his staff, we also needed to find an old woman, two old men and a group of schoolchildren.

'No problem, Miss Mary. I have a big family. We get everyone you need.' Mr Tang promised and then negotiated another cash deal to get everyone to the studio and back, which involved the hire of a mini-bus with a driver, who also happened to be his nephew.

On Sunday morning I met with a costume designer, a props buyer and a set designer at a café in Soho so we could go through the storyboard together and make lists of everything we would need for the shoot. The wardrobe lady told me when the film industry first started, all the costumes were provided by the actors themselves, so this is what we should do this time, especially as there was so little time. She would talk to each of our cast members and go through their own clothes first but also grab anything she thought might be usable from her usual sources. I thought the props would be much harder to locate but was informed most of them could be bought in Chinatown and what she couldn't hire we could buy. The set design was simple as I had come up with some very cost-effective ideas where every set could be utilised more than once.

The voice-over session with Bernard Hill went like a breeze, as he was such a professional. As soon as it was over, I drove down to Bray to spend the night at a B&B, so I could be at the studio when the cameraman arrived in the morning and reassure him despite having 17 set-ups, we could manage them all in one day as long as we followed my meticulous plan.

Mike Garfath had been the DOP on Mike Hodges' movie *A Prayer For The Dying* starring Bob Hoskins and Alan Bates, so I knew I was in good hands but I needed him to feel he was too, so while the crew unloaded their gear, I went through the storyboard with him and explained what I had in mind. I then suggested he allow me to act as my own camera operator, so he could start lighting the next set-up while I directed the scene he had already lit. My idea was by leap-frogging in this way, we would get everything we needed without having to go into overtime. I could tell Mike wasn't convinced but was willing to give it a go.

The first shot was of a group of young Chinese children dressed in matching school uniforms, standing on a large square of paving stones laid out on the studio floor. On my cue, all they had to do was to look up at me behind the camera, which was mounted on a crane looking directly down at them, and smile and wave at the same time. They got it right the first time but I decided to do three takes, so I had a choice in the edit. For the second set-up, I adjusted the camera position so the lines in the paving stones were at a different angle and then filmed an old man wearing a conical straw hat cooking on a portable stove with a wok. From above his hat and the stove made two circles, which slightly overlapped until I asked the man to look up and smile. We then placed a large tarpaulin over the paving stones and tipped four wheelbarrow loads of earth onto it. The standby props man placed half a dozen cabbages on the ground which from my high vantage point looked as though they were firmly planted in the soil and then three men dressed as farmers pretended to work in the mini-mock-field before looking up at an imaginary plane flying overhead. With the three high-angle shots completed in less than an hour, Mike now started to believe my plan might actually work and gave me an encouraging pat on the back. The next set up was of an old woman holding two baskets full of colourful flowers, and behind her was an old market stall with a couple of straw bags and some additional garlands hanging from it, so it looked like she was in a genuine street market. We then filmed an elderly chef spinning noodles in front of a cauldron of boiling water, and an old man doing calligraphy on a scroll. The rest of the shots were filmed against a chromakey blue screen, so I could add archive images of the Forbidden City and the Great Wall in the online edit.

Much to Mike's amazement, and I suspect a certain amount of

relief, we finished the shoot without going into overtime and judging by the smiles, shaking of hands and laughter of the Chinese 'actors' as they piled into the mini-bus, they had all enjoyed the day too.

As I knew this might be the last time I would get to work with Ken and Mary, saying goodbye to them was hard. They had not only given me my first break as a commercial's director but had also given me other opportunities since then so I owed them both a huge debt of gratitude.

A few days later, I got a call from a friend of a friend of Mike McCartney who had been part of the Liverpool satirical band The Scaffold and was famous for writing two hit singles *Thank U Very Much* and *Lily the Pink*. Mike also happened to be Paul McCartney's younger brother as well as a terrific black and white photographer, so when they were growing up, he was in the perfect position to take photos of the early days of the Beatles. My friend, knowing I had a few contacts in the publishing world, had mentioned this fact to Mike's friend and after a few calls a lunch meeting was arranged in Soho. I liked Mike straight away as he was a lovely man and a great raconteur. I also loved his iconic images so as I had a friend in the publishing world, I offered to introduce Mike to him and eventually a deal was agreed and his wonderful photos were published in a coffee table book called *Remember*. When Mike gave me a first-edition copy of the book, I was flattered to discover he had given me an honorary mention in the foreword.

In late August, Eric Clapton released a live double album called *Unplugged.* The acoustic re-working of Layla was delightful but the cover of Bo Diddley's *Before You Accuse Me* was the track which got into my bloodstream and I spent ages trying to learn how to play the licks. I wished I could afford a Martin 000-42 like Clapton had. I also wished I could play like him... but neither was likely to happen anytime soon.

Mike Oldfield released *Tubular Bells 11* on the last day of the month. I liked it a lot more than the original as it was a reinterpretation rather than a re-mix. It was hard to believe almost 20 years had elapsed since he recorded his landmark album. Another album from 1973, was *Brain Salad Surgery* by Emerson Lake & Palmer. I had first seen ELP at the Isle of Wight Festival in August 1970 so getting the chance to see them again in October 1992 was a magical musical bookend. This time the venue was the Royal Albert Hall and I went with my friend Emma who was a huge fan. It was a memorable gig and Keith Emerson showed off his keyboard wizardry to the max, especially on *Tarkus* and *Lucky Man*. Greg Lake showed he still had a great voice on *Still... You Turn Me On* and Carl Palmer got a chance to show off his incredible drumming skills during the encore on Aaron Copeland's *Fanfare for the Common Man,* which also contained a generous helping of Leonard Bernstein's *America* and Dave Brubeck's *Rondo* thrown in the mix for good measure. My ever-lasting memory of the show is the image of Keith Emerson stabbing his Hammond organ to an early grave with some Nazi knives, allegedly given to him by the legendary Motörhead frontman and bassist Lemmy Kilmister who once said, 'Home is in here (tapping his temple). Where you live is just a geographical preference.'

I couldn't have agreed more, so at the end of October, I decided to fly 'home' to Australia.

*When it comes to luck, you make your own.*

Bruce Springsteen

## CHAPTER 13: MY COUNTRY

The first thing I did when I got back to Sydney was to find out what albums had been released by Australian bands while I had been away. I have never been able to walk out of a record shop without buying at least one album and this time was no exception. I bought *Earth and Sun and Moon* by Midnight Oil, which had some strong tracks on it but the one which meant the most to me was *My Country* purely because of the title. Going through immigration using my Australian passport reminded me of how lucky I was to have dual-nationality allowing me to fly in and out of 'my country' whenever I wanted.

Two days later, I had a meeting with a Canadian producer called Sandy McCauley who offered to represent me in Australia, which I gratefully accepted as I knew she was well respected by all the top advertising agencies and therefore my chance of getting work was much higher than trying to do it on my own. Sandy warned me it might take a while before we got our first gig as Australia was still coming out of recession, so it looked like I was back in the 'hurry up and wait' mode I now knew so well.

At the weekend I moved into a two-bedroom duplex in the leafy suburb of Cremorne. It was a wonderful place to live as every morning I woke up to the sound of laughing kookaburras and melodious magpies. I would then walk to Balmoral Beach to swim in the sea, followed by a coffee at my favourite café, while chatting to the locals about everything and nothing at all. After doing this daily routine for a couple of weeks, I soon got fit and started to get my tan back, which I'd lost while in the UK.

Although I now had some extra income coming in from the sales of my photos, the amounts were quite small and sporadic so when my old mentor Edwin popped in to see me and asked if he could rent my spare room whenever he was in town, I readily agreed as it would help me cover the cost of the rent.

Before leaving the UK, I had transferred all my overseas earnings into my Aussie bank account, so I wasn't too worried about not having any regular income for a while, but just in case I was ever in financial strife again one day, I decided it might be wise to set up an emergency fund. This simple act was enough to help me put aside my past scarcity mindset and make me feel less anxious about having to survive on the smell of an oily rag again, so at the weekend I bought myself a second-hand car.

As I wanted to know how my UK earnings would affect my tax situation in Australia, I rang my accountant only to discover he had died while I had been away. The secretary told me his son had recently taken over the business and would like to continue doing my tax returns as long as I was happy with this arrangement but if so, they would need me to sign a couple of legal documents. When I gave her my new address, the secretary told me she lived in the same suburb, so instead of me having to go to their office, she could bring the documents home with her after work and I could sign them there and then she would then bring the signed copies back to the office in the morning. When I got to her flat, the secretary explained the papers had to be signed in front of a witness who wasn't a member of staff at the accountancy firm, so she had asked her flatmate to do it.

This was the moment when Leah walked into the room... and into my life.

The first thing I noticed was her beautiful smile. She also had a mischievous twinkle in her eyes and a happy-go-lucky personality, which I was immediately attracted to.

Two days later, I asked Leah out on a date. Having messed up my last relationship so badly, I was a bit cynical about the possibility of ever finding love again but, despite being quite a lot younger than me, we hit it off and she agreed to be my girlfriend. We both liked the same kind of music, which was a big plus from my point of view as it was fun having someone to share my passion with. Leah's current favourite album was *Us* by Peter Gabriel but this might simply have been due to the title and how she was feeling about 'us' at the time. The tracks I liked the most were *Come Talk to Me* and *Blood of Eden,* which both featured duets by Gabriel and Sinéad O'Connor who had a unique quality to her voice.

For my birthday, Leah bought me the latest Hunters & Collectors album *Cut*, which had some great original songs on it including *Holy Grail* and *True Tears of Joy,* both written by singer-songwriter Mark Seymour, whose intense voice works perfectly on top of the band's unique sound, a rock-cocktail of guitar, bass and drums with a twist of mini-brass section consisting of trumpet, trombone and French horn.

I also received an illustrated book in the post called *The Tale of Veruschka Babuschka* from my American friend Marcia, which she had kindly dedicated to me on the inside of the cover. We had first met at our mutual friend Veruschka's party when she and her husband Rich were living in Sydney but as the couple now lived on Vashon Island near Seattle, I thought it unlikely I'd ever see them again, which was a pity as I was very fond of them.

As Leah and I wanted to have Christmas Day with our friends, we managed to persuade Larry, the owner of Rosie's, one of our favourite restaurants in Neutral Bay, to cook a lovely turkey dinner with all the trimmings for a dozen of us all sitting at the same table. His wife Rosie and their two children acted as our waiters and then sat down with us to eat, so it felt like one big extended family. After pulling our crackers and donning silly paper hats, Baggers told his obligatory Tommy Cooper joke, 'Two cannibals were eating a clown. One said to the other: 'Does he taste funny to you?' I expect the groans from the rest of us could have been heard on the other side of the harbour.

On New Year's Eve, we went sailing on Sydney Harbour with our Pommy mates Baggers and Colin. When it started to get dark, we moored the yacht near Cremorne Point so a few of our mutual friends could join us onboard to watch the midnight fireworks display along with thousands of other revellers all crammed on and around the harbour. As we watched the impressive pyrotechnics exploding overhead, I realised it wasn't the fireworks but the interspersed black gaps between them which provided the real beauty. However, the simple act of seeing so much light come out of the darkness gave me

456 *My Country*

a new hope for the new year.

My first music gig of 1993 was also the first time WOMADelaide was established as a standalone event. The outdoor music, arts and dance festival was held at the Botanic Park between the 19th-21st of February. Hugh and I had agreed to go together because we both wanted to see WOMAD founder Peter Gabriel, who was going to be the headline act, but we were also keen to see Yothu Yindi. When they came on stage the crowd broke out into spontaneous applause to acknowledge Mandawuy Yunupingu, the Aboriginal band's singer-songwriter and front man as he had recently been crowned Australian of the Year. They were followed by the South African supergroup Mahlathini and the Mahotella Queens who sang in Zulu but we were enjoying the incredible beat so much, the lyrics were a bit lost on us. A wonderful Ugandan singer called Geoffrey Oryema appeared a bit later and we were amazed by his impressive voice ranging from baritone to falsetto.

When Peter Gabriel came on stage, he started his set with *Across the River* followed by *Shakin' the Tree* and then sang a few tracks from his album *Us*. *Steam, Blood of Eden, Solsbury Hill* and *Sledgehammer* all went down well but it was *Biko,* which got the most crowd participation especially after Peter turned his microphone towards the audience and told us, 'The rest is up to you!'. He then left the stage followed by each band member one by one until drummer Manu Katche was left on his own to take 'us' to the end while we all continued to sing the chorus. Being part of a mass choir, all singing in time, if not in tune, was a wonderful moment and made us feel like we were part of one enormous tribe of like-minded souls, connected by the magic of music. At the end of the song the ecstatic crowd gave a huge cheer and as I looked around, I could see quite a few people with tears running down their cheeks. The power of this musical moment still makes me smile at the memory. The band did one encore appropriately called *In Your Eyes.* We came back to the festival the following day to see *Not Drowning, Waving* who had three musicians with them from Papua New Guinea. The powerful percussive crescendo to *Sing Sing* remains one of the most thrilling climaxes to a piece of music I have ever heard.

While I was still in Adelaide, Sandy rang to tell me she had got a commercial for me to direct the following month. I was relieved, as this would allow me to start re-building my film career one brick at a time. Almost literally, as the job was for Lego.

The script featured a ten-year-old Indiana Jones wearing his trademark Fedora and leather jacket, discovering an underground Egyptian Tomb complete with a Tutankhamun mask and gold treasure, all made entirely from pieces of Lego. Les Parrott, our DOP lit the sets to look like scenes from *Raiders of the Lost Ark,* which was impressive considering our limited budget. After the shoot, Les told me he had spent three weeks filming The Beatles in 1970 during the making of their album *Let It Be*, as part of Lindsay-Hogg's film crew.

'I didn't realise it was music history at the time,' he confided, 'it was just a job!'

Over the next two months, Sandy and I worked on a series of commercials for Nature's Way vitamins, working with cameraman Steve 'Dobbo' Dobson, known for his exceptional lighting, and Jim Frazier, known for his innovative special lens system. The quirky style we came up with together was perfect for the client's needs and the shoot was one of the most fun I had ever worked on. After the TVCs had appeared on television, Sandy got a call from another advertising agency who wanted us to make a similar series of 'weird and whacky' Ads for Yates to promote their garden products, so we used the same winning combination of talent and got an equally unorthodox and unconventional look for their commercials too.

Although I'd had plenty of work recently, I decided it might be a good idea to have another skill to fall back on, just in case the industry went through another quiet patch, so I went back to college and took a three-month freelance travel writing and photography course at the Australian School of Journalism, which I thoroughly enjoyed as it was a challenge.

On the 29th of May, I took Leah to see Midnight Oil at the Sydney

Entertainment Centre. Their setlist included *Beds Are Burning, Dreamworld, The Dead Heart* and my current favourite *My Country*.

The following month I received a call from a company called Wildfire who offered me two corporate videos to direct, so I asked Sandy if she would mind me doing them. She had no problem with it at all and told me their timing couldn't have been better as she wanted to take a holiday to see her family in Canada. One of the videos was for a pharmaceutical company and the other for P&O. I asked Steve Newman, who shot the commercial in Kuala Lumpur with me, if he would like to film them and it ended up being a most enjoyable experience. The music was composed by a lovely chap called Paul Smith who became an instant friend because we shared the same passion for music.

In October, I got a call from the Australian current affairs show *60 Minutes* as they wanted to do an interview with Jim Frazier and wanted me to direct a sequence for them using Jim's specialist lens system. The presenter was well-respected journalist Richard Carlton who Jim and I liked straightaway, as he was honest and told us he knew nothing about wildlife filming so wanted our help to make his story work.

Richard told us his story about Jim was going to be called *The Lensman* and his opening words would be, 'Chances are you've never heard of Jim Frazier but in the world of motion pictures, this shy Australian is a star. And he's got an Emmy to prove it. He's a cameraman and director of films that have astounded filmgoers with their casts of angry, spitting and biting characters. Jim makes wildlife pictures and his specialty is filming those creepie crawlies the rest of us run from. He's so expert in the field that he's made his own lenses - lenses so revolutionary that Hollywood wants to buy them.'

As Richard wanted a montage of images which had been shot with Jim's lens system to cover his narration, I gave him a copy of my documentary *Sounds Like Australia* and Jim gave him some archive footage of him receiving his Emmy award, so they could use them in the edit later and then we prepared for our shoot in the studio...or 'double garage' as it was usually called when not filled to the roof with everything from aquariums to zoom lenses with macro capability.

'What we're going to do is put a funnel web up here,' Jim said teasing poor Richard who had unadvisedly admitted he was terrified of spiders, which is why Jim, being the wicked man he was, had decided to film one in the foreground with Richard in the background, so both the funnel web and presenter were in focus at the same time. When the spider suddenly jumped in the foreground, Richard screamed and ran away to the studio's far side, making Jim and I laugh out loud.

The following day, Richard asked me to direct a short sequence utilising the specialist lens system, which would feature him talking to camera while being served a plate of chargrilled octopus and then being poured a glass of chardonnay at Tony Bilson's famous fish restaurant right next to Sydney Harbour. It was great fun and although we did the shoot for free, we were treated to a fabulous seafood lunch afterwards.

Two days later Leah and I went to see John Williams, Paco Pena and Inti Illimani at the Sydney Opera House, which she loved and then we went on to a bar in Kings Cross for a nightcap. In the morning, I felt terribly hungover, which was due to the nightcap turning into an 'all-nighter', so when the phone rang, I didn't feel like getting up to answer it. However, when it rang a third time, I realised whoever was calling was intent on speaking to me, so I dragged myself out of bed, and crawled into the living room. The call was from Sandy to tell me we had just been hired to produce two commercials for Omon, the most creative advertising agency in Sydney at the time.

The TVCs were for Natural Gas and the quirky scripts depicted two famous artists who might not have become famous if it hadn't been for their use of natural gas in their studios. The first spot featured a young Picasso, when he still had hair, pacing up and down in front of one of his more realistic portraits sitting on an easel. Dissatisfied with his artwork he takes the canvas down and puts it into a washing machine to clean off the paint so he can re-use it. While this process is happening, Pablo takes a hot shower. When he re-appears, he opens the washing machine and takes out the canvas frame. But instead of it being completely clean, the hot wash has made the old portrait melt so it now resembles one of the modern portraits the artist became famous for with both eyes on one side of the face. The last shot was of Picasso who looks very happy with the result as he has now found his unique style. The second advert featured a young Salvador Dali in his studio painting a realistic but rather boring clock. After he turns up the gas heating, the clock melts and starts to look like one of his surreal paintings.

Having been to Dali's house a couple of years earlier and studied the surreal artist's life and work in great detail since then, I had a fairly good idea of what I wanted the set to look like but after we hired a very talented art director called Sean, I threw away my amateur scribbles as his designs were far superior and he was able to make the sets of both artist's studios look exactly how they would have done at the time the artists were alive.

After buying every book we could lay our hands on to give us a better idea of what Picasso and Dali looked like when they were aged thirty and hired casting agent Toni Higginbotham to find us our very own Pablo and Salvador. When we did a camera test in costume and full make-up, it was amazing how close the two actors looked to the photos we had of the real artists. Picasso was the hardest to get approved by the client, as most of us remember him when he was old and bald and not with a mop of dark hair as he was when he was younger but Dali was much easier, as with the famous moustache in place, he already looked the part and as the actor had taken the time to study the artist's exaggerated movements from the film clips, we had shown him, it felt like a young Dali was standing right in front of us.

Our DOP Gary Wapshott used Jim Frazier's special lens system to film some ants crawling over a stopwatch in the foreground and Dali working on a painting in the background making sure both were in focus. We did the edit at Animal Logic who were able to make the clock on Dali's studio wall look like it was melting in the same way as one of his famous paintings using computer graphics.

When the client saw what we had been able to achieve he said, 'That's surreal man!' completely unaware of his unintentional pun but the rest of us fell about laughing.

Sandy and I did three more commercials together before Christmas and then I flew back to the UK to attend my mother's 70th birthday party. It was lovely to see my Mum again and I was moved when she told me she thought my father would have been proud of me for not giving up and finally turning things around. I also had time to see some of my old friends at the pub once or twice while I was there. Although I had stayed in touch with them all by mail over the years, I loved catching up with them as a group and talking about old times. Sharing happy memories with my mates not only allowed me to re-experience those moments with them but also reminded me of how far I had come since then.

I got back to Sydney on the 7th of January 1994 and the following day I went down with a nasty fever. Leah nursed me through the night and when I regained full consciousness, she told me I had been talking in my sleep, so I told her about the delirious dream I'd had.

*'I was driving along a gravel road in an old MG, like they had in the 1930s. As I turned the bend, I could see an old stone cottage on the edge of a cliff with the sea glistening in the distance. I was on the west coast of Scotland. It was remote and really beautiful. As I got closer, I noticed there was smoke coming out of the chimney. Someone was at home. As I pulled the car into the driveway, I was greeted enthusiastically by a friendly but rather ancient cocker spaniel. Then the front door opened. Imagine my shock when I was suddenly standing in front of my father. I ran up to him and gave him a huge hug. My father then took me inside and told me this was where he had been 'living' since I had last seen him. I couldn't wait to ask him questions about the war and what it had been like to be a Spitfire pilot. He told me nobody could possibly imagine what hell it is to have enemy gunfire aimed directly at you unless you experience it for yourself. Each day you wake up and wonder if today will be your last, so you have to live for the moment and make the most of every day.*

# 462    *My Country*

*'Not much point in making plans and worrying about the future laddie!' he said with a smile as he headed towards the kitchen, presumably to put the kettle on. I looked around his study and noticed a pair of binoculars and a row of bird identification books on the window sill. The view of the ocean through the window was breathtaking. After a couple of minutes my father still hadn't returned, so I went to find him. But he had vanished into thin air and there was no sign of him or his faithful canine companion. I was completely devastated. No sooner had I found him than he was gone again.'*

Telling Leah about my dream made me feel quite emotional but also gave me a sense of peace, as I now had somewhere 'visual' to go whenever I wanted to connect with my father, or at least my image of him.

On the 24th of February, we went to see Victor Borge at the Sydney Opera House. The Danish comedian had recently turned 85, so I was a bit concerned Leah might find his sense of humour a bit old-fashioned but I needn't have worried, as within minutes the comic genius had the whole audience in stitches and we had tears running down our cheeks. After a few hilarious jokes and playing the piano like a virtuoso, he did his famous phonetic punctuation routine and also did his clever inflationary language sketch where any word which sounded like it had a number in it would now be double its value. For example. A sentence like, 'I *ate* a *ten*derloin with my *fork*' would now be 'I *nine* an *eleven*derloin with my *five*-k. And so on and so *fifth*.' By the end I was in *eighth* heaven and Leah was *three*.

I also took Leah to see Peter Gabriel when he came to Sydney in March on his *Secret World* tour. His setlist was much the same as at WOMADelaide but this time he included *Family Snapshot* and *Shock the Monkey*. When I told Leah I had first seen the ex-Genesis frontman in 1972 she looked at me aghast and said, 'I was only three years old then!'

The following month, I took her to see Jethro Tull at the State Theatre. Seeing them perform *My Sunday Feeling, For a Thousand Mothers* and *So Much Trouble* made me feel like a teenager again but my happy childhood memories were soon quashed when after playing *Too Old to Rock'n'Roll but Too Young to Die,* Leah leant over and whispered in my ear, 'Hey old man, did they write that one for you!'

The reminder of our age difference made me wince. It's hard enough keeping a relationship going at the best of times but when your partner is considerably younger than you, you come to a point when you realise their hopes and dreams for the future might be a bit different to yours...but not wanting to ruin the present I chose not to spoil it by asking.

The next series of commercials I got to direct were for the State Bank and they proved to be quite a challenge but enormous fun to do. The scenarios included an extra-long sausage dog in an extra-long kennel, a tortoise with a second-floor extension on top of its shell and a pair of cockatiels sitting in a small cage, which suddenly became twice the size. The most amusing commercial featured two white mice, one sitting by a miniature swimming pool in a tiny deckchair and the other slipping down a slide into the pool. My modelmaker friend Roger Gillespie made all the miniature sets and Malcolm McCulloch was the DOP and it was mainly due to their exceptional talent the commercials won a Gold Mobius Award as well as a Certificate for Outstanding Creativity at the New York International Advertising Awards as well as finalists at the Montreux Film Festival. As a reward for my part in the awards, I bought *The Division Bell* by Pink Floyd. David Gilmour's fiancée Polly Sampson, who was a novelist, co-wrote some of the songs including *What Do You Want From Me*, which I quite liked but still preferred and missed the clever and thought-provoking lyrics of Roger Waters. Gilmour's guitar solos on *Poles Apart, Marooned, Coming Back to Life* and *High Hopes* were all of the highest order and it was hard to choose my favourite one even after numerous plays.

In April, I had to fly to Darwin in the Northern Territory to do a recce for a British natural history film company called Zebra Films who wanted me to find locations where they could film half a dozen scenarios for a documentary series, they were producing about people who had been in dangerous situations with wild animals but survived the ordeal. The first one was a recreation of how a woman had survived a crocodile attack while paddling her canoe in Kakadu. I took photos of the actual attack spot and then found an almost identical location which had clear fresh water and made sure there were no saltwater crocodiles, so they could safely recreate the canoe tipping scene with a local actress playing the part of the survivor. Finding an actress willing to do this stunt was harder than I thought but luckily for me, a local filmmaker's wife agreed to do it. I also had to find a female stunt driver to *almost* crash a car because she had seen a huge huntsman spider on the inside of the windscreen. Apart from the stunt woman I also found a second-hand car dealer and was able to get permits for the crew to do the stunts from the right authority.

In May, Leah and I went to see B.B. King at the Sydney Entertainment Centre. 'The King of the Blues' seemed to have got even better with age and seeing the twinkle in his eyes, it was obvious the thrill hadn't gone for him quite yet and 'Lucille', the name he gave his semi-hollow Gibson guitar, was still the love of his life.

The next morning, Sandy called me to let me know Nature's Way had liked our previous work for them so much they had come back with another script. This one featured two hummingbirds, which had to hover over two flowers, one on each side of the screen, and dip their long beaks into them at exactly the same time. Roger made the two puppet-hummingbirds about fist-size and then mounted them on hollow metal rods, so the wires which operated the animatronics could be hidden inside them. We would then make the rods 'invisible' at the online stage by painting them out. As hummingbirds beat their wings 10-15 times a second, we had to work out how to film the model birds so they looked as though their wing flaps were realistic. I say 'we' but it was our clever cameraman Steve who calculated the correct frame rate. I wouldn't have had a clue how to do it.

The day after we finished the edit, I got a call from a friend who was now the editor of a brand-new international travel magazine, asking me if I wanted to finally put my diploma in travel writing and photography to use by providing two glossy magazine articles for them. They wanted one about the ancient sites in Java and the other about how Lombok was being hyped as the new Bali. They also needed me to provide some photos for both stories.

'What's the catch?' I asked, knowing my friend wouldn't have come to me first if there wasn't one. I was right to have made the assumption. The catch was there were no actual fees involved but the good news was all my travel expenses would be paid for, so a week later, after doing some intense research on the locations I was about to write about, I was on a plane and on my way to Bali for the third time in my life.

For my first night I was treated to a bit of luxury as I was given a room at the Grand Hyatt in Nusa Dua, which was very swish and everything was brand new. The hotel complex had landscaped tropical gardens, numerous waterfalls and lagoons and even had its own stretch of pristine beach. I suspect it cost a wee bit more than the Losmen I had stayed at in 1977.

In the morning, I caught a flight to Jakarta to connect with another plane which took me to Yogyakarta and then hired a local guide to take me to the 9th Century Brambanan Temple, which is the largest Hindu temple in Indonesia. The locals called it the Temple of the Slender Virgin, which I thought was intriguing so asked my guide if he knew why. He told me the ancient story of Princess Loro Jonggrang who was given to Prince Bandung as a bride after he had defeated her father in battle. However, she would only agree to the wedding if he could build a thousand temples before sunrise, so the Prince called on the help of the spirits. Nine hundred and ninety-nine temples were built overnight but when the spirits saw the first glimpse of dawn, they stopped working. As the Princess didn't want to marry the Prince, she had summoned her supporters to start a huge bonfire to the east of the temples, which fooled the spirits into thinking it was sunrise, so they left early thus saving her from her fate. But when the Prince discovered he had been fooled, he didn't take kindly to her trick and turned her into stone.

Having now got a wonderful story to write about, we then drove to Borobudur, the largest Buddhist monument in the world, completed in 825 AD. From the top the views were spectacular so I took some photos, including one from behind the head of one of the 504 Buddha statues with Mount Merapi in the background. I then flew back to Bali and connected with another flight to Lombok. The mostly Muslim island was known to have some excellent beaches, so I hired a moped and took myself to one called Kuta, which was a bit confusing as it was also the name of the most popular beach in Bali. The Lombok one was much smaller and had course white sand, which crunched underfoot but it was a pretty spot and the sea was crystal clear so I had a quick swim. On the way back to my hotel I saw a dozen women all wearing bamboo hats working in a paddy field, so I stopped to take some photos. As soon as I had my camera out of my bag, a group of schoolchildren surrounded me and told me they wanted me to take their photo as well, so I duly obliged and got some shots I knew the magazine editor would love.

My final location was Senggigi, which was the main hub, or at least would become one when more tourists came to the island in the future. In the evening, I went to a bar for a Sundowner and heard a young Indonesian playing acoustic guitar and performing songs by The Beatles, The Beach Boys and Bob Dylan. As there was a second guitar sitting on a stand right next to him, I pointed at it and he nodded, so I picked it up and started jamming with him. After *Blowin' in the Wind,* he sang *All Along the Watchtower,* so I turned up the volume, channelled my inner Hendrix and did my best to play a solo 'similar' to the one Jimi did on *Electric Ladyland.* Little did the small audience of mainly tourists know they had just witnessed the only performance of *Acoustic Ladyland.*

When I got back to Sydney, Leah picked me up from the airport and on the drive home she told me she had left her job while I was away but she now couldn't afford the rent for her flat, so asked if she could move in with me. Thinking she only meant until she found another job, I agreed straight away but when I asked her what she wanted to do next, meaning what kind of job she would like to find, her answer was not what I was expecting.

What she wanted was to settle down and start a family.

*Uncertainty is the refuge of hope.*

Henri-Frédéric Amiel

## CHAPTER 14: TIME TO MOVE ON

'Why now?' I asked Leah, 'You are still so young, don't you want to have a life of your own first and do all the things you won't have time to do after having a baby?'

'Well, I may be young but you're not.' Ouch! She had me there, 'Well, let's just say you're not getting any younger,' my broody girlfriend added kindly… if a little late.

The truth was, I wasn't sure whether I wanted to be a father. I loved Leah and knew she would make a wonderful mother but something was holding me back. Perhaps it was because I had no idea how to be a father, having lost mine when I was only three. After he died, my siblings, who were a lot older than me, were sent to boarding school during the term, so my mother treated me more like an only child until they came home for the holidays. I would then often stay with friends, so she could do things with my brother and sister without having to compromise what they wanted to do because of having a small child with them. It must have been very hard for my mother to cope with three children on her own without having a regular income to provide for us, so her unenviable situation may well have been one of the reasons I was scared of being unable to provide for my own family… if I ever had one, which because of the unpredictable nature of the film industry seemed a little foolhardy.

I loved working as a freelancer because it gave me flexibility, but the one thing I never really got used to was the constant uncertainty of when the next pay cheque would appear. As a single man it wasn't too much of a problem for me, as I could live hand to mouth until work picked up again or try my luck elsewhere, but as a father with a young family neither of those options would be viable and I would have to stop working in my chosen profession and get a 'proper job'.

Leah wasn't the only person who wanted a baby. Sandy had recently decided she was going to adopt a child from an orphanage in Bolivia, so had asked our mutual friend Annie Hughes to step in to run her company while she was away. As I already knew Annie from my time at Ashenhurst-Hughes, this temporary arrangement suited everyone but unfortunately things didn't work out the way we all hoped and we didn't get any paid work for the next three months at all. Quite why this happened was a mystery as Annie and I made a good team and quoted on some big-budget commercials but unfortunately none of them came to fruition. It looked as though the agencies would only work with me if Sandy was acting as my producer so when she rang one day to let us know she would be away for at least another month, Annie and I had a chat and agreed it was time for us to both move on and look for a source of income elsewhere.

My first port of call was the Department of Social Security to find out if I was entitled to any unemployment benefits, which I hadn't been in the past but after the recession the rules had changed so it was worth finding out what they were. After waiting for an hour to be seen by someone in authority, a rather officious young woman informed me there was a new initiative called Newstart, which had been introduced three years earlier, but there were strict rules to encourage job seekers to look for alternative employment. She then said something, which changed the course of my life dramatically.

'We can't do anything, until you admit you have failed.'

I couldn't believe what I had heard. I already felt embarrassed and ashamed just for being there but to tell me I had to admit I was a failure to her face was a step too far.

I looked into her eyes searching for her soul…but they were empty.

Despite having had some success with my career in the past, even winning a few awards along the way, the long gaps with no income still haunted me and her words struck home, as they were intended to and I went into an instant downward spiral.

I should have sought some professional help again but instead I went to the nearest pub, and by the time I got home, I was drunk as well as depressed. Perhaps I should have just taken a couple of Paracetamol and gone straight to bed but as Leah was still up, I ended up telling her what had happened and how I felt like a complete failure and therefore wasn't fit to be a father. I then made matters worse by telling her I thought we should split up so she could be free to find someone else who was worthy of her love and have a baby with them instead.

What followed was a heart-wrenching scene with both of us crying like babies, although the irony was lost on both of us at the time.

When I eventually sobered up and realised what a terrible mistake I had made, it was too late. Leah moved in with her parents and our relationship was over.

I spent the next few days feeling utterly miserable as I had ruined everything.

I needed to be in my safe place now more than ever and chose *Endangered Species* by Lynyrd Skynyrd to help me get through the pain of the breakup. The album featured unplugged versions of *Saturday Night Special and Sweet Home Alabama*. There was also a cover of the Elvis Presley song *Heartbreak Hotel*, which was ironic as I was currently a guest at the very same establishment.

As walking and listening to music at the same time always makes me feel better, I decided to make a brand-new mix-tape and go for a long walk. My pick-me-up playlist started with *Face the Day* by The Angels followed by *With Or Without You* by U2 and *Nothing to Fear* by Chris Rea, which were all suitably melancholic and then added *Running Up That* Hill (A Deal with God) by Kate Bush, *Don't Give Up* by Peter Gabriel and *Dream On* by Aerosmith to lift my spirits, as those powerful songs had done for me in the past. I then thought some Rock N' Roll with a bit of attitude was in order so added *Start Me Up* by The Rolling Stones, *Rising Sun by* Cold Chisel and *The Jean Genie* by David Bowie to the mix and ended it with *Jigsaw Puzzle Blues* by Fleetwood Mac as it always makes me smile. By the time I got home, I was in a much better frame of mind and although I was still feeling sad, I was now able to start making plans for my future... albeit on my own.

Feeling a bit unsure of what to do next but needing to do *something*, I decided to try my luck using my travel writing and photography skills. After going through all my slides and selecting what I considered were my top ten transparencies and photocopying the articles I had written about Indonesia, I made an appointment to meet the picture editor at Random House, to ask him if his publishing company needed any travel photos for any of their books. By pure coincidence, he was just about to produce a series of high-quality coffee table books and needed some very specific travel images of the USA, UK and France. They wouldn't be able to afford my travel costs but would be willing to pay me a reasonable rate for any of the photographs they published and even if I only managed to get half of them, the money I earned from selling them should be enough cover my travel expenses, so I thought it was worth giving it a go. Quite where this sudden optimism came from, I have no idea but now feeling a sense of hope rather than hopelessness, I sublet my flat to my muso mate Paul for the next six weeks and flew to America.

I arrived in L.A on the 8th of September 1994 and spent the first night with my musical mate Mars, who had just released an album called *The Eleventh Hour*, which was labelled 'music from the future' in one of his many positive reviews. I then flew to San Francisco and stayed with Geof and Jana again for a couple of nights. When I told them I was going to take some photos at the Lambert Bridge Vineyards, a small, family-owned winery located in the heart of Sonoma County's Dry Creek Valley, they asked if they could come with me. The endless rows of vines in the early morning sun made for some great landscape shots and after I had enough exterior shots, we went inside and had a private 'wine-tasting experience' in their cellar room. Geof took a sip of the 1992 Chardonnay, swirled it in his mouth and then after spitting the wine into a bucket gave us his opinion, 'To me it tastes of apple, pear and tropical fruit aromas layered in butter, caramel, vanilla cream, cloves and oak.'

'Wow! That's impressive,' Jana said to Geof, 'How can you tell from just one sip?'

Her husband picked up the bottle and replied, 'I read the blurb on the bottle first!'

On the way back to San Francisco we stopped off in Mill Valley for a quick cuppa with my friends Mark and Suzanne and then drove to Baker Beach so I could take some photos of the Golden Gate Bridge at sunset, which was an unusual pink on this particular night due to the humidity and complimented the orange vermillion of the bridge.

When I got to New York, I caught up with Andy, the agent who had tried to get me a job at ILM a couple of years earlier. While eating the best pastrami on rye sandwich I had ever eaten, he told me it was unlikely I would be offered any work in Hollywood until I had already worked for someone else in America and the best way to make this happen would be to find a smaller film company who were willing to help me apply for an O1 Visa, which would allow me to work in the States for a given period of time and then if one of the big studios wanted to hire me at a later date, they wouldn't have to concern themselves with my visa and this would increase my chances of success. It was great advice and now having a brand-new option to explore gave me plenty to think about.

In the afternoon I took some more photos for the publisher, ticking each famous landmark off my list after I had been to each one. Central Park, SoHo, Times Square, The Empire State Building, Rockefeller Center and the World Trade Center. The view of Manhattan from the observation deck on the 107th floor of the South Tower was quite spectacular. Looking down over the edge to get some photos of the street action below, the pedestrians looked like ants and the yellow cabs like toys. Five minutes later I was back at street level and hailing a 'toy' to take me back to my hotel.

I arrived in the UK on the 17th of September and spent the first few days catching up with my family and friends. Their emotional support was just what I needed and when it was time to leave I felt re-energised and ready to continue my journey.

After taking the train up to London, I spent the morning taking photos of tourist sites like Big Ben, The Palace of Westminster, Tower Bridge and The Tower of London and then flew to Paris in the afternoon where I took photos of the La Tour Eiffel, Notre Dame,

L'Arc Triomphe and Pont Neuf at twilight. It had been a long tiring day but I had now ticked enough photos off my list to cover the expense of my trip.

When I had finished my *petit déjeuner*, I took myself to the Louvre for a much-needed infusion of art and culture. I then popped in to one of the production companies I had been to before on my last trip to Paris to say *Bonjour* to the owner to ask if he had time for a coffee. Unfortunately, he was away on business but his production manager was available and asked me if I would like to have a coffee with her instead.

Marie-Cecile had long dark hair and the kind of smile, which made it impossible for me not to smile back. She spoke English well but with a French accent, which I thought was rather sexy. After talking to her for only a few minutes it was obvious she was well-educated and seemed interested in discussing both art and music. When I felt I had taken up enough of her time I stood up to leave, thanked her for the coffee, and just as we got to the front door of their office, she asked me if I would like to come to her parent's house after work to have a glass of champagne and then go to a TV recording of Cyndi Lauper being interviewed and singing a few of her hit songs. After agreeing a time and making sure I had written down her address and phone number correctly, I then bent down and kissed the back of her hand in the way I had seen done by gallant gentlemen in old-fashioned movies. Thankfully, she took my spontaneous action as a sign of respect, as I had intended it to be and then I went back to my hotel to get ready for a night out.

After drinking a couple of glasses of French champagne on the roof of her parent's house we took a taxi to a TV studio in the centre of Paris. I hadn't taken much notice of Cyndi Lauper when her hits were first on the radio but hearing *Heure Après Heure* and *Vrai Couleurs* being sung in French and with no accompaniment was a completely different kettle of *poisson.* She was... *merveilleuse.*

I had enjoyed Marie-Cecile's company but doubted we would ever see each other again... but I was wrong. Two days after getting back to the UK, she rang me to ask if I would like to spend the weekend in Brussels with her, so I immediately said *Oui,* as I had never been to Belgium before and thought I might be able to get some more photos for Random House while I was there, which would make the trip tax-deductible. Although, I have to admit this wasn't the first thing I'd had on my mind. Even when I landed in Brussels three days later, I still had no idea whether Marie-Cecile just wanted some company with a new friend or had more in mind but when I checked into the Hotel Les Tourelles, I saw she had only booked one room, so my hopes were high.

As Marie-Cecile's flight wasn't due to land for another hour, I had a quick nap. Just as I was dozing off, there was a knock on the door and when I opened it, Marie-Cecile was standing there with an elf-like grin on her face. She kissed me on both cheeks, as they do in France, and then hugged me in the way old friends do when reuniting after a long time apart rather than as potential new lovers, so I responded accordingly and tried not to show my disappointment.

After some chit-chat about both our journeys there, she told me she had booked somewhere unique for dinner, which she thought I would like to see, as La Quincaillerie had once been an ironmongers shop but was now a stunning brasserie and oyster bar. The first thing I noticed was the green metal staircase right in the middle of the restaurant which split in two halfway up to get to the first floor. The place had a great ambience but I couldn't eat most of what was on their menu, as I am allergic to molluscs, so while she ate half a dozen oysters, I ate some white fish in a white wine sauce instead.

When we got back to our hotel, Marie-Cecile told me she wanted a long soak in a bubble bath, so I went in search of an affordable bottle of champagne.

After I returned, I poured two glasses of bubbly and then gently knocked on the bathroom door in amorous anticipation. I then heard her giggle to herself before saying, 'Entrez s'il vous plait!'

We stayed in bed until about 10 am and then ventured out to find somewhere suitable for breakfast. After a short walk we found a cosy brasserie which overlooked the Grand Place and while we ate we talked about what else we had in common apart from both working in the film business. When we discovered we were both fans of Hergé's Adventures of Tintin, we took a taxi to the Hergé Musee just outside the city. The museum was an incredible tribute to the creator of Tintin. As a present Marie-Cecile bought me *Flight 714 to Sydney*, which was the twenty-second volume of the series. This priceless gift opened up a conversation about whether she would like to come to Australia for a holiday and if so, if she would like to stay with me. When she said, '*Pourquoi pas pour Noël?*' I replied, 'Forget about this Noel fella. Why not come for Christmas?' The sound of her giggle made my heart skip a beat.

I flew back to Sydney in mid-October and two days after I got home, I sold a hundred of my photos to Random House, which covered the cost of all my travel expenses easily, making the risk of taking the trip more than worthwhile. As I hadn't bought any albums for a while, I treated myself to Bryan Ferry's *Mamouna*, which was his first record of original material in seven years and I enjoyed his old Roxy Music cohort Brain Eno's subtle but effective contribution to the mix. My personal favourites were *Don't Want to Know, Your Painted Smile* and *The 39 Steps,* which contains the lyrics 'Where do we go from here. I wish I knew.' Me too, I thought as I sent a fax to Marie-Cecile, which is how we agreed to stay in touch because it was so much cheaper than using the phone. Despite the irritating noise of the machine waking me up in the early hours because of the time difference, I looked forward to receiving her handwritten messages. We did call each other from time to time too but kept our calls to a minimum because of the cost. However, hearing her infectious giggle was as essential as it was expensive.

On the 3rd November, I turned 40, and as my old friend Hugh would be turning the same age two days later, we decided to share a birthday party as we had done for our 21st and many other times since. Hugh gave me Tom Petty's new album *Wildflowers*, which had a track on it called *Time to Move On,* which couldn't have been more appropriate.

'What lies ahead, I have no way of knowing but under my feet, baby, grass is growing It's time to move on, time to get going.' It was time to take Mr. Petty's advice.

A week later, Paul Ibbetson, who owned one of the top production companies in Sydney, asked me to come on board as one of his directors. I had all but given up on ever working on TV commercials again, so this unexpected opportunity was a godsend.

The first TV commercials I directed for Ibbetsons were for a brand of Asian cup noodles. The concepts were quirky, so right up my alley. The first featured a very well-dressed customer in a specialised restaurant, which served bicycles... as food. In the script, the waiter served the customer a pedal crank arm as a main course with a side of washers and bolts, which we made out of white chocolate and painted them with edible silver colouring. The two actors did a splendid job and hammed it up perfectly and although the whole thing looked very weird, it worked.

The other commercial featured a man riding a black stallion in the Australian Outback. After a short ride he dismounted and yelled 'Cooeee!' so ear-piercingly loud his horse reared up on two legs, his faithful cattle dog hid behind a log and a couple of cockatoos sitting on a fallen branch squawked and madly flapped their wings. The last shot was of the man sitting by a campfire and eating cup noodles with his dog and horse by his side. We hired Heath Harris, who had been the horse wrangler on *The Irishman*, the movie I had worked on in 1977, as the man with no name and he brought his own horse. The cattle dog was called Kane and was a star in the making, as he had done numerous TV commercials so was already a true pro. The two cockatoos flapped their wings and squawked on command when offered a nut, so getting the animals to do their thing was relatively easy but finding the right location had been a lot harder.

As we couldn't afford to film in the actual Outback, we had to cheat and film the spot in an empty car park on the Northern beaches and place the camera so low on the ground we could only see sand and dirt and not the upmarket houses on the hills in the distance. An Uluru-look-alike-rock was then added into the background during the edit using CGI at Videolab. We had to use their impressive computer skills again after our Asian client had seen the rushes, as the tip of one of Heath's fingers was missing from a past accident at a sawmill, and they didn't like this 'deformity', so we had to replace it by duplicating the perfect finger next to it and then place it over the missing tip frame by frame. It worked so well you couldn't see the join. When we told Heath he wasn't impressed at all and as the client walked away he gave him the finger but which one, I can't remember.

Marie-Cecile arrived in Sydney two days before Christmas. It was lovely to see her and after five minutes it felt as though no time had passed since we had last seen each other. We spent Christmas Day with my Pommy mates and on Boxing Day, we watched the start of the 50th Anniversary of the Sydney to Hobart race from a great vantage point in Mosman. 370 yachts took part, so it was quite a sight.

We flew to Hobart on New Year's Eve and arrived in time to see some of the yachts arrive at Constitution Dock. 'Tasmania' took line honours, which was a bit of a coincidence, but it was 'Raptor', which won the overall title. The fireworks at midnight were spectacular and a great way to start 1995.

The first stop on our mini adventure of Tasmania was at Port Arthur. The former convict settlement had also once been a busy dockyard where prisoners were taught the skills required for shipbuilding, so when they were freed, they could find work in their profession elsewhere. We explored the grounds on our own and I was amazed at how well preserved some of the old buildings were. It was easy to imagine what it must have been like to be imprisoned there in those incredibly tough times. Absolute hell.

When we arrived in Ross it looked like a typical English village…but with sunshine. Ross Bridge was constructed by convicts, so it would have been a crime not to see it, and I was very glad we did as it was breathtakingly beautiful and the craftsmanship was exemplary. We booked a charming cottage called Church Mouse, which was self-contained and had a decent cooker, so after we had unpacked, we went to the local store to buy some food so we could make our dinner. Marie-Cecile bought some champagne and candles to put on the table and we had a very romantic evening. In the morning, we drove our hire car to a place called Honeymoon Bay. The half-moon shaped beach in Freycinet National Park was as pretty as a picture but as it was very windy, we didn't go for a swim and 'got lost in the right direction' instead, as I like to call my sudden spontaneous decisions when driving without any time restraint. I have always enjoyed going left when you are supposed to turn right, just to see what I am missing. Quite often they are the roads less travelled for a very good reason, as there is Sweet FA to see, but sometimes you get lucky and strike gold, or as in this case, nine miles of golden sand near a tiny town called Dolphin Sands. Looking out at the saturated blue ocean, it felt like we had just found one of Tassie's best kept secrets.

The decision to base ourselves at Ross for a few nights proved to be a good one, as it was well placed for each of our chosen expeditions. The Freycinet Peninsula had only taken us about 90 minutes to get to and our next destination, Mt Field National Park, took less than 2 hours. The three-tiered Russell Falls were suitably impressive, although not in full flow as there hadn't been much rain recently. Walking through the rainforest past huge eucalyptus and tall ferns to get to the waterfalls was magical and made us feel very small by comparison, but I have always found it does you a power of good to be humbled by nature from time to time.

Strahan, pronounced Straw-n, is on the west coast of Tasmania. As it was so calm when we arrived, I suggested we go on a cruise down the Gordon River. The tannin in the water allowed for mirror image reflections of the magnificent scenery on either side of the boat and I was able to get some decent photos. We passed through Hell's Gates, the narrow and shallow entrance to Macquarie Harbour. It got its name from some convicts who were imprisoned on nearby Sarah Island, who described it as 'The entrance to hell!'

Thankfully our next destination was the exact opposite and absolute heaven. When we got to Cradle Mountain, we checked into the luxurious Lemonthyme Wilderness Retreat. To get to our log cabin we had to walk under a fern canopy, which felt like we were entering into another Kingdom. The cabin was much larger than I had expected and had some steep wooden steps leading up to the entrance. Sitting on the veranda right next to a huge pile of already chopped wood for our fire, was a Rufous hare-wallaby, which was so tame it allowed us to stroke it. We had been informed at reception there were several pretty bush walks available to explore and as one of them was named Champagne Falls, which was the obvious place for us to go to first. We walked past a myriad of myrtles and mosses and as we got closer to the falls, the noise of it cascading got louder and louder. When we finally reached the spot, we both felt the hike had been well worth the effort. It felt very romantic to kiss each other while listening to the sound of a waterfall.

In the morning we drove to Dove Lake directly beneath Cradle Mountain and it was like walking into a picture postcard. It was more than likely I had taken an almost identical photo to the one many other tourists had taken at the same spot in the past and would continue to take in the future. I found the thought rather reassuring for some reason. Another tourist took a photo of the two of us, which made the romantic and magical moment immortal... or at least for our lifetime.

On the way to Deloraine, we stopped off at Mole Creek to visit the Trowunna Wildlife Sanctuary, as I wanted to see what was being done to save the Tasmanian Devils. Sadly, a horrible facial tumour disease had been killing many of these marvellous marsupials on the island over the last few years, and it was sad to see how the contagious cancer had caused nasty lumps around their mouths making it hard for them to eat. It was truly tragic and I had to take my hat off to the wonderful and compassionate people who were doing their best to try and save them. Tasmania's thylacine, better known as the Tasmanian tiger, became extinct in 1936 so it was vital for the island not to lose another species.

As soon as we were back in Sydney, I had to attend a pre-production meeting for a commercial for Ajax. Geoffrey Simpson, who had recently shot the movie *Little Women,* was our DOP so I couldn't have been in better hands. To make the commercial look stylish, we built a brand-new kitchen in a studio with a raised black and white square tiled floor, so we could film the actress playing the housewife mopping the tiles at ground level while her dog looked on. As the product was supposed to look like a mini-tornado, we decided we would add an animated whirlwind over the live action in post-production. One of the shots called for the tornado to interact with the dog, so what we needed was to get a reaction from it which would make the viewers laugh but not hurt the animal in any way. In the end, we agreed with the animal trainer it would be safe to use an industrial strength fan and swivel it left to right in the same direction as the cartoon tornado would be seen moving once it was animated. When we filmed the shot, the dog's hair stood on end and it looked hilarious. It might have been a little cruel but I am glad to say we got it in one take and everyone, bar the poor dog, was happy.

After saying *Au revoir,* Marie-Cecile flew back to France and we had no idea whether we would ever see each other again. Our holiday romance had been like two ships meeting in the night. I just hoped they weren't the Mary Celeste and the Titanic.

*The future belongs to those who believe in the beauty of their dreams.*

Eleanor Roosevelt

## CHAPTER 15: FOR ALL THE COWS

The first few months of 1995 were a mega-music-fest for me as I got to see so many great artists one after the other. I saw Midnight Oil, Hunters & Collectors and Crowded House on *The Breaking of the Dry* tour in January. Georgia bluesman Tinsley Ellis and Bryan Ferry in February and ELO 2 in March. To top off an already amazing start to the year, I then saw The Rolling Stones at the Sydney Cricket Ground in April. I was interested to see how Darryl Jones, who replaced Bill Wyman on bass after he left the band in 1993, fitted in but I needn't have worried, as he was the perfect choice. And at the end of the month, I saw an amazing double-header with the Doobie Brothers and Foreigner on the same bill.

In between all these wonderful gigs, I directed half a dozen commercials, including a series of six for Sunbeam Selections, who wanted to promote dried fruit as the healthier alternative to sugar-filled sweets. We filmed them all at Narrabeen, a beachside suburb north of Sydney, and the cast included a lifeguard standing at the edge of a seawater pool, a backpacker hiking over some large rocks, a goalkeeper leaning against a goalpost, a cyclist riding on a dirt track, and a skier with a broken arm in a sling, sitting on the veranda of a mock ski lodge covered in fake snow. It was a very enjoyable shoot to work on as Les Parrott was the DOP and we managed to get our favourite crew on board, who we had got to know so well over the years it was a bit like having a family reunion.

Two days after the job was approved, I was on a plane to London sitting in Business Class with a glass of champagne in my hand. I hadn't suddenly won the lottery, but it felt as though I had, as my travel costs were being paid for by Oxford Scientific Films, who had rung me two days earlier to ask me to direct a commercial for them. When a familiar-looking man sat down next to me, I was pleasantly surprised to see it was Tris Miall, the producer who I had worked with at Golden Dolphin and Film Australia. It had been a long time since we had first worked together on *The Mystery of the Full Moon* and *Sounds Like Australia*. My career had experienced a lot of ups and downs since then but Tris had gone from strength to strength and most recently produced one of Australia's most popular movies *Strictly Ballroom* directed by Baz Luhrmann.

As soon as I got to the UK, I went to the OSF office in London to discuss the script with Paddy Carr, their producer, and Steve Downer, the in-house cameraman. The commercial was for Ispat Steel and although it would only be shown in India, it would be screened in cinemas all over the country as well as on national television, so it would be seen by millions of people. Ispat had two integrated steel plants in the state of Maharashtra but instead of flying there to film in the real plants, they wanted us to create a miniature one in the studio. When Paddy showed me a photo which depicted molten metal being poured from a giant ladle in a steel plant for reference, I realised this was going to be a tricky project and it would take all our imagination, intuition and ingenuity to make it work. How on earth could we create a model of a mini steel plant which looked like the real thing in just three days? It seemed impossible... but I have always loved making the impossible possible and was confident Steve and I we would find a solution...eventually.

Before we drove up to Long Hanborough, to brief the crew, I rang Marie-Cecile in Paris to tell her where I was and what I was doing for the next few days. To my delight she told me she was between jobs so would take the next flight to the UK and then hire a car so she could be at The Bear Hotel in Woodstock in time for dinner.

When we arrived at the studio, Simon and Neil, who had worked with Steve many times before, were already there waiting for us. Together, we created a miniature steel plant out of a variety of odds and sods, including a small stainless-steel bucket, which looked uncannily similar to the ladle used for transporting liquid steel in the real factory and a few unidentified bits of plastic, which had once belonged on an Airfix model of the Bismark. After adding a secret ingredient to a gallon of orange juice to give it more viscosity and then filming the liquid being poured in slow motion from one bucket to another, we thought it looked uncannily like molten metal, so this was a promising start. It was all a bit Heath Robinson but this is what boffins do and thankfully do very well.

When I got to The Bear, Marie-Cecile had already checked in, had a bubble bath and was now drinking a glass of chilled champagne and reading her book in our King-size four-poster bed with two Queen-size pillows behind her for support. I had to admire her style. My femme fatale certainly knew how to look after herself royally.

'It's called multi-tasking!' she said with a huge grin on her face. I took a sip of champers from her glass, put her book on the bedside table and then finally got my wish to share a four-poster bed with someone else.

In the morning, I let Marie-Cecile sleep in and drove the short distance back to the OSF studio to begin shooting the commercial. The short journey gave me time to reflect. I would have loved to have had a more serious relationship with this beautiful French woman but she was at a stage in her career where she was just starting to become really successful, having recently made the step-up from production manager to producer, so she wasn't interested in moving to Australia at this moment in time and I wasn't interested in living in France either, so although we both cared for each other, there was little chance of us ever having a future together.

Having resolved the problem of creating a mini steel plant we now needed to work out a way of making it look life-size and soon realised the only way this could be achieved was to have some humans actually in the shot, so after taking some careful measurements of lens distance, tripod height and light direction, we moved the camera to another part of the studio and filmed Simon and Neil, now wearing overalls and hardhats, in front of a black background. We then did the online edit at Framestore, a post-production house in London, and 'placed' our two 'steelworkers' into our mock steel plant. The final composite was surprisingly convincing, so much so the client thought we had filmed everything at a real steel plant in India.

After everything was done and dusted, Marie-Cecile and I headed south to visit my parents. While we were there, I got a call from Australia to tell me my animator friend Peter Luschwitz had suddenly died of a heart attack while playing a game of squash. I was upset and thought about cancelling the rest of my trip to fly back for his funeral but as we were expected at a wedding in the South of France at the weekend and our flights and hotel were non-refundable, in the end I decided to stick to my original plan.

After flying to Nice, Marie-Cecile and I drove a hire car to Monaco to get a taste of the French Riviera and then went across the border to Sanremo to get an idea of what the Italian Riviera had to offer. I wasn't particularly impressed with either and wondered whether a trip to Torbay in Devon, considered the English Riviera, would have been just as much fun. It would have been a lot cheaper.

The wedding was held in the glorious Cathedrale Notre Dame in Grasse. I first met Dianne, the bride, in a jacuzzi in Sydney when I was housesitting in 1989 and we stayed friends ever since. We also had quite a few mutual friends so it was lovely to catch up with them at the reception afterwards. When we got back to Paris, I took Marie-Cecile out to a posh restaurant to celebrate her 30th birthday. Over dinner, we decided it would be fun to go on another mini-adventure together and chose the Loire Valley. There are around 40,000 châteaux in France. 300 in the Loire region alone. We agreed 2 would be enough.

On the way to Château d'Angers we passed some spectacular poppy fields, so stopped by the roadside to take some photos, which I thought the publishing house in Sydney would buy off me when I got back to Sydney. When we arrived at the Château, I was surprised to discover it wasn't a house at all but a 13th-century castle with 17 impressive towers. Inside there was a collection of medieval tapestries, which were remarkable. Château de Chenonceau was much more what I'd had in my mind. It was an amazing piece of architecture and had a series of eye-catching arches which straddled the River Cher and well-groomed gardens screamed photo opportunity from every angle.

After saying *Au revoir* at the airport, we went our own ways once more but as we had formed such a good bond since we'd first met, I knew we would stay friends for the rest of our lives and always keep in touch.

On the flight back to Australia, I thought about all my past relationships and wondered why I hadn't been able to maintain any of them. The brief encounters I'd had in my youth hadn't required any commitment, which had suited both parties at the time. The more serious relationships I'd had since then had nothing to do with feeling comfortable with short-term 'no strings attached' commitments or were sexually convenient in any way, although my nomadic lifestyle had certainly affected the longevity of them. The only times I had really struggled in a relationship had been when I had been anxious about the lack of work and felt I couldn't handle the weight of responsibility, which is why the break ups hurt so much and why I had felt such a failure, especially afterwards when I realised, I may have made the wrong decision. I came to the conclusion my dream of working in Hollywood must have been more important to me than my relationships, and perhaps it was always thus. This unpleasant realisation didn't sit comfortably with me at all and wasn't something I wanted to dwell on too deeply either.

As soon as I got back to Sydney, I rang Peter Luschwitz's widow Bronnie to offer my condolences and ask her if I could be of any help. Peter had been working on an animated TV commercial for Westfield Shopping Centre starring Bugs Bunny just before he died, and as he was the only Australian animator trusted by Warner Brothers to reproduce their characters to the high standard they demanded, there had initially been a problem. However, as my friend had been mentoring a young animator right up to his untimely death, Bronnie had managed to persuade the client to let him finish the animation but wanted me to direct the live-action background plates for her, which I was happy to do.

After the job was approved, I got a letter from my cousin Elmar in California inviting me to a big family reunion in late August. The time seemed to fly by and before I had time to do any other work, I was jetting my way to L.A yet again. It was lovely to see my American family again and to spend some quality time with them. As I remembered one of my younger cousins had loved the grunge band Nirvana, before their singer Kurt Cobain committed suicide, I asked him what new band he was into now.

'The Foo Fighters man... they're fucking awesome!' he replied enthusiastically and then seeing my blank expression said, 'Like, you've heard of Dave Grohl yeah? Nirvana's drummer? Well, it's like his new band and...and... they're fucking awesome!'

'So, you said,' I responded, 'Can you play me the album?'

'Like, for sure man!'

After hearing the whole album played at full volume, I had to agree with my cousin's review. The future of rock and roll was in safe hands. *For All The Cows* took me right back to the time when I smelt like teen spirit and was playing my guitar in our shed at the bottom of the garden next to a field full of Friesian cows. I had come a long way since then.

On my way to the airport the next day, a red sports car drove past us and on the boot, or the trunk as Americans call it, was the funniest bumper sticker I have ever seen.

'I Wanna Be Barbie. That Bitch Has Everything!'

I have always found it fascinating how humour can vary so much around the world. The English seem to be far more self-deprecating than their American cousins, who adamantly refuse to see themselves in a bad light, whereas Aussie humour is much drier and more sarcastic. They often take the piss out of themselves while abusing you at the same time. It's considered a sign of affection. Aussies may not be politically correct and their delivery can be quite crude but they know how to tell a good joke and I was treated to a doozy by the bloke sitting next to me on the flight to Seattle.

'Two men are taking a walk in the outback when they see a dingo sunning itself on a large flat rock. After a while, the dingo sits up, doubles over and starts licking its balls. One of the men sighs and says, 'I wish I could do that.' The other man replies, 'You can give it a go mate, but for Fuck's sake pat him on the head first, he looks bloody fierce to me!''

An hour after landing in Seattle, the city where the Foo Fighters originated from, I was on a ferry heading to Vashon Island to meet my friends Rich and Marcia, whom I had first met in 1982 when they were dressed as Wild Bill Hickok and Calamity Jane at a costume party. When they moved back to America, I thought I might not ever see them again, so I was quite emotional when the time came to step onto the island and into their welcoming embrace. Over a cuppa and some of Marcia's homemade cookies, she told me she was still getting royalties from *Wombat Stew*, her best-selling children's book, which she had written when they were living in Sydney, and Rich was writing original songs, which although would never be top ten hits, were much better than a lot of what was currently passing itself off as music on the radio. It gave me great pleasure to hear him sing his own material, as he had a soothing melodic voice and his guitar picking was exquisite. In the evening we had a jam while watching the sun slowly sink into the ocean.

Magic hour is the period just before sunrise and just after sunset when the sun is not visible but its light is diffused evenly. In the movie industry and photography world, the term is used a lot as it is the best time of day to get the very best light, so when I discovered there was a company called Magichour Films in Seattle, I was keen to meet them.

In the morning, I took a ferry across to the mainland and after a quick call to make sure I would be welcome, I went to the Magichour office and instantly made four new friends. John, Dan, Brett and Jorge.

John was in charge of the business end of the company and Dan was a director like me and also into music, so we got on like a house on fire. Brett was a writer who also loved music and had a wicked sense of humour, and Jorge, pronounced 'Whore-hay' not 'George', as I had incorrectly done after reading his name off the business card, was their in-house cameraman. After seeing their impressive showreel I knew I wanted to work with this exciting, proactive and friendly team and after they saw my showreel, Dan asked me if I could extend my stay in the US and act as their visual effects consultant on a project for the Compaq computer corporation. John quickly added they wouldn't be able to pay me an actual fee, as I wasn't officially allowed to work in the States but I could sleep in his spare room for the duration of the shoot and they would cover all my food and travel expenses while I was working with them. I immediately said yes as it was a 'no brainer', as the Americans like to say.

Dan was very well-prepared, so the shoot went like clockwork. Most of the visual effects were done at the editing stage at a local post-production house called Post Modern. They were more than up to the task and it was a very easy and enjoyable experience. We completed the project on the 3$^{rd}$ of October 1995, which just happened to be the same day Orenthal James Simpson, better known as OJ, was acquitted of two counts of murder, despite the significant forensic evidence against him.

The following week, I was back in Australia directing a commercial for the agriculture company Monsanto. The client wanted my DOP Graham Lind and I to film it in 'a suburban garden in full bloom' but as it would be at least another three weeks before the spring flowers had bloomed naturally, we had to cheat by buying over two hundred cut flowers from three different florists. After hiring a small army of helpers to collect, plant and arrange the flowers to look as natural as possible, the garden, which had been devoid of any life a few hours earlier, now looked good enough to be featured in a glossy magazine. Two weeks later, there were colourful spring flowers everywhere and the jacarandas were also in bloom. Seeing rows of jacaranda trees completely covered in lavender-blue flowers is a spectacular sight, especially when you are fortunate enough to witness their mesmerising purple haze clashing with the red roof tiles behind and between them.

In mid-November, I flew to Thailand for some R&R and then on to Paris to see Marie-Cecile for a couple of days. On our last night together, we discussed how lucky we were to be able to do the kind of work we loved so much and how we wouldn't be able to do it if we had settled down and had a family. Our international love-affair had been like a couple of fireflies living life to the full and as brightly as possible right until their short lives were over. 'We'll always have Paris!' I said to Marie-Cecile trying to impersonate Humphrey Bogart saying his famous line from the movie *Casablanca*.

'And Bruges, Nice, Sydney, Hobart…and Oxford!' she replied with a giggle giving me one last hug before I got into a taxi to take me to the airport.

I then flew to the UK to spend Christmas with my parents and with the money my mother gave me, I bought the CD of *Roots to Branches* by Jethro Tull, which I thought was much more melodic than their previous album. I particularly liked the acoustic guitar into on *Beside Myself* and the melancholic melody of *Another Harry's Bar*.

Before leaving home, I showed my mother my latest showreel, which included a short montage of all the commercials I had directed over the last five years edited to music. Feeling rather pleased with the result, I thought she would be proud of her clever son but instead, she said, 'It's taken you an awfully long time to have so little to show for all your hard work!' I couldn't help but laugh. Mum was quite right and now with my ego firmly put back in its box, I drove up to London to spend New Year's Eve with Mops.

On the 5th of January 1996, I flew back to Seattle to see my friends at Magichour Films who had agreed to apply to the American government on my behalf to get me an O-1 Visa, which would allow me to work in the USA on specific projects if I was able to prove I possessed a '*demonstrated record of extraordinary achievement in the motion picture or television industry and has been recognized nationally and internationally for those achievements.*' To my surprise, my 'achievements' were considered enough to tick all the right boxes and my visa was approved, which meant I could now work with Magichour whenever they needed me. I was finally edging closer to working in Hollywood but before I could turn my dream into a reality, I had to return to Sydney, as according to the many messages on my answer machine, my services were suddenly and unexpectedly in demand.

February was bonkers as I was asked to direct five different commercials in a row. The one I enjoyed doing the most was a rather quirky one for Radio Rentals. The script called for a young man with a 14-inch square television set attached to his neck where his head would normally be and his face had to be seen on the 4:3 aspect screen talking to camera. Our modelmaker Roger custom made a lightweight hollow monitor, so the actor could wear it like an oversized motorbike helmet and then placed a piece of thick cardboard painted chromakey green over the screen area. After lunch, we filmed a close-up of the actor saying his lines to camera against a black background and then all we had to do was combine the two elements in post-production, using the four corners of the cardboard green screen to ensure the image of the man's face fit inside the television set perfectly every time he moved. It looked a bit weird but it worked beautifully.

My housemate Paul and I went to see Robert Plant and Jimmy Page perform at the Sydney Entertainment Centre on their *No Quarter* tour on the 25th of February. The ex-Led Zeppelin members started their set with *Babe, I'm Gonna Leave You* and *Celebration Day* and ended it with *Black Dog* and *Rock and Roll.* It was a magical night from start to finish. The pair of ageing rockers were accompanied by a group of excellent musicians from the Middle East, which gave their songs a new twist, especially on *Kashmir* and *Gallows Pole* but the loudest cheer of the night was when the band did a cover version of The Doors song *Break On Through (to the Other Side).*

My next job began after receiving a call from Australian TV presenter Don Burke, best known as the host of his own horticultural show *Burke's Backyard.* When he asked me if I would direct a 90-minute TV Special for him called *Wild Sex,* I wondered if it was a wind-up by one of my mates, as the date was the 1st of April, but it was a genuine offer.

When I first met Don, it was obvious his knowledge of animal sexual behaviour was on par with my own. In other words, what we both knew would fit on the back of a butterfly wing with room to spare. As far as anything to do with horticulture, Don knew his Dicots from his Monocots and when it came to vegetable patches, he certainly knew his onions, but when it came to natural history facts it was a different matter, so I rang Densey Clyne for her advice, as she had done a number of segments for his show. After she told me she was the one who had recommended me to Don, she suggested I talk to a woman called Karen McGhee, as she was not only considered one of the best natural history researchers around but was also a respected writer. Don wasn't convinced we needed her but let me have my way and the next day Karen and I started working on the script.

It was fascinating to learn about the different ways animals reproduce and the diverse kinds of sexual behaviour they have including, monogamy, polygamy, and promiscuity to name but a few. Karen shared some interesting facts about how mammals, reptiles, amphibians, birds and insects find their mate, about their courtship rituals and what apparatus they had, like the echidna which has a bizarre four-headed penis and a snail which is hermaphroditic, with both male and female genitalia. It soon became apparent whatever we humans like to do behind closed doors, the animal kingdom has been there done that already plus a few extra behaviours which made my eyes water. For instance, there is a male spider which castrates itself mid-coitus, which is not for the fainthearted.

With my brain now full of fun fornicating facts, I was ready to start filming but the night before our first shoot, Don's producer rang to tell me they had decided to postpone the shoot until September. I wasn't too fussed, as Jim Frazier and I had been asked to do another freebie, so I could now concentrate on this instead. The shoot was for the NRMA, an organisation which offered roadside assistance as the AA does in the UK. The script featured an echidna, which had quills about two inches long and very sharp, so we had to wear thick gloves before handling the animal. It was a fun shoot to do and after we had finished Jim asked the client the question, 'What eats, roots, shoots and leaves?' Having heard this joke a dozen times before I kept quiet, and if our client also knew the answer she kindly pretended not to and politely laughed when he said, 'A male koala.' He then turned to me and said, 'Seriously though mate, make sure you include the mating call of the koala in Don's film, as the deep grunting bellow they make can be heard for miles.'

In the evening, I saw Melissa Etheridge at the State Theatre on her *Your Little Secret* tour. She started her set with *An Unusual Kiss* and her intimate interaction with the audience continued throughout the evening right up to *Bring Me Some Water* when she poured a bottle of water over her adoring fans standing at the front of the stage. They lapped it up.

On the 28th of April, 35 people were massacred and 23 others were wounded at the historic site of Port Arthur when lone gunman Martin Bryant deliberately opened fire on them. It was hard to imagine how Australia's worst mass shooting could have happened here, as it had felt so peaceful when Marie-Cecile and I had visited the former prisoner colony on our trip to Tasmania the previous year.

There is no set time to recover after such a distressing event and everyone deals with grief and trauma in different ways. For me, music has always been my refuge but this time the psychological distress of the shocking massacre and the collective disturbance it had on the whole country made me prefer silence, so I went for long walks on my own and tried to re-connect with nature. However, after a week with no music I'd had enough and needed it back in my life, so I bought a ticket to see Jethro Tull at the State Theatre on their *Roots to Branches* tour. Ian Anderson had hurt his leg when the band were in Peru so the poor chap had to perform the entire show sitting in a wheelchair. Despite the obvious pain he was in, he carried on like a trouper and sang *Thick as a Brick* and *Aqualung* as well as two of the tracks off his solo album *Divinities: Twelve Dances with God* called *In the Grip of Stronger Stuff* and *In the Moneylender's Temple,* which both went down well with the audience and received an appropriate sitting ovation.

A few days after the concert, I had to fly to Mount Isa in the Gulf country region of Queensland, as I had been commissioned by an international travel magazine to take some photos of a cattle muster in full swing. This unexpected photography gig allowed me to catch up with Alison, one of my old friends from the New Forest, who had been living in the mining town for quite a few years. Through her, I met Kelly Dixon, an award-winning bush poet, author of *From West of the Scrub* and prestigious songwriter, including one for Slim Dusty called *Leave Him in the Longyard.* Kelly and his wife Marion lived in Camooweal, about a two-hour drive west of Isa and after showing me around the area, he told me where I could get some good shots of some brolgas, if I came back on my own nearer sunset. Watching the birds dance was a thing of rare beauty. As I took some photos of the brolgas, they bowed, bobbed weaved and leapt in the air like ballerinas.

After crossing the border into the Northern Territory early the next day, I parked next to the police station in Avon Downes, as this was where the helicopter pilot had suggested we meet before he flew me out to the Barkly Downs to cover the muster. When a Robinson-22 landed in the nearby field, I saw the pilot take the passenger door off and then ask one of the coppers to look after it for him while we were away, so it didn't get nicked.

'You won't need to shoot through glass now and your pictures will be a million times better I promise you.' The pilot said and then added, 'My name's Larner and I've done loads of musters before so you're in safe hands mate don't worry.' Once we were airborne, I told him I'd been on quite a few chopper flights before. 'Not like this one mate, I can assure you!' He was right. I had never been on such an exhilarating helicopter ride before. One minute we were so close to the cattle I could have lent out and touched one on its back and the next we were so high I could see the curve of the horizon. Taking photos of a dozen men on horseback droving 1600 head of cattle in the dust was one of the most exciting experiences I have ever had. It felt like I had suddenly been transported back in time to witness a group of cowboys herding cattle on their ranch in the Wild West. One of the pilot's jobs is to guide any stragglers towards the herd, so when we dropped down and hovered directly above some cattle standing in a dam, I knew this would be a good opportunity to get some spectacular shots. We were so close to the water the downdraft of the blades made waves, which in turn made the cattle leave the dam and head for dryland.

'Sometimes they get amongst the trees, and you have to get so low you put yourself in danger of getting caught in the branches,' Larner informed me, 'so don't lean out to take piccies until I tell you it's safe, okay mate?' He only had to tell me once.

When the muster was over, we flew back to the station and just before the drovers dis-mounted I persuaded them to line their horses up in a row and throw their hats up in the air at the same time. They all laughed at me but I didn't care, I got a terrific shot of them and as the travel magazine used it as a double spread my remuneration was also double, so I had the last laugh.

*I may not have gone where I intended to go,*
*but I think I have ended up where I intended to be.*

Douglas Adams

## CHAPTER 16: FULL CIRCLE

On the 25th of July 1996, I went to see *The House of Blues* tour at The Gorge Amphitheatre in George, about a half hour's drive from Seattle. First on were The Fabulous Thunderbirds with Kim Wilson on vocals and blues harp. Blues legend Buddy Guy was up next and his unique guitar style was mesmerising to watch and a joy to hear, especially on *Damn Right, I've Got the Blues.* Joe Cocker was the headline act and he sang all his well-known hits but with a blues twist, which made each song sound better for me than ever before.

The reason I was back in America was to help my friends at Magichour Films promote their company by taking their latest showreel to various advertising agencies in Seattle, San Francisco, Vancouver and New York and showing it to the creative teams at each one. I was more than happy to do these 'go sees' for them and as they paid my travel expenses it was more like a holiday than work. By a stroke of serendipity, Lynyrd Skynyrd would be performing on Long Island at the same time I was on the East Coast, so I got two tickets, one for me and one for Andres their representative in Manhattan.

As soon as I arrived in New York, I took a cab to Andres' office and after a quick chat he suggested we go to a nearby bar, so he could tell me about agencies he had lined up for us to see in the afternoon and have a drink at the same time. When a couple of his friends who looked like supermodels waved at him, he beckoned the women to join us at our table. It was fairly obvious they both fancied him, as their eyes hardly left his face for a moment. I hadn't noticed it when I had first met him at his office but now he was flirting with his admirers, I could see why they had such a crush on him. Andres bore a striking resemblance to the Spanish actor Antonio Banderas, whom I had seen in the entertaining Robert Rodriguez movie *Desperado.* When I finally managed to drag him away from his female fan club, we spent the rest of the day showing the Magichour reel to some of the top advertising agencies in the Big Apple.

After a couple of 'after work' drinks, we then made our way by public transport to the outdoor amphitheatre at Jones Beach on Long Island. The Doobie Brothers were on first and got the crowd going with their excellent vocal harmonies and exciting virtuoso guitarists, so by the time Lynyrd Skynyrd came on stage it felt like we were all part of the biggest beach party in the world. After a bit of pushing and shoving we got right to the front of the stage, which allowed me a much better view of the two new guitarists in action. I had seen Hughie Thomasson twenty years earlier with The Outlaws but I had never seen Rickey Medlocke before, so it was great fun to watch them trade sublime licks with each other. Skynyrd started with *Workin' for MCA* and ended with *Sweet Home Alabama* before doing their usual encore *Freebird*, which I thought was the best version I'd ever heard.

When I got back to Seattle, my friends at Magichour were all in high spirits because they had just got a couple of new jobs to do. To celebrate, we went out for dinner and then on to a cocktail bar for a nightcap, which is where I heard *No Code*, the latest album by Pearl Jam, for the first time. It wasn't really my cup of tea except for a song called *Off He Goes* written by their vocalist Eddie Vedder, which tells the story of someone who feels they are a useless friend to those they care about because they are always on the move.

Hearing this rather sad song reminded me to send some postcards before I left the States. It's hard to maintain good friendships over time and distance but despite my nomadic ways, I was pretty good at staying in touch with my mates and I always remembered their birthdays without fail every year.

I got back to Sydney on the 1st of September and started work on *Wild Sex* four days later.

The idea of the 90-minute film was to take the viewer on a journey through the animal reproductive process, finding a mate, courtship, apparatus and 'the act', while unravelling some of the mysteries of the sexual world, including taboos. Our first subject was a spotted hyena, also known as a laughing hyena, which we filmed at Perth Zoo in

Western Australia. The females have functional penises, which they not only pee with but also use to sign, mount males and other females in an act of dominance, and also give birth through. While we were at the Zoo, we also filmed Don talking to camera about a mixture of Australian, Asian and African animals and then flew to Dubbo Zoo in New South Wales to do similar setups there, including getting a shot of the presenter standing in the same enclosure as a tapir from South America.

Filming Toby, as the tapir was called by the zoo staff, proved to be the funniest moment on the entire shoot because just as Don was saying his lines to camera, Toby suddenly got an enormous erection, which was so impressive his prehensile penis looked more like a fifth leg and was actually touching the ground. As Don was completely unaware of what was happening right behind his back, we had to keep ourselves from laughing until he had finished saying his lines. To make matters worse the end of the tapir's willy then suddenly swelled up like a brick, which made the camera crew giggle like naughty schoolboys. When we pointed at Toby's massive member, Don turned around and nearly fell over as he was laughing so much.

When we got back to Sydney, we spent a day filming at Taronga Zoo and another at the Australian Reptile Park in Gosford where we got some footage of two red-bellied black snakes entwined around each other's bodies while they mated and a couple of lizards doing what their keeper described as a 'cloaca kiss', but nothing we saw there came anywhere close to seeing Toby the tapir's turgid tackle in Dubbo!

After playing Don some of my housemate Paul's original music he was suitably impressed and agreed he could compose the music for *Wild Sex*, which he did brilliantly as I knew he would. Once the film was completed and had gone to air on Channel Nine in Australia, I finally had some time to think about what I wanted to do next.

I had been very fortunate over the last few months to earn some decent money while combining my love of film, photography and music with travel at the same time but although I was currently at the top of a circle, I knew only too well how easy it was to be at the bottom again, so decided it was time to have a meeting with my accountant to find out what my financial situation was and make some plans for the future.

Over a tax-deductible business lunch, he told me I had now saved enough to get back on the property market and advised me to buy an investment, so a week later I bought a two-bedroom flat in Mosman and was able to rent it out almost immediately.

Having had an up-and-down relationship with money over the years, it felt very satisfying to finally be in a position to no longer have the kind of financial stress I had experienced in the past. I wasn't rich by any means but at least I was now able to get past the unhealthy scarcity mindset, which had been so damaging to my mental wellbeing.

A week after becoming a landlord, I received an invite from one of the publishing houses who had bought some of my travel photos, to a literary lunch they were having. Their guest speaker was Bill Bryson, author of *Neither Here nor There: Travels in Europe,* so I couldn't wait to go as his book had made me laugh out loud more than once. Hearing him tell the assembled crowd some amusing anecdotes made me laugh again but at least this time I had company. I wished I could be as eloquent as Bill but his way with words was unique. After his hilarious speech, I joined the queue to get an autographed copy of his latest book *Notes From a Small Island* while smartly dressed waiters served drinks and canapes to the guests. When I finally got to meet the author, I asked him if he was going to write a book about Australia. 'Oh yes most definitely,' he replied, 'but I have a couple of others in the pipeline which I have to finish first.'

A lady of considerable fragrance who had been standing behind me in the queue, now tried to elbow her way past me to get to him, and as she did so she said in a rather loud and pompous voice, 'Bill's prolific, you know,' as though it was an intimate secret, which only she was privy to, so unable to resist I quipped, 'Oh, in that case don't let him go near the vol-au-vents, they have cheese in them!' I have no idea whether Bill heard me or not but as I shook his hand and wished him luck with his latest book, I noticed he had a slight smirk on his face, although in retrospect it might have just been a grimace after getting an unwelcome close-up whiff of the over-bearing woman's overly-sweet smelling perfume.

On the 24th of November, Crowded House bid *Farewell to the World* on the forecourt of the Sydney Opera House or to at least 100,000 of their closest friends who made it to the event anyway. As I had already arranged to meet my old friend Steve Twiggs wife Karen and her daughters Julia and Nicola for dinner at The Waterfront, we missed the supporting bands while we were eating but after we had finished our meal, we were able to find a safe spot to stand and watch the rest of the concert. My favourite moment was when Neil Finn's brother Tim joined the band to sing *Weather With You* and *It's Only Natural.* The encore was *Don't Dream It's Over* but sadly, it was for them…at least for now.

I felt blessed to have such good friends all over the world and loved it when any of them visited me in Australia, as well as when I got to see them in their own countries, so when Nikki, my assistant when we were both at Oxford Scientific Films, told me her employer in Botswana had told her she could invite a couple of friends to go on safari with them I leapt at the chance and after a quick stop-over in Johannesburg caught a connecting flight to Maun where Nikki and her partner Dave were there to meet me at the airport.

The first thing I noticed after we disembarked was the powerful smell of wild sage.

Our generous hosts were wildlife filmmaker Tim Liversedge and his wife June who had lived on the southern edge of the Okavango Delta for years. Tim had been a game warden and riverboat captain before becoming a natural history film cameraman and Nikki had recently been editing a film for him about the Marsh lion pride of Botswana.

The Okavango Delta is one of the world's largest inland deltas and unlike other deltas which lead to the ocean this one floods onto open land so its form is ever-changing. As we motored down the delta, I hoped the tiny boat we were in was more stable than it looked, especially after Tim had warned us Nile crocodiles are known to be quite aggressive.

The first wild animals I saw were a female hippopotamus and her calf, or rather their heads, which we could see just above the surface. When Tim told us hippos have incredibly powerful jaws and extremely sharp teeth, which could easily chop us in half in one bite, I decided it might be wise to hold on to the rail in front of me a little tighter.

I was so busy taking photos of a huge Nile crocodile sunning itself on the bank, I nearly missed the action taking place right behind me. An African fish eagle was attacking a white-backed heron. Its squawk sounded like someone screaming. Tim explained it was a territorial dispute. We then spotted a brightly coloured Southern carmine bee-eater, which was stunning but very small, so I was glad that I had brought a decent zoom lens with me.

As the sun got lower, the sky started to turn orange and I took my first African sunset. But there was much better to come. When it finally set, the sun was a luminous bright yellow and the sky was a dark tangerine colour. It was truly magnificent and the following morning was just as spectacular, with the addition of layers of mist on the Delta surface, which was a little eerie but beautiful. As we watched the hippos rise out of the mist, it was hard to imagine just how dangerous they can be.

Flying a Cessna from Maun to the Meremi Game Reserve only took us 45 minutes, but was well worth the cost as when I looked out of the window I could see elephants and giraffes walking below us, so was able to get some snaps of both species. After landing in what felt like the middle of nowhere, one of the local rangers drove us around the reserve in a jeep and while we were being chauffeured in comfort we saw impala, roebuck, zebra, buffalo, baboons and a variety of colourful birds. When we came to a halt to look at a jackal, I leant out of the jeep in an attempt to take a better photo of it and as I did so I heard the ranger say very calmly, 'Ladies and gentlemen, may I suggest you keep all parts of your body inside the vehicle.' I was about to ask why but when I looked behind me, the reason was obvious. A pack of lions were so close to us we could have touched them... or rather worryingly vice versa.

We stayed the night at Okuti Camp right by the Maunachira River, which flows through the Zakanaxa Lagoon. There were seven reed huts along the river bank and we had one each to ourselves, which was very luxurious. After a superb meal by the campfire, our ranger told us what he swore was a 'true' story about a tourist who had a close encounter there one night. The elderly man had walked out of his tent for a pee in the middle of the night and started to urinate on a nearby tree. But was slightly bemused when the now steaming tree started to move away from him mid-pee, so he rushed back to his tent to put on his glasses before investigating what he had just witnessed. When he came back outside, he realised to his horror the tree had been a hippo.

On our next safari we saw some giraffes, a waterbuck, a warthog, a chameleon and a very colourful bird called a lilac-breasted roller but no elephants at all but later in the evening we finally saw a large male attempting to push down a tree, so I took a couple of photos. Nikki then tapped me on my shoulder and said, 'I think you are going to want to see this.' When I turned around, I saw 200 elephants all walking towards us. It was a once-in-a-lifetime experience and one I would never forget.

In the morning, Nikki, Dave and I flew to Zimbabwe for a couple of days to see the famous falls which Dr Livingstone had discovered in 1855 and being a Brit had named after his Queen, or at least this is what I presumed. Before Livingston's discovery of the Victoria Falls, the Kalolo-Lozi people called them Mosi-oa-Tunya, which translates as 'the smoke that thunders.' Unfortunately, the day we went there they more like 'the tap that trickles', mainly due to the exceptionally low amount of rainfall they'd had in the area recently, so we were more than a little disappointed and after taking some photos decided to go back to our rather posh hotel a bit earlier than planned for a drink or three at the bar. The Safari Lodge Hotel, although a little pricey was well worth it, as beneath the back deck was a huge waterhole where we could watch all kinds of wildlife as they came there at dusk for a drink, while we sipped our G&Ts at a safe distance.

After returning to Maun to say thank you to our hosts we flew to Cape Town. Nikki and Dave stayed with some friends and I explored the capital on my own, which gave me the chance to go for long walks and listen to some music again. I spent Christmas Day on my own but on Boxing Day, Nikki, Dave and their friend Andrea picked me up and we drove to Hout Bay, where we took a short cruise to see the huge colony of Cape fur seals on Duiker Island. Seeing so many of them so close was invigorating. We then went for a swim at Llandudno beach, which must be one of the cleanest anywhere in the world. The white sand looked like new and if it hadn't been for the fact the ocean was so cold, we would have happily spent the rest of the day there but instead, we drove to Boulders Beach to take photos of a colony of endangered African penguins who were so used to humans I was able to take some close-up without disturbing them. In the evening, we went to Hemmingway's Nightclub to meet some of Nikki's other friends for a jol, as the South Africans call a party. Some of the men were wearing black dinner jackets and white shirts, making them look remarkably similar to the penguins we had seen earlier.

Still feeling a little hungover, a small group of us drove out to the Chamonix vineyard in Franschhoek the following day to have lunch together. We were served ostrich steaks, which tasted more like venison than chicken, and drank a superb 1995 Cabernet Sauvignon, which tasted intense and rich, which you'd need to be if you bought it by the bottle rather than by the glass. We had a lovely time and got the giggles when Dave tried to pronounce Chamonix and Franschhoek with his broad Scottish accent. Imagine Sean Connery trying to flirt with 'Meesh Munnypinny' after a few bevvies and you'll get the picture.

I flew back to Sydney on the 5th of January 1997, but I was only there for a couple of weeks before flying to Vancouver, as Magichour Films had asked me if I would be willing to base myself there for three months in an attempt to get some more TV commercial work for them, so with no work on the horizon in Sydney I agreed.

When I arrived in Vancouver, I took a taxi to English Bay where the company had rented a small furnished flat for me for the duration of my stay. It was a stone's throw from Stanley Park, which soon became the location for my daily walks, and as it was also close to the ferry, I took one to Granville Island every Saturday morning to explore the food market and treat myself to a peameal bacon bagel with maple mustard. The unsmoked lean bacon had been rolled in cornmeal before being fried, and the mustard was a mixture of stone-ground and yellow mustards with a dash of maple syrup and black pepper. Irresistible!

On the 1st of March my life turned upside down once again when I rang my answer machine in Sydney to see if there were any messages for me and immediately wished I hadn't, as one of them was to let me know my friend and mentor Edwin Scragg was dead.

I sat in my apartment staring at the wall in total shock for what felt like hours. I couldn't believe he was gone. I was also angry at the way his life had ended. Having survived being caught in the middle of one of Australia's worst-ever bushfires while filming the heroics of the firemen, survived leaning out of a helicopter while filming the mangroves below with only me holding his belt to save him from falling, and survived filming inside a giant container as a ton of raw sugar was emptied on top of him just so he could get the best possible shot, it seemed unlikely he would end up losing his life while simply pruning a poinciana tree in his garden. Edwin hadn't seen the power line hidden behind one of the branches he had been trimming, which stretched between the branch and a telephone line, so when his shears touched the wires, he was electrocuted and died instantly.

After I had recovered sufficiently from the shock, I rang his wife Jane to offer my condolences and to let her know that I wouldn't be able to attend the funeral but would be thinking of her and their two girls. After I had put the phone down, I let the tears flow. Edwin had been more like a big brother to me, so it felt like losing part of my family. I would miss him terribly and always be grateful for him teaching me so much over the twenty years we knew each other. Thank you, Scragg.

Edwin's untimely death brought back memories of my friends Alastair and Peter who had also meant so much to me. Losing someone you love hurts like hell but the experiences you shared never die and become treasured memories and remembering those wonderful times is what gets you through the worst until you can move on again.

A few days after receiving the news about Edwin, I flew to Calgary to show the Magichour showreel to an agency there who had a TVC script they wanted a quote on. While I was there, I caught up with my old kindergarten friend Phil who had been living there for quite some time and being the 'outdoorsy' chap he is, loved being so close to the Rockies. In an attempt to cheer me up, Phil took me to see Lake Louise and as it was completely frozen and covered in snow, we were able to walk from one side to the other. He then took me to Banff, which was very attractive and had a mixture of restaurants, gift shops and old hotels. It also had a sweet shop or 'sweet shoppe' as the sign above the doorway read. After buying a mixture of homemade fudge, chocolates and candies, we went back to Calgary by which time there weren't many left.

'Some things never change!' Phil said laughing at me for grabbing the last of the sweets. By pure coincidence *Some Things Never Change* also happened to be the title of Supertramp's tenth album and as Phil was a big fan of the band, he had bought a copy the day it was released. The opening track *It's a Hard World* had some lyrics which made me smile and also gave me a sense of hope. 'Should be some mail for me soon from Hollywood. When the phone rings, could be big things, anytime. Operator is there somethin' wrong with this line.' Although I hadn't been offered any work in Hollywood yet, I felt I was getting a little closer to my quest and it was just a matter of time.

Meanwhile, Jim Frazier's Panavision lens system was about to take Hollywood by storm.

Three days after I got back to Australia, Jim asked me to direct a video for him which showed off its capabilities, as it now had three revolutionary features. It could hold everything in focus from the front of the lens to infinity, had a swivel tip so the lens could move in any direction without moving the camera, and also had a built-in rotator which allowed the image to rotate inside the lens without spinning the camera. The demonstration video was sent wherever the lens went, including to a couple of up-and-coming American directors called Steven Spielberg and James Cameron. I believe they have done quite well since then. We called the video *All The Right Moves* and it helped Jim negotiate a deal with Panavision, the largest lens manufacturer in the world. The rest is movie folklore.

On the 14th of April, I got to meet B.B. King. The King of the Blues was playing at the Hordern Pavilion on his *How Blue Can You Get?* tour. At the end of the show, I went backstage and when I shook B.B. King's hand, he asked me if I played the blues, so I told him I had tried to learn some of his licks but wasn't very good yet and would never be able to play as well as him. He looked me straight in the eye and said, 'Just keep practicing and don't try to play like me. Just be yourself...and don't forget to *feel* the blues.'

I was just about to go for my daily walk when I received a call from the UK to let me know Ken Friswell had died after a short illness. I was very upset as Ken had taught me so much and been such a good friend to me. Losing two of my mentors in such a short space of time really upset me and I needed some time and space to think about them privately, so I went for a long walk and listened to Aerosmith's album *Nine Lives* on my Walkman. The track which resonated with me the most was *Full Circle*, as the lyrics seemed rather appropriate. 'In time. We're all gonna trip away. Don't piss heaven off. We got hell to pay. Come full circle.'

It certainly felt as though my life had come full circle. Not in a negative way where you come back to where you first started and have to begin all over again but in a positive way where you have completed a circle and have earned the right to go to the next level and start another whole new circle rather than have to do another lap of the original. But before I embarked on anything new, I decided to fly to the UK to see my family and friends. My mother was sad to hear about Edwin and Ken's untimely deaths. As she had met them both, she could understand my grief but wouldn't allow me to wallow in it for too long and suggested I go to the pub to catch up with some of my old mates and find out what they had been up to lately. Jerry was now living in Cornwall but back for the weekend to see his family. Nicol had recently become CEO at The British Racing and Sports Car Club (BRSCC), which was the ideal job for him, as he was so passionate about racing. Jon G was working a tax consultant. Mike was travelling all over the country as a salesman in the motorcycle trade, and Vicki was enjoying her new job at an advertising agency in London. I felt blessed to have such loyal friends both here and all over the world. It was like having an extended family.

On the 8th of June Nicol drove me to Wembley Arena in his Ford RS Cosworth to see Jean-Michel Jarre. The French musical genius performed tracks from his two Oxygene albums, Equinoxe, Chronologie and Magnetic Fields and the laser show was incredible. Two days later, I saw Supertramp at the Royal Albert Hall with Emma whom I had last seen at the same venue when we went to see ELP together.

Supertramp started the concert with *It's a Hard World* and also performed *Breakfast in America, Bloody Well Right, School* and *Crime of the Century* but something was missing, or rather someone. Roger Hodgson whose voice was so unique, he was irreplaceable.

While I was in London, I also got to see Steve Winwood at Shepherds Bush Empire with Mops, who had let me use her spare room again. Steve's autobiographical set included *Gimme Some Lovin'* from when he was with The Spencer Davis Band, *Can't Find My Way Home* when he was with Blind Faith and *The Low Spark of High Heeled Boys* when he was with Traffic. The following morning, I popped into a post-production house in Soho called Framestore to say hello to their CEO Sharon, as I had promised to do for my friend Felicity who worked at another post-facility in Sydney. Sharon told me Framestore had recently merged with the Computer Film Company

(CFC) and were now doing a lot of visual effects work on some big-budget movies in both the UK and USA. When she asked me what I had been up to lately, I told her all about the commercials and docos I had directed over the last couple of years and how I now had an O-1 Visa, which allowed me to work in America.

'So, let me get this straight,' she said writing down notes as she spoke, 'you have experience working with animals and visual effects and also have an O-1 visa?'

'Yes, that's right, but the visa only allows me to work on specific projects for the length of the project.' I replied.

'In that case, I think I have the perfect job for you.'

Sharon then told me how Steven Spielberg, Jeffrey Katzenberg and David Geffen had launched DreamWorks SKG in 1994 and Framestore-CFC had just been hired to work on one of their movies called *Paulie*, which featured a talking parrot who recounts his travels, searching for the little girl, who was his original owner, to a Russian janitor who tries to help him find her. The director was a young man called John Roberts and his DOP was Tony Pierce-Roberts, who had shot the Merchant Ivory films *Room With a View* and *Howards End,* which had both been nominated for an Academy Award. The cast included Tony Shalhoub, Gena Rowlands, Cheech Marin, Buddy Hackett and Jay Mohr, who was also supplying the voice of Paulie. But they had one major problem… the parrot.

DreamWorks had hired the same team who had created the brilliant animatronic dinosaurs for *Jurassic Park* to make a robotic parrot but unfortunately it looked …like a robotic parrot. After the second week of the shoot, an executive decision had been made to ditch the animatronic version, as it looked unconvincing, and only use real parrots, which were being trained by Boone's Animals for Hollywood. Boone Narr was one of the most well-renowned animal trainers and wranglers in the movie business, so if anyone was going to get the parrots to 'act' it would be him and his dedicated team.

The original plan had been to program Jay's voice into the robotic parrot so it would say its lines correctly every time it was filmed but as this was no longer an option, Framestore-CFC had devised a clever way of replacing the real beak of the parrot with a computer generated one, so Jay's voice could still be used and the beak would speak in perfect sync, so the reason they wanted to hire me to be their visual effects set supervisor was to ensure the correct elements were shot for every single take. As there would now be approximately 300 shots, which required 'beak-replacement' or some other visual effect, it was now going to be a much bigger job than they had originally thought.

Before leaving Sharon's office, I signed a contract and was given the address of the serviced apartment they had rented for me in West Hollywood, which had its own gym and swimming pool, and I was also given the number of a young man who would drive me to the set every morning and bring me back to my accommodation every night.

After my meeting was over, I rang my Mum to tell her the news and she told me how proud she was of me for never giving up, especially after all the ups and downs in my erratic career, 'It's all down to your resilience and perseverance, so well done darling!'

'And a good deal of luck too Mum,' I said truthfully.

'You've made your own luck. Now go and enjoy the rewards,' My mother replied and then added, 'and don't forget to write!'

Four hours later I was on a Jumbo on my way to L.A. While sitting in business class and drinking a glass of champagne, I couldn't stop smiling. After all the hard work I had done over the years and the personal sacrifices I had made, my dream of working in Hollywood was finally about to come true.

A couple of hours into the flight, I needed a pee and when I was inside the tiny toilet cubicle, I saw the crow's feet around my eyes in the reflection of the mirror. It was hardly surprising I had so many wrinkles considering all the stress and anxiety I had experienced when work had been thin on the ground, from the grief of losing so many friends and mentors as well as fighting the odd bout of depression. But I knew they were also caused by laughter as I'd had a great deal of fun along the way, which reminded me of what my youngest niece had said to me the last time I saw her. Pointing at the corners of my eyes, she asked, 'What are all those lines on your face?'

'They're called laughter lines,' I replied, but I could tell by the look on my niece's face she wasn't completely satisfied and after a lengthy pause decided to ask another question, 'You do have an awful lot of them Uncle Jamie ... What was so funny?'

## THE END

*Life is like a jigsaw puzzle, you have to see the whole picture,*
*then put it together piece by piece!*

Terry McMillan


## CODA
(An Italian musical term that means 'conclusion of a dramatic work'.)


Looking back and re-living my musical memories side by side with my rollercoaster film career and numerous travel adventures, while making many wonderful friends along the way, has been a cathartic experience and helped me solve the complicated jigsaw puzzle of my life. Writing my story has also helped me put everything into context and allowed me to measure my worth by who I am not what I have. I don't need to have fame or fortune to feel successful. For me, travelling the world, experiencing other people's cultures and values, while indulging in my passion for music, has been more than 'enough'.

Once I was in Hollywood, I realised the process I'd put myself through of evolving, learning new skills and seeing life through a different lens had brought its own rewards. Now I was on a movie set surrounded by a huge crew in L.A I could finally see the big picture.

The irony was not lost on me.

If this book can act as a guide, or a tool, to help just one other person navigate their journey through life, or inspire someone to take responsibility for their own actions, or become more resilient and decide not to give up when the going gets tough, or be curious rather than judgemental of others, then it will have been worth sharing my hopes, fears and dreams in print.

I found it incredibly hard to write about the relentless verbal and physical abuse I experienced as a schoolboy and the periods of self-doubt and depression I suffered when I was older, but forcing myself to go through it all again has helped me have a better understanding of where each of the jigsaw pieces fit and why they still mean something to me today.

Losing my father when I was three had profound consequences on my life and was probably the key reason for my occasional bouts of melancholia but by witnessing my mother listen to sad music to comfort her through her grief I was also given the antidote, albeit only in my subconscious, and as a result music became my safe place and has been ever-present ever since, providing solace when I was bullied at boarding school and immense joy when I was backpacking around the globe having the time of my life.

Working as a freelancer meant I was my own boss, so after each successful job I rewarded my staff (me!) with a new album as a pat on the back, which created another positive connection to music and contributed to my well-being. When I finally realised my dream, it felt like I had come full circle - from a boy full of self-doubt and pessimism to a man brimming with self-confidence, optimism and hope.

On each of my adventures, I discovered qualities I never knew I had. Resilience and perseverance are at the top of the list but it was my self-deprecating humour, which had always come to the rescue in awkward social situations. Making fun of myself was also good for my mental health as it reduced my anxiety levels immediately and still does to this day. My best trait is the willingness to make mistakes. My ability to make them was never in question! I have gained far more from my failures than I have from my successes, which has not only made me more patient with myself but also with others, and certainly less quick to judge. Making mistakes is inevitable. The trick is to learn from them as quickly as you can.

When I did finally get to work in Hollywood it was 1997, the same year Duran Duran released *Electric Barbarella* on the internet, making it the first-ever digital single to be sold in this way. I bought my first mobile phone a year later, a Nokia 5110, but didn't get my first computer, an iMac, until 1999. Life changed for us all once we started using this technology, but not necessarily for the better.

Perhaps this is why music is so important to us. It doesn't matter what else changes, hearing the songs we loved when we were younger allows us to travel back in time to when we first heard them and re-live those special moments.

After taking a trip down memory lane and listening to the soundtrack to my life as I wrote this auto-audio-biography, *Free Bird* by Lynyrd Skynyrd remains my favourite song but the B-side, as it was in 1968 when it was the flip side of *Albatross* by Fleetwood Mac, is the uplifting *Jigsaw Puzzle Blues* written by Danny Kirwan.

I must also give a special mention to *The End*, the last song recorded by the Beatles during the recording of *Abbey Road*. I have always loved Ringo's drum solo and the way John, Paul and George took turns doing their guitar solos and traded riffs. The Fab Four inspired millions of young people like me to find light in moments of darkness through music and for this alone, they have my eternal gratitude.

My obsession with music continues to this day. I have been lucky enough to see many of my favourite rock bands perform live again including AC/DC, Lynyrd Skynyrd, Jethro Tull and The Rolling Stones, as well as blues legends John Mayall, Peter Green, Buddy Guy and Joe Bonamassa and prog rock bands such as The Flower Kings, Spock's Beard and Transatlantic.

I still love listening to new music and discovering new talent. The two bands who excite me the most today are Måneskin from Italy and The Warning from Mexico. These young and talented musicians make me want to turn up the volume, jump up and down in the air, make the sign of the devil's horns and scream 'Hell Yeah!', so Grazie and Gracias for making me feel twenty-one again!

Over my long career, I have been lucky enough to travel all over the world and work with some truly talented people from completely different backgrounds and a diverse range of cultures, many of whom have become lifelong friends who share my insatiable passion for music and appreciate its importance to our health and wellbeing. One of them once said to me, 'You may not be a millionaire Jamie, but you are rich in friends.' That'll do me.

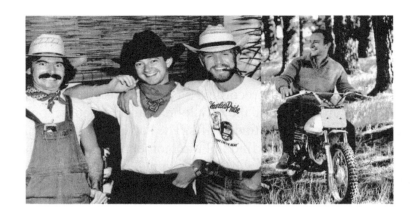

Jamie '*Boomerang*' Robertson

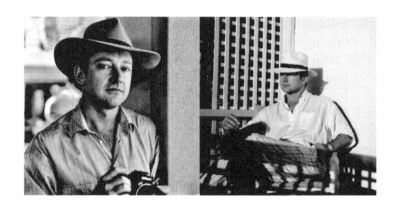

# A-Z LIST OF CONCERTS (1970-2024)

\#      10cc READING FESTIVAL 1974

**A**

AMERICA THE OVAL CRICKET GROUND LONDON 1971
ATOMIC ROOSTER THE OVAL CRICKET GROUND LONDON 1971
+ BOURNEMOUTH 1972
ANGE READING FESTIVAL 1973 + LONDON 1976
ABBA ADELAIDE 1977
AIR SUPPLY ADELAIDE 1977
AC/DC LONDON 1980 + SYDNEY 2010
AVERAGE WHITE BAND LONDON 1980
THE ANGELS SYDNEY 1982
AUSTRALIAN CRAWL SYDNEY 1982
BRYAN ADAMS SYDNEY 1984
AEROSMITH SYDNEY 1990
ARENA LONDON 2005 + SOUTHAMPTON 2022

**B**

JOAN BAEZ THE ISLE OF WIGHT FESTIVAL 1970
BLACK WIDOW THE ISLE OF WIGHT FESTIVAL 1970
BLACK SABBATH BOURNEMOUTH 1971 + 1973
JACK BRUCE HYDE PARK FREE CONCERT 1971
+ With CHARLIE WATTS BIG BAND (Cello) RONNIE SCOTTS LONDON 1985
+ With ULTIMATE ROCK SYMPHONY MELBOURNE 2000
DAVID BOWIE BOSCOMBE 1972 + SYDNEY 1983 + 1987
THE CHRIS BARBER BAND READING FESTIVAL 1973
ANDY BOWN READING FESTIVAL 1973
BAD COMPANY (Paul Rodgers Ex-Free) CHARLTON FC LONDON 1974
JOHN BALDRY READING FESTIVAL 1974
BARCLAY JAMES HARVEST READING FESTIVAL 1974
MAGGIE BELL (Ex-Stone the Crows) CHARLTON FC 1974 LONDON
ERIC BURDON READING FESTIVAL 1974
BE BOP DELUXE BOURNEMOUTH 1976 + LONDON 1978
BRAND X (Phil Collins Ex-Genesis on Drums) LONDON 1976
BLACKFEATHER ADELAIDE 1977
KATE BUSH LONDON 1979
BLONDIE LONDON 1980
ART BLAKEY (Drums) RONNIE SCOTTS LONDON 1985
ELVIN BISHOP SYDNEY 1986

JIMMY BARNES (Ex-Cold Chisel) SYDNEY 1987 + 1999
GEORGE BENSON LONDON 1988
ROY BUCHANAN SYDNEY 1988
THE BLACK SORROWS MELBOURNE 1989**
LONNIE BROOKS (with Donnie Brooks) MELBOURNE 1990
BONDI CIGARS BLUES ON BROADBEACH 2007
OLI BROWN LONDON 2009
DANNY BRYANT LONDON 2014
BIG BIG TRAIN LONDON 2015 + 2017 +2023
BLACKBERRY SMOKE BRISTOL 2018
JOE BONAMASSA SYDNEY 2019

## C

CACTUS THE ISLE OF WIGHT FESTIVAL 1970 (Carmine Appice – Drums)
CHICAGO THE ISLE OF WIGHT FESTIVAL 1970
CHICKEN SHACK BROCKENHURST 1970
LEONARD COHEN THE ISLE OF WIGHT FESTIVAL 1970
CAMEL BOURNEMOUTH 1971 + READING FESTIVAL 1974
CURVED AIR BOURNEMOUTH 1971 + READING FESTIVAL 1972
+ LONDON 2018
CAPABILITY BROWN READING FESTIVAL 1973
CARAVAN BOURNEMOUTH 1973 + LONDON 2018
COMMANDER CODY READING FESTIVAL 1973
KEVIN COYNE READING FESTIVAL 1974
THE CHIEFTANS SYDNEY 1977
CHEAP TRICK BOSTON 1978
ALBERT COLLINS SYDNEY 1986 + (With Jack Bruce on Bass) LONDON 1991
ERIC CLAPTON SYDNEY 1987+1990 + WINTERSHALL 1989
+ LONDON 1992 (With Elton John) (Guest appearance by Bonnie Raitt) + BRISBANE
2007
ROBERT CRAY SYDNEY 1987 + LONDON 1988
ALICE COOPER MELBOURNE 1990 + With Ultimate Rock Symphony 2000
JOHNNY COPELAND MELBOURNE 1990
CROWDED HOUSE MELBOURNE 1990 + LONDON 1992 + SYDNEY 1995
+ 1996
JOE COCKER SEATTLE THE GORGE 1996
CALIFORNIA GUITAR TRIO LONDON 2003
CANNED HEAT BLUES AT BROADBEACH 2007
JOE CAMILLERI EUMUNDI 2008
KATE CEBRANO NOOSA 2009
TIJUANA CARTEL NOOSA 2009 + PEREGIAN 2009** + COOLUM 2009

## D

MILES DAVIS THE ISLE OF WIGHT FESTIVAL 1970
DONOVAN THE ISLE OF WIGHT FESTIVAL 1970
THE DOORS THE ISLE OF WIGHT FESTIVAL 1970
DEEP PURPLE BOURNEMOUTH 1971 + 1974 LONDON 1999
DIRE STRAITS LONDON 1979 + 1985 (Hank Marvin played on Going Home)
+ SYDNEY 1986 + 1991
DEVO SYDNEY 1982
THE DIVINYLS SYDNEY 1982
DRAGON SYDNEY 1982
IAN DURY & THE BLOCKHEADS LONDON 1985
JOHNNY DIESEL SYDNEY 1987
THE DOOBIE BROTHERS SYDNEY 1995 + JONES BEACH NEW YORK 1996
DREAD ZEPPELIN (Reggae Led Zep with Elvis Impersonator) L.A 1997
ROGER DALTREY (The Who) With Ultimate Rock Symphony MELBOURNE 2000
DREAM THEATER CARDIFF 2007
DAMANEK SWINDON 2018
DIM GRAY LONDON 2023

## E

EDGAR BROUGHTON BAND BROCKENHURST 1970 + READING
FESTIVAL 1972
EMERSON LAKE PALMER THE ISLE OF WIGHT FESTIVAL 1970
+ BOURNEMOUTH 1972 + LONDON 1992
ELECTRIC LIGHT ORCHESTRA READING FESTIVAL 1972
+ (ELO 2) SYDNEY 1995 + (JEFF LYNNE'S ELO) LONDON 2015
JON ENGLISH ADELAIDE 1977 + SYDNEY 1981
THE EURYTHMICS (Dave Stewart & Annie Lennox) SYDNEY 1987
TINSLEY ELLIS SYDNEY 1995
MELISSA ETHERIDGE MELBOURNE 1990 + SYDNEY 1996
TOMMY EMMANUEL SYDNEY 1998 + BRISBANE 2000
+ BATH 2024 (Guests Molly Tuttle + Mike Dawes)
ENCHANT LONDON 2015

## F

FAMILY (Roger Chapman) THE ISLE OF WIGHT FESTIVAL 1970
+ BOURNEMOUTH 1971 + 1973
FREE (Paul Rodgers) THE ISLE OF WIGHT FESTIVAL 1970
THE FACES (Rod Stewart) THE OVAL CRICKET GROUND LONDON 1971
+ BOURNEMOUTH 1971+ READING FESTIVAL 1972 +1973
FORMERLY FAT HARRY HYDE PARK FREE CONCERT 1971

FOCUS BOURNEMOUTH 1972** + READING FESTIVAL 1972 + 1974

FUMBLE READING FESTIVAL 1973 + 1974 + BROCKENHURST 1975

GEORGIE FAME & THE BLUE FLAMES READING FESTIVAL 1974

THE FABULOUS POODLES LONDON 1976

BRYAN FERRY (Roxy Music) ADELAIDE 1977 + SYDNEY 1995
(Phil Manzanera + Chris Spedding – Guitars. John Wetton – Bass. Paul Thompson – Drums)

PETER FRAMPTON with David Bowie SYDNEY 1987 + With Ultimate Rock
Symphony MELBOURNE 2000

FLEETWOOD MAC (With Rick Vito Lead Guitar) LONDON 1988
+ MELBOURNE 1990

FAIRPORT CONVENTION LONDON 1988

FOREIGNER SYDNEY 1995

THE FABULOUS THUNDERBIRDS SEATTLE THE GORGE 1996

THE FLOWER KINGS LONDON 2003 + 2004 + 2007 + 2012 + 2018
+ SOUTHAMPTON 2023

DALLAS FRASCA NOOSA 2007 + 2009

FAR FROM SAINTS BATH 2023

# G

THE GROUNDHOGS THE ISLE OF WIGHT FESTIVAL 1970 + BOURNEMOUTH
1973

GENESIS (Peter Gabriel) BOURNEMOUTH 1972 + 1974 READING FESTIVAL 1972
+ 1973 + SOUTHAMPTON 1973 + (Phil Collins) SYDNEY 1986

GOOD HABIT READING FESTIVAL 1972

ARLO GUTHRIE CRYSTAL PALACE GARDEN PARTY 1972

RORY GALLAGHER (Taste) READING FESTIVAL 1973

GREENSLADE READING FESTIVAL 1973 +1974

GRYPHON READING FESTIVAL 1974

PETER GABRIEL (Genesis) LONDON 1978 + 1980 + ADELAIDE 1993
+ SYDNEY 1994 + LONDON 2023

RENEE GEYER SYDNEY 1982

GOANNA SYDNEY 1982

GYAN MELBOURNE 1989**

BUDDY GUY SEATTLE THE GORGE 1996 + SYDNEY 2014

PETER GREEN (Ex-Fleetwood Mac) LONDON 2000

GEORGE with KATIE NOONAN BRISBANE 2000

GANGgajang SYDNEY 2016 + CABOOLTURE 2019 + NOOSA 2019

## H

**RICHIE HAVENS** THE ISLE OF WIGHT FESTIVAL 1970
**HAWKWIND** BROCKENHURST 1970
**JIMI HENDRIX** THE ISLE OF WIGHT FESTIVAL 1970
**ROY HARPER** HYDE PARK FREE CONCERT LONDON 1971
**TIM HARDIN** READING FESTIVAL 1973
**JON HISEMANS TEMPEST** READING FESTIVAL 1973
**HUMBLE PIE** (Steve Marriott +Clem Clemson) CHARLTON FC LONDON 1974
**DR HOOK** MELBOURNE 1977
**STEVE HACKETT** (Ex Genesis) LONDON 1980 + RAH 2013
(With John Wetton, Ray Wilson, Nad Sylvan + Roine Stolt) + SOUTHAMPTON 2009
(With Nick Beggs - Bass) + BASINGSTOKE 2015 (With Nad Sylvan + Roine Stolt –
Guitar + Bass)
**HUNTERS & COLLECTORS** SYDNEY 1995
**HUMAN NATURE** SYDNEY 1998
**ROGER HODGSON** (Ex Supertramp) SYDNEY 2013
**HASSE FRÖBERG MUSICAL COMPANION** LONDON 2015


## I

**IRON BUTTERFLY** BOURNEMOUTH 1971
**INCREDIBLE STRING BAND** BOURNEMOUTH 1972
**ICEHOUSE** SYDNEY 1981 + 1987
**INXS** SYDNEY 1981 + 1982 + 1991 + (With Jon Stevens) BRISBANE 2001
**INTI ILLIMANI** (With John Williams and Paco Pena) MELBOURNE 1990 +
SYDNEY 1993


## J

**JETHRO TULL** THE ISLE OF WIGHT FESTIVAL 1970 + BOURNEMOUTH 1971
+ 1972 + SOUTHAMPTON 1974 + LONDON 1973 + 1978 + 1980 + 1980 + 1988 + 1989
+ 1992 + 1999
+ BRISTOL 2006 + GLASGOW 1992 + SYDNEY 1977 + 1994 + 1996 + 2011 +
BRISBANE 2005
+ (IAN ANDERSON'S JETHRO TULL) LONDON 2014 + BASINGSTOKE 2015
**BERT JANSCH** SYDNEY 1977
**ELTON JOHN** SYDNEY 1984 (Guest appearance with Robert Plant) + SYDNEY 1986
+ 1998
(With Billy Joel) + LONDON 1992 (With Eric Clapton) (Guest appearance by Brian May)
**BILLY JOEL SYDNEY** 1987 + 1998 (With Elton John)
**JUNKYARD** MOUNTAIN VIEW USA 1991 + BRISTOL 2018
**JAY Z** BRISBANE 2010

# 522      *A-Z List of Concerts*

## K

KRIS KRISTOFFERSON THE ISLE OF WIGHT FESTIVAL 1970
KING CRIMSON HYDE PARK FREE CONCERT 1971 + BOURNEMOUTH 1971 +
1972
JONATHAN KELLY READING FESTIVAL 1972 + BOURNEMOUTH 1972
LEO KOTTKE LONDON 1979
B.B. KING SYDNEY 1989 +1994 +1997
KILLING HEIDI MELBOURNE 2000
PAUL KELLY BRIBIE ISLAND 2004
MARK KNOPFLER (Ex Dire Straits) BRISBANE 2005

## L

LINDISFARNE THE OVAL CRICKET GROUND LONDON 1971
+ BOURNEMOUTH 1972 + READING FESTIVAL 1973 + CHARLTON FC 1974
RONNIE LANE (Ex Faces) READING FESTIVAL 1974 + LONDON 1980
LED ZEPPELIN LONDON 1975
LITTLE FEAT CHARLTON LONDON FC 1976
LITTLE RIVER BAND SYDNEY 1982
LYNYRD SKYNYRD MOUNTAIN VIEW CALIFORNIA 1991
+ LONDON 1992 + JONES BEACH NEW YORK 1996 + L.A 1997 + 2019 + SYDNEY
2014
LARKIN POE BRISTOL 2022
AYNSLEY LISTER FROME 2023

## M

RALPH MCTELL THE ISLE OF WIGHT FESTIVAL 1970
MELANIE THE ISLE OF WIGHT FESTIVAL 1970
JONI MITCHELL THE ISLE OF WIGHT FESTIVAL 1970
THE MOODY BLUES THE ISLE OF WIGHT FESTIVAL 1970
+ LONDON 1979
MOTT THE HOOPLE THE OVAL CRICKET GROUND LONDON 1971
+ BOURNEMOUTH 1973
MAN READING FESTIVAL 1972 + BOURNEMOUTH 1975 + LONDON 1976
MUNGO JERRY READING FESTIVAL 1972
JOHN MARTYN READING FESTIVAL 1973 + SYDNEY 1977
MEDICINE HEAD READING FESTIVAL 1973
GEORGE MELLY READING FESTIVAL 1973 + 1974
MOTHER GOOSE SYDNEY 1977
MEMPHIS SLIM (PIANO) LONDON 1976
MACHINATIONS SYDNEY 1982

MEN AT WORK SYDNEY 1982
MENTAL AS ANYTHING SYDNEY 1982
MODELS SYDNEY 1982
MONDO ROCK SYDNEY 1982
THE MOTELS SYDNEY 1982
MEATLOAF LONDON 1985
BROWNIE MCGHEE WELLINGTON 1987
MIDNIGHT OIL LONDON 1988 + SYDNEY 1993 + 1995 + BRISBANE 2017
JOHN MAYALL (Buddy Whittington) LONDON 2000
GARY MOORE LONDON 2001 + 2007
NEAL MORSE LONDON 2006
NEAL MORSE BAND LONDON 2022
KATE MILLER-HEIDKE EUMUNDI 2007
STEVE MILLER BAND SYDNEY 2013
CHARLIE MUSSELWHITE (Harmonica) SYDNEY 2014
MARILLION BATH 2021
MOSTLY AUTUMN SOUTHAMPTON 2023

**N**

STEVIE NICKS (Fleetwood Mac) SYDNEY 1986
NOISEWORKS SYDNEY 1987
NOT DROWNING, WAVING ADELAIDE 1993 + SYDNEY 1994

**O**

OSIBISA CRYSTAL PALACE GARDEN PARTY 1972
JOHNNY OTIS & The Three Tons of Joy READING FESTIVAL 1972
THE OUTLAWS CHARLTON FC LONDON 1976

**P**

PENTANGLE THE ISLE OF WIGHT FESTIVAL 1970
THE PRETTY THINGS GUILDFORD 1970 + 1976
PROCUL HAREM THE ISLE OF WIGHT FESTIVAL 1970 + BROCKENHURST 1971
PINK FLOYD BOURNEMOUTH 1972 + LONDON 1974 + SYDNEY 1988
ROBERT PLANT SYDNEY 1984 (Guest appearance by Elton John on Treat Her Right)
THE POLICE SYDNEY 1984
THE PRETENDERS SYDNEY 1987

PACO PENA MELBOURNE 1990 + SYDNEY 1993
TOM PETTY & THE HEARTBREAKERS LONDON 1992
ROBERT PLANT & JIMMY PAGE (Ex-Led Zeppelin) SYDNEY 1996
POWDERFINGER BRISBANE 2001
PENDRAGON LONDON 2018

## Q

QUINTESSENCE THE OVAL CRICKET GROUND LONDON 1971
QUEEN BOURNEMOUTH 1974

## R

TERRY REID with DAVID LINDLEY
ROXY MUSIC CRYSTAL PALACE GARDEN PARTY 1972
+ BOURNEMOUTH 1973 + 1974 + LONDON 1979 + BRISBANE 2001 + LONDON 2022
REFUGEE READING FESTIVAL 1974
RENAISSANCE BOURNEMOUTH 1974
LOU REED CHARLTON FC LONDON 1974
THE ROLLING STONES LONDON 1976 + SYDNEY 1995 + BRISBANE 2003
CHRIS REA WELLINGTON 1987 + LONDON 2003
BONNIE RAITT LONDON 1992
PAUL RODGERS With Ultimate Rock Symphony MELBOURNE 2000

## S

JOHN SEBASTIAN THE ISLE OF WIGHT FESTIVAL 1970
SLY AND THE FAMILY STONE THE ISLE OF WIGHT FESTIVAL 1970
STEELEYE SPAN BOURNEMOUTH 1971
SUPERTRAMP BROCKENHURST 1971 + BOURNEMOUTH 1974 + LONDON 1997
STATUS QUO READING FESTIVAL 1972 +1973 + LONDON 1976 + MELBOURNE 1977
+ LONDON 1979 + 1981 + 1991 + 2019
THE SENSATIONAL ALEX HARVEY BAND BOURNEMOUTH 1972
+ READING FESTIVAL 1973 + BOURNEMOUTH 1973 + CHARLTON FC LONDON 1976
STACKRIDGE READING FESTIVAL 1972 +1973 + LONDON 2015
STONE THE CROWS CRYSTAL PALACE GARDEN PARTY 1972
STRAY READING FESTIVAL 1972
STRING DRIVEN THING READING FESTIVAL 1972

SUTHERLAND BROTHERS & QUIVER READING FESTIVAL 1972 +1974
SPENCER DAVIS READING FESTIVAL 1973
THE STRAWBS BOURNEMOUTH 1973
STRIDER READING FESTIVAL 1973 + 1974
STREETWALKERS (Roger Chapman) CHARLTON FC LONDON 1976
ROD STEWART (The Faces) ADELAIDE 1977 + LONDON 1978
SUPERCHARGE SYDNEY 1977
SANTANA LONDON 1978 +1989 + SYDNEY 2013
BOB SEGER & THE SILVER BULLET BAND LONDON 1980
SIMON & GARFUNKEL SYDNEY 1983
SKY LONDON 1980 + SYDNEY 1984
THE SUNNYBOYS SYDNEY 1984
SIMPLE MINDS SYDNEY 1986 + LONDON 1989
BRUCE SPRINGSTEIN & THE E STREET BAND LONDON 1988
ARTURO SANOVAL (Trumpet) RONNIE SCOTTS LONDON 1989 + 1992
SPLIT ENZ MELBOURNE 1990 + BRISBANE 2006
KENNY WAYNE SHEPHERD L.A 1997 + SYDNEY 1998
SEBASTIAN HARDIE SYDNEY 2003
SYMPHONY X CARDIFF 2007
SEASICK STEVE SYDNEY 2009
JOANNE SHAW TAYLOR LONDON 2009 + SYDNEY 2013 + 2014
SPOCK'S BEARD LONDON 2013 + 2014 + 2018
ANGUS & JULIA STONE LONDON 2014
SOUTHERN EMPIRE SWINDON 2017


**T**

TASTE (Rory Gallagher) THE ISLE OF WIGHT FESTIVAL 1970
TEN YEARS AFTER THE ISLE OF WIGHT FESTIVAL 1970
+ READING FESTIVAL 1972
TINY TIM THE ISLE OF WIGHT FESTIVAL 1970
TANGERINE DREAM SOUTHAMPTON 1971 + LONDON 1978
THIRD EAR BAND HYDE PARK FREE CONCERT LONDON 1971
ROBIN TROWER BROCKENHURST 1971 + LONDON 1973 + ADELAIDE 1977
+ SYDNEY 1995
TIR NA NOG BOURNEMOUTH 1972
THIN LIZZY READING FESTIVAL 1974
TRAFFIC (Stevie Winwood) READING FESTIVAL 1974
TRAPEZE READING FESTIVAL 1974
THE TOURISTS (Dave Stewart & Annie Lennox) LONDON 1979
BILLY THORPE With Ultimate Rock Symphony MELBOURNE 2000

WALTER TROUT LONDON 2003
THE TANGENT LONDON 2003
THEM CROOKED VULTURES LONDON 2009
(John Paul Jones, Dave Grohl, Josh Homme)
TRANSATLANTIC LONDON 2010

## U

UNCANNY X-MEN SYDNEY 1982
U2 BRISBANE 2010
UNITOPIA ADELAIDE 2010

## V

VINEGAR JOE (Robert Palmer & Elkie Brooks) READING FESTIVAL 1972
STEVIE RAY VAUGHAN LONDON 198

## W

THE WHO THE ISLE OF WIGHT FESTIVAL 1970 + THE OVAL CRICKET
GROUND 1971
+ CHARLTON FC 1974 + CHARLTON FC 1976
TONY JOE WHITE (Cozy Powell) THE ISLE OF WIGHT FESTIVAL 1970
ROY WOODS WIZARD READING FESTIVAL 1972
WILD TURKEY (Glenn Cornick Ex-Jethro Tull) BOURNEMOUTH 1972
EDGAR WINTER CRYSTAL PALACE GARDEN PARTY 1972
WISHBONE ASH BOURNEMOUTH 1973 + LONDON 1980 + FROME 2022
CHARLIE WATTS ORCHESTRA Ronnie Scotts LONDON 1985
(Jack Bruce Cello-Bass. Courtney Pine Saxophone)
JOHNNY WINTER SYDNEY 1986
JOHN WILLIAMS MELBOURNE 1990 + SYDNEY 1993
STEVE WINWOOD (Ex-Traffic) LONDON 1999
WOLFMOTHER SYDNEY 2010
WHOLE LOTTA LOVE - LED ZEPPELIN CELEBRATION SYDNEY 2016
STEVEN WILSON (Ex-Porcupine Tree) LONDON 2016
THE WAIFS TARONGA ZOO SYDNEY 2019

## X

## Y

YES GUILDFORD 1970 + SOUTHAMPTON 1971+ BOURNEMOUTH 1973 + SYDNEY 2003

## Z

ZZ TOP SYDNEY 1987

## THE ISLE OF WIGHT FESTIVAL 1970

- BLACK WIDOW
- THE GROUNDHOGS (Tony Mcphee - Guitar)
- TERRY REID with DAVID LINDLEY
- TASTE (Rory Gallagher -Guitar)
- TONY JOE WHITE (Cozy Powell – Drums)
- CHICAGO
- FAMILY (Roger Chapman – Vocals)
- PROCUL HAREM (Gary Brooker - Keyboards)
- CACTUS (Carmine Appice – Drums)
- JOHN SEBASTIAN
- JONI MITCHELL
- MILES DAVIS
- TEN YEARS AFTER (Alvin Lee - Guitar)
- EMERSON, LAKE & PALMER
- THE DOORS (Set Started At 2am on 30th August)
- THE WHO
- SLY AND THE FAMILY STONE
- MELANIE
- KRIS KRISTOFFERSON
- RALPH MCTELL
- FREE (Paul Rodgers–Vocals + Paul Kossoff–Guitar)
- DONOVAN
- PENTANGLE
- THE MOODY BLUES
- JETHRO TULL
- JIMI HENDRIX
- JOAN BAEZ
- TINY TIM
- LEONARD COHEN
- RICHIE HAVENS

## HYDE PARK FREE CONCERT **1971**

- JACK BRUCE
  (Chris Spedding - Guitar - Graham Bond - Keyboards, Art Themen –
  Saxophone
  and John Marshall – Drums)
- KING CRIMSON (Boz Burrell – Vocals and Bass)
- ROY HARPER
- FORMERLY FAT HARRY

## CONCERT FOR BANGLADESH THE OVAL LONDON 1971

- THE WHO
- THE FACES (Rod Stewart)
- ATOMIC ROOSTER
- AMERICA
- MOTT THE HOOPLE
- QUINTESSENCE
- LINDISFARNE

## CRYSTAL PALACE GARDEN PARTY 1972

- ROXY MUSIC (Bryan Ferry and Eno)
- STONE THE CROWS (Maggie Bell)
- EDGAR WINTER (Rick Derringer – Guitar)
- OSIBISA
- ARLO GUTHRIE

## READING FESTIVAL 1972

- EDGAR BROUGHTON BAND
- CURVED AIR
- ELECTRIC LIGHT ORCHESTRA
- THE FACES (Rod Stewart)
- FOCUS
- GOOD HABIT
- GENESIS (Peter Gabriel)

# 530 — A-Z List of Concerts

- JONATHAN KELLY
- MAN
- MUNGO JERRY
- JOHNNY OTIS & THE THREE TONS OF JOY
- STACKRIDGE
- STATUS QUO
- STRING DRIVEN THING
- STRAY
- SUTHERLAND BROTHERS & QUIVER
- TEN YEARS AFTER (Alvin Lee –Guitar)
- VINEGAR JOE (Robert Palmer & Elkie Brooks – Vocals)
- ROY WOODS WIZARD

READING FESTIVAL 1973

- RORY GALLAGHER
- GREENSLADE
- CAPABILITY BROWN
- ALQUIN
- COMMANDER CODY
- THE FACES
- LINDISFARNE
- ALEX HARVEY BAND
- FUMBLE
- ANDY BOWN
- STRIDER
- THE CHRIS BARBER BAND
- STATUS QUO
- GENESIS
- JON HISEMANS TEMPEST
- MEDICINE HEAD
- STACKRIDGE
- SPENCER DAVIS
- TIM HARDIN
- ANGE
- JOHN MARTYN
- GEORGE MELLY & THE FEET WARMERS

## SUMMER OF 74 - CHARLTON FC

- THE WHO
- HUMBLE PIE (Steve Marriott)
- LOU REED
- BAD COMPANY (Paul Rodgers)
- LINDISFARNE
- MAGGIE BELL

## READING FESTIVAL 1974

- ALEX HARVEY
- 10cc
- FUMBLE
- CAMEL
- TRAFFIC
- RONNIE LANE
- GREENSLADE
- THIN LIZZY
- SUTHERLAND BROTHERS & QUIVER
- TRAPEZE
- GEORGIE FAME & THE BLUE FLAMES
- JOHN BALDRY
- FOCUS
- ERIC BURDON
- BARCLAY JAMES HARVEST
- REFUGEE
- GRYPHON
- STRIDER
- GEORGE MELLY
- KEVIN COYNE

532 *A-Z List of Concerts*

CHARITY CONCERTS

OZ FOR AFRICA 1982
SYDNEY ENTERTAINMENT CENTRE

- INXS
- RENEE GEYE
- THE ANGELS
- MONDO ROCK
- LITTLE RIVER BAND
- GOANNA
- UNCANNY X-MEN
- AUSTRALIAN CRAWL
- MEN AT WORK
- DRAGON
- ELECTRIC PANDAS
- DO RE MI
- MODELS
- I'M TALKING
- MACHINATIONS
- MENTAL AS ANYTHING

PICNIC BY THE LAKE 1989
WINTERSHALL ESTATE, SURREY

Featuring BAND DU LAC
ERIC CLAPTON
STEVE WINWOOD
GARY BROOKER
PHIL COLLINS
MIKE RUTHERFORD
ANDY FAIRWEATHER-LOW
DAVE BRONZE
HENRY SPINETTI
MEL COLLINS
VICKY & SAM BROWN & MARGO BUCHANAN

THE ULTIMATE ROCK SYMPHONY 2000
MELBOURNE COLONIAL STADIUM

- ALICE COOPER
- ROGER DALTREY
- PETER FRAMPTON
- PAUL RODGERS
- BILLY THORPE
- JACK BRUCE
- GARY BROOKER
- NIKKI LANBORN
- SIMON TOWNSEND
- ZAC STARKEY
- GEOFF WHITEHORN
- JAZ LOCHRIE
- 'RABBIT' BUNDRICK

# Quote Sources

*60 Minutes Australia.* "The Australian cameraman who revolutionised the film industry". https://www.youtube.com/watch?v=xORxhVDb-NU

A.A. Milne. *Winnie The Pooh.* Methuen, London 1926.

Alexander Pope. An Essay On Criticism, 1711.

Allen Collins and Ronnie Van Zant. *Free Bird.* 1973.

B.B. King. *The Charlotte Observer,* p. 2D, October 5, 1997.

Bill Nelson. *Panic in the World.* 1978.

Black Sabbath. *War Pigs.* 1970.

Bob Dylan. *Open the Door Homer, Basement Tapes,* Bob Dylan and The Band, 1975.

Bruce Springsteen. *Lyrics from Lucky Town by Bruce Springsteen,* 1992.

Carew Paprit. *The Legacy Letters: His Wife, His Children, His Final Gift,* King Northern Publishing, 2013.

Charles F. Glassman. *Brain Drain – The Breakthrough That Will Change Your Life,* RTS Publishing, 2009.

Dalai Lama (Vol. 1, Chap. 13). *Advice on Dying: And Living a Better Life,* Atria Books, 2002.

Dalai Lama (Vol. 2, Chap. 11). *The Book of Joy: Lasting Happiness in a Changing World,* Cornerstone 2016.

David Gilmour and Pete Townshend. *Love on the Air.* 1984.

Denis Waitley. *Denis Waitley's Little Green Book of Inspiration,* Barnes & Noble Books, New York, 1995.

Douglas Adams. *The Long Dark Tea-Time of the Soul,* William Heinemann, 1988.

*Easy Rider.* 1969.

Echo & The Bunnymen. *Thorn of Crowns.* 1984.

Elbert Hubbard. *Loyalty in Business: One and Twenty Other Good Things,* p.29, Cosimo, Inc, 2005.

Eleanor Roosevelt. Quoted in *Providence Journal-Bulletin,* 8 June 1994.

Farhan Akhtar. Interview with *The Indian Express,* September 2017, https://images.dawn.com/news/1178489

Freddie Mercury and Peter Straker. *I'm Going Slightly Mad.* 1991.

Hans Christian Andersen. *Hans Christian Andersen's Complete Fairy Tales,* Canterbury Classics, 1913.

Henri-Frédéric Amiel. *Amiel's journal; the Journal intime of Henri-Frédéric Amiel,* p. 368, 1890.

Henry David Thoreau. *Walden,* publ. by Ticknor & Fields, USA, 1854

Ibn Battutah.*The Travels of Ibn Battutah,* Picador, UK, 2002.

Joan Miró, Joan Miro: Selected Writings and Interviews, Editing by Margit. Rowell, Thames and Hudson, 1987.

536 *Quote Sources*

Jonas Salk. Address on receiving the Nehru Award (10 January 1977), *Virginia Woolf Quarterly* (1977), Vol. 3, p. 11.

Joseph Campbell (Vol. 1, Chap. 11). *Myths to Live By*, Viking, USA, 1972.

Joseph Campbell (Vol. 1, Chap. 9). *Follow Your Bliss Conversations with Bill Moyers,* Vanderbilt University, 1989.

Joseph Campbell (Vol. 2 Chap. 7). *A Joseph Campbell Companion: Reflections on the Art of Living, Harper Collins 1995.*

Joseph Campbell (Vol. 2, Chap. 12). *The Hero's Journey (On Living in the World),* Harper & Row 1990.

Joseph Campbell (Vol. 2, Chapter 3). *A Joseph Campbell Companion: Reflections on the Art of Living*, Harper Perennial 1991.

Laura Ingalls Wilder. *These Happy Golden Years*, Harper & Brothers, USA 1943.

Lemmy Kilmister."Interview with Fiona Sturges". *The Independent,* 2005

Lin Yutang. *The Importance of Living,* Reynal & Hitchcock, Inc. 1937.

Lionel Stander. Interview with *Playboy* magazine, December 1967.

Lionel Stander.'Lionel Stander…that's who', by Helen Lawrenson, *Esquire: The Magazine For Men*, p. 182, December 1967.

Marrk Callaghan. *Sounds of Then (This Australia).* 1985

Michael ONeill. *Road Work: Images and Insights of a Modern Day Explorer,* self-published, 2021.

Neil Finn. *History Never Repeats.* 1981.

Neil Murray and George Rrurrambu. *Blackfella/Whitefella.* 1985.

Paulo Coelho. *Aleph*, Harper Collins, Brazil 2011.

Plato. *Wordsworth Dictionary of Musical Quotations*, 1991, p. 4.

Prince. *Let's Go Crazy*. Purple Rain. 1984.

Ray Davis. *Waterloo Sunset.* 1967.

Ronnie Van Zant and Gary Rossington. *Simple Man.* 1973.

Roy Buchanan. PBS Documentary introducing Roy Buchanan. 1971.

Rusty Wright and Linda Raney Wright. *Secrets of Successful Humor.* San Bernardino, CA: Here's Life Publishers 1985, p. 182.

Saint Augustine. Attributed to Augustine in *Select Proverbs of All Nations*, by Thomas Fielding (John Wade), p. 216, 1824.

Sarah Dessen. *Just Listen*, Viking, USA, 2006

Simple Minds. *Waterfront.* 1984.

Søren Kierkegaard. *Repetition: An Essay in Experimental Psychology*, C.A. Reitzel, Denmark, 1845.

Steppenwolf, *Born to be Wild*, 1968.

Terry McMillan. *A Day Late and a Dollar Short*, Berkeley Pub. Group 2002.

Terry Pratchett. *Shall Wear Midnight,* Discworld series, Doubleday 2010.

Theodore Roosevelt. *Theodore Roosevelt on Bravery: Lessons from the Most Courageous Leader of the Twentieth Century*, p.13, Skyhorse, 2015.

Tom Petty. *Time to Move On.* 1994.
Tommy Cooper. "The best quotes", by Michael Hogan, *The Guardian*. April 22, 2014
Walter Elliot. *The Life of Father Hecker*, The Columbus Press, New York, 1891.

# Acknowledgements

I would like to thank…

My inspirational mother for encouraging me to be 'me' and to never ever give up.

My family and friends dotted all over the world, including the ones who are no longer with us. I feel truly blessed to have known you.

My old art teachers Miss le May and Mr. Jones for encouraging me to use my intuition.

My mentors Mike Reed, Edwin Scragg, Alastair Macdonald, Ken Friswell and Jim Frazier for the opportunities they gave me and the knowledge they passed on to me.

The many talented DOPs and tireless film crews who made me look better than I really am. It was a privilege to work with you all.

And finally, Rob Fisher for his much-needed editing advice and for understanding why it was important for me to write this book in the first place.

Thank you to all of the above for enriching my life and giving me so many happy memories.

My life wouldn't have been half as much fun without you in it.